Kettlebell 365

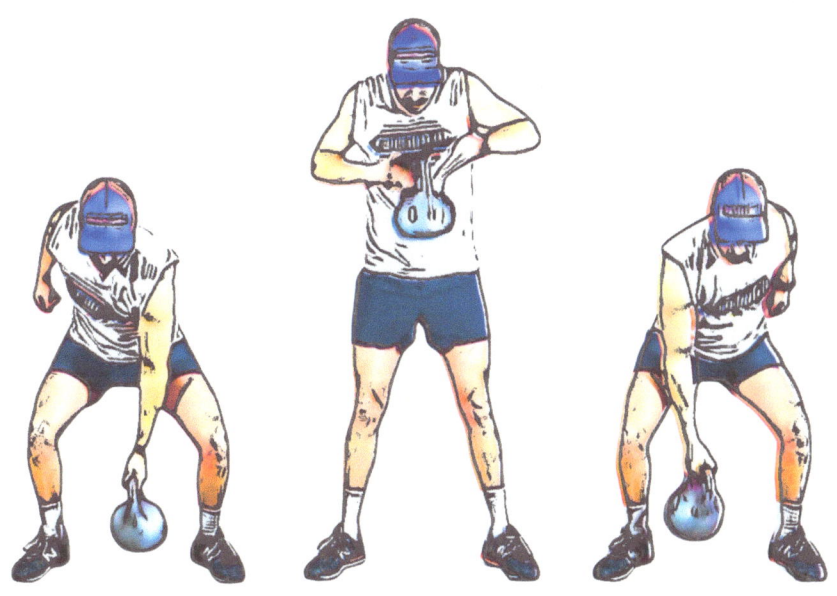

THE ULTIMATE KETTLEBELL EXERCISE LIBRARY

365 Kettlebell Movements to Build Strength, Improve Your Health and Train Athleticism

©2025 PRO KETTLEBELL

www.prokettlebell.com

A Note from the Authors

When we decided to create Kettlebell 365, we gave ourselves a very specific challenge:

Send an email with a kettlebell exercise every day of the year.

Not 50 great exercises.
Not 100 days.
A new exercise prescription every day of the year.

That requirement alone shaped everything that followed. It forced us to go deeper than surface-level variety and to think in terms of foundational movement patterns, intelligent variations, and meaningful combinations. We weren't interested in novelty for novelty's sake.

Every exercise had to earn its place, and at the end of the year we had the lineup and a video how-to for the 365 moves in this book.

Built on Principles, Expanded Through Variation

All 365 exercises in this book—whether static, singular, or complex combinations—are rooted in the same foundational kettlebell movements. The challenge was not inventing new ideas but exploring those ideas thoroughly and responsibly.

We examined:

- How hinges can be expressed in multiple ways
- How presses, pulls, squats, carries, and rotations can be varied
- How movements can be combined without losing intent
- How patterns can evolve while remaining teachable and repeatable

The result is a library that provides variety without abandoning structure.

Just as important as what's included is what's excluded.

There are many kettlebell exercises and combinations you may notice are not present in this book. That omission is intentional. If a movement did not provide enough return for its risk, complexity, or coaching demand—especially in group or shared training environments—it did not make the cut.

Designed for Real Training Environments

Nothing in Kettlebell 365 is theoretical and it was created for how people actually train.

That includes training at home—often with one kettlebell or a single pair—but it also includes gym floors, group classes, and coached environments where clarity, safety, and repeatability matter even more.

Kettlebell 365 is not about showing absolutely everything you can do with kettlebells or only including the best kettlebell-specific exercises. It's a collection of tested and proven exercises you can use to get a comprehensive workout when kettlebells are the chosen tool.

Thank you for training with us.
— Amber & Nikolai

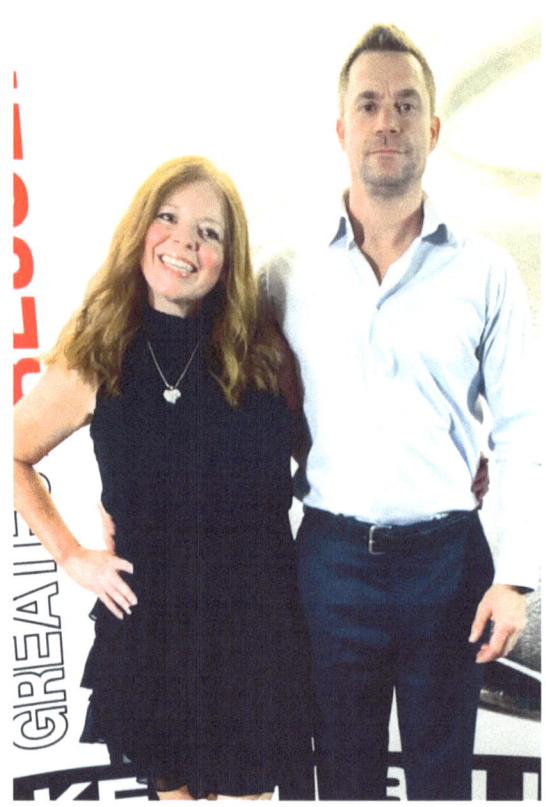

Amber & Nikolai Puchlov
Founders, Pro Kettlebell

THE ULTIMATE KETTLEBELL EXERCISE LIBRARY

Table of Contents

INTRODUCTION		6-12

SECTION 1	PAGE	UPPER BODY
	14	Presses
	25	Push-Ups
	28	Rows
	30	Curls, Compounds & Miscellaneous

SECTION 2	PAGE	LOWER BODY
	43	Squats
	56	Lunges
	68	Compounds & Miscellaneous

SECTION 3	PAGE	CORE & MORE
	73	Sit-Ups, Twists & Crunches
	85	Core-Focused Planks
	88	Windmills

SECTION 4	PAGE	FULL BODY / COMPOUND POWER & CONDITIONING
	93	Swings
	101	Cleans
	110	Snatches
	116	Jerks

SECTION 5	PAGE	FULL BODY / COMPOUND STRENGTH & CONDITIONING
	121	Deadlifts
	127	Plank Combinations
	130	Thrusters & Get-Ups
	135	Walks, Holds & Carries

SECTION 6	PAGE	SPECIALTY EXERCISES
	141	Agility
	145	Mobility

SECTION 7	PAGE	COMPLEXES
	151	Combination Sequences

GLOSSARY	173	INDEX	174
WORKOUTS	178		

TERMINOLOGY

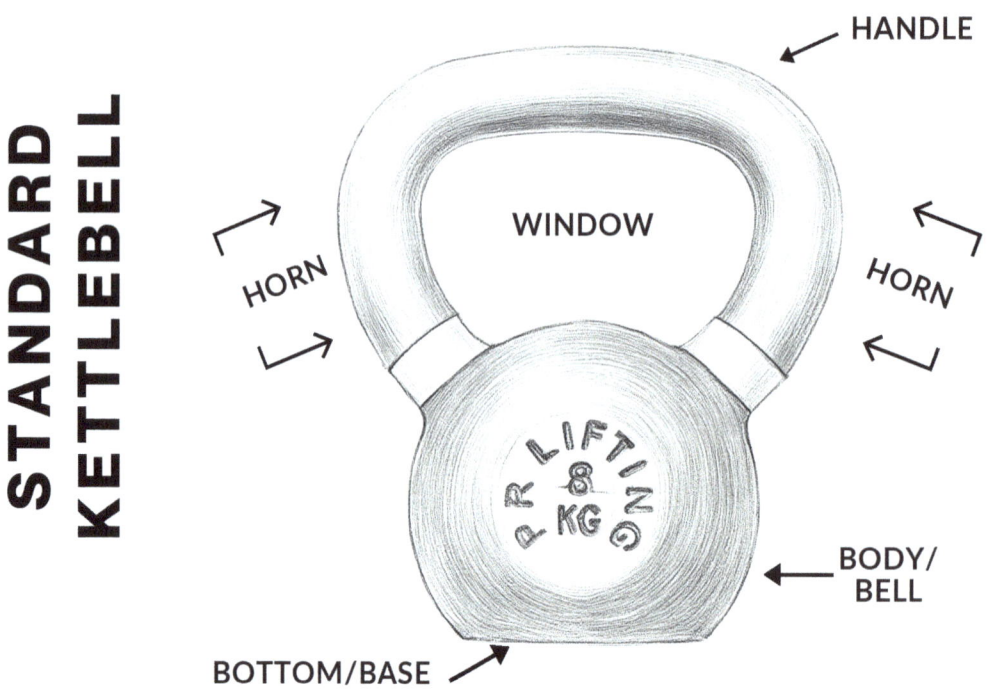

STANDARD KETTLEBELL
- HANDLE
- WINDOW
- HORN
- HORN
- BODY/BELL
- BOTTOM/BASE

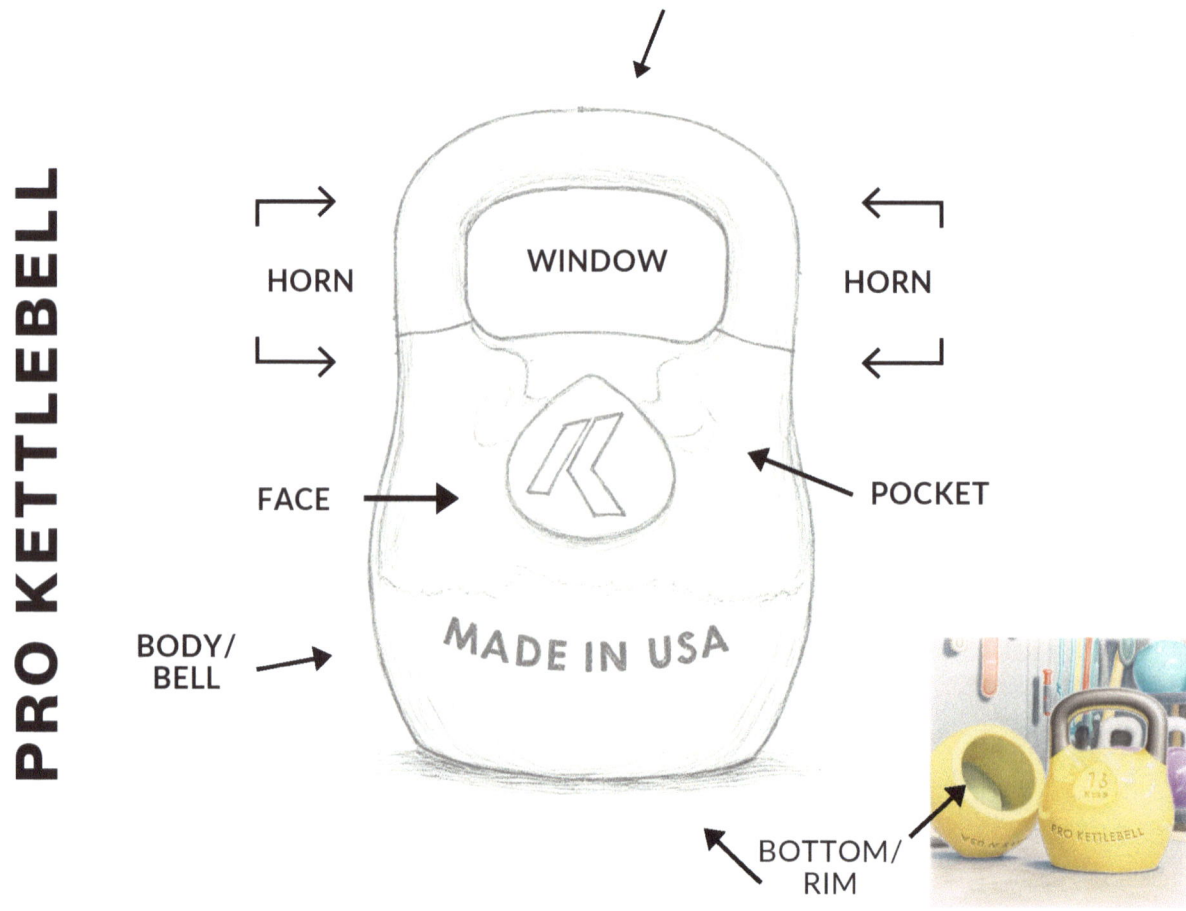

PRO KETTLEBELL
- HANDLE
- WINDOW
- HORN
- HORN
- FACE
- POCKET
- BODY/BELL
- BOTTOM/RIM

Efficiency. Athleticism. Kettlebells for Life.

Welcome to **The Ultimate Kettlebell Exercise Library**—a complete, categorized reference of 365 kettlebell movements designed to build strength, improve mobility, sharpen coordination, and elevate your overall fitness.

This isn't just a collection of cool lifts. It's the distilled knowledge of thousands of hours coaching real people, in real time.

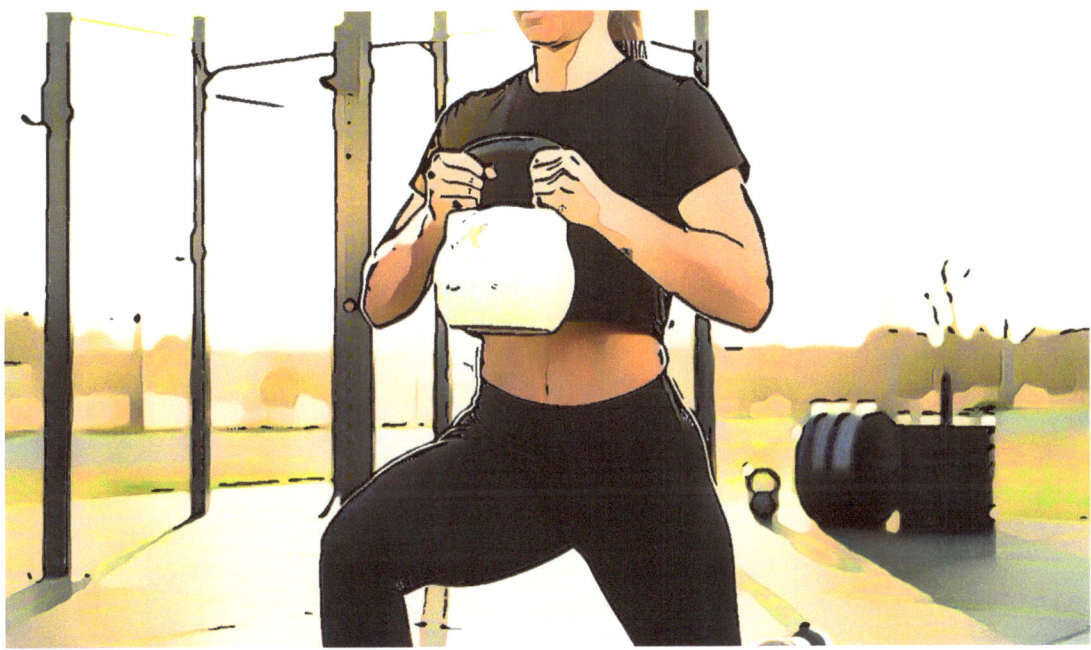

Kettlebell training is one of the most efficient ways to train the human body.

- Strengthen **multiple muscle groups** at once
- **Boost cardiovascular output** without needing to "do cardio"
- Enhance **joint health** through full-range, dynamic movement
- Train **mobility and stability** while lifting weight
- Develop **explosive athleticism**, even if you're not an athlete

Whether you're swinging for endurance or pressing for power, every rep delivers full-body benefit. The kettlebell's offset load and dynamic nature demand—and reward—precision, intention, and control.

How this Library Works

Each exercise includes clearly labeled details—movement pattern, technical difficulty, recommended load, speed (RPM), and a direct URL to its corresponding video instruction on prokettlebell.com—so you can instantly understand how to perform it and how to use it effectively in your training.

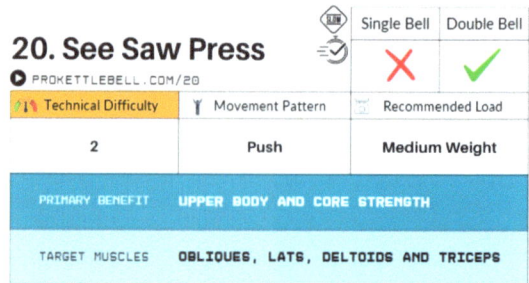

Exercise Categories

Exercises in this book are grouped by region—Upper Body, Lower Body, Core, Ballistics, and more—but kettlebell training rarely isolates a single muscle. Most movements are full body by nature, and the "target muscles" listed simply highlight the primary areas involved, not the only ones. This is the magic of kettlebells: **true isolation is nearly impossible.**

Within each category, exercises are listed alphabetically and organized by technical difficulty level to help you progress smoothly and confidently.

Technical Level Isn't a Value Judgment

A Level-1 exercise isn't "beginner"—it's just less technical to perform. Some of the simplest movements, like the goblet squat, are also the most effective and humbling. We use technical levels to guide planning—not to rank the value of a movement.

 ## Recommended Speed

Speed in kettlebell training is determined in one of two ways:

1. **The amount of time taken between repetitions while the kettlebell is still** (this is how speed is measured in ballistic lifts like swings, cleans, snatches, and jerks—RPM/reps per minute)

2. **The actual speed at which your body moves with the kettlebell** (used for grinds and non-ballistic movements)

Ballistic lifts cannot be performed "slow." A swing or snatch is always a fast-twitch action. You can apply more force to make it slightly faster, but the difference is minimal—the movement will always be explosive by nature. Just like a ballistic push-up, you might not complete many reps per minute, but every rep must be executed with speed.

Grinds, on the other hand, can be intentionally **slow-twitch, medium,** or **fast** depending on the goal, the format (circuits, AMRAPs, strength sets), and the safety of the exercise.

The speed icons in this book indicate the safest and most effective pace for each movement—whether it belongs in fast conditioning work or should be performed at a slower, strength-focused tempo.

Recommended Load

Kettlebells are incredibly versatile, but no single weight is perfect for every movement—or every part of your body. Your legs can safely lift **2–4×** more than your shoulders, your posterior chain thrives under heavier loads, and your shoulders need far more precision and stability. That's why the bell that feels great for swings or deadlifts might be unsafe overhead, and the one that feels right for presses may not challenge your lower body at all. Across warm-ups, mobility, rehab, conditioning, strength, and skill work, your body performs best when each movement is paired with an appropriate load.

If you only own one or two bells, you can still train effectively. In this book, each exercise is labeled light, medium, or heavy and paired with a recommended pace to help you make the most of whatever equipment you have:

- **Conditioning:** typically, lighter + faster
- **Strength or hypertrophy:** typically, heavier + slower

These guidelines are here to help you choose smartly—but your body, your mechanics, and your safety always come first. Listen to them.

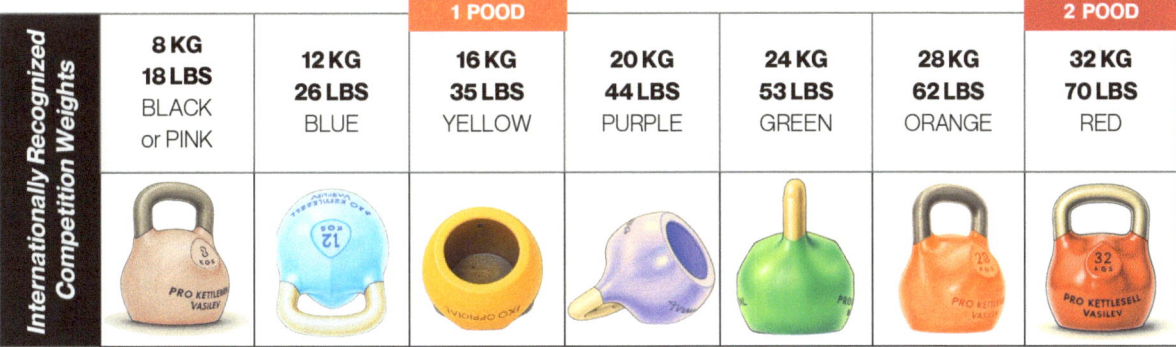

PRO KETTLEBELL

The Four Cornerstones of Pro Kettlebell Technique

LOOSE GRIPS, NO RIPS & YOU'LL HIT THE GOAL WITH MAX CONTROL #1

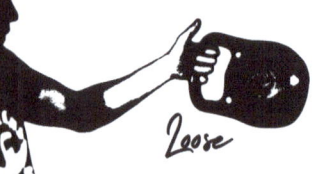

Every exercise in this book starts with picking up the bell—even if it's just to move it.

Death-gripping the kettlebell can cause hand tears, overuse injuries like tennis elbow, and prematurely end your workout.

A tight squeeze has its place, but as a general rule: learn to loosen up. This protects your skin and improves dexterity for movements that demand it.

KEEP THOSE BELLS WITHIN FRAME & YOUR RACK'S GOT GAME #2

The rack position is a foundational posture in kettlebell lifting, where the bell rests against your forearm and biceps at chest height. Mastering it matters. Keep your hands close enough toward center that the kettlebell(s) stay inside your frame—this creates maximum stability and a solid platform for any lift.

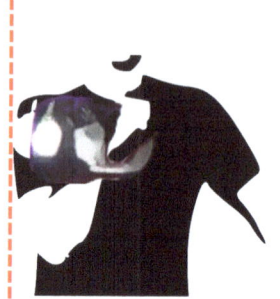

#3

MASSES STACKED? SAFETY IN-TACT

There are exceptions, but as a general rule, keep your center of mass aligned with the kettlebell's center of mass during holds and non-swinging or ballistic movements.

You're strongest and most stable when the kettlebell's weight is stacked over multiple joints, allowing your body to support the load efficiently.

SWING WITH CONNECTION FOR BACK PROTECTION #4

Keep the bell high between your legs and maintain full arm-to-body contact—from wrist to armpit—through the entire back swing and until the bell rises past your knees on the upswing. This arm–body connection (the A-B-C of the kettlebell swing) ensures the legs, glutes, and hips—not the back—absorb the load on the drop and drive the power on the ascent. In both directions, remember: **your lower body is the engine; your arms are just the steering wheel.**

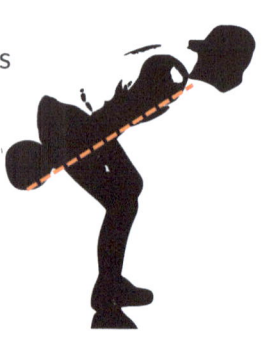

House Rules

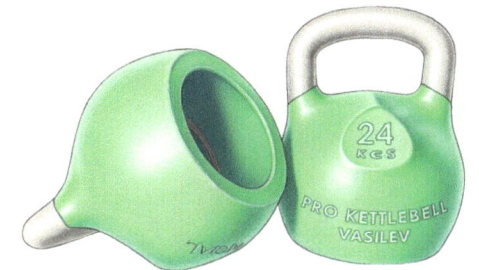

Prepare Your Body

- Take off rings, watches and loose jewelry.
- Wear flat-soled athletic shoes—or go barefoot if you prefer.
- Choose snug workout clothing.
- Warm up your **muscles and joints** prior to intense or heavy weight exercises.

Treat Every Kettlebell Like It's Heavy

- Whether it's 4kg or 32kg, every kettlebell deserves the same respect. Even a light bell can cause injury if you lose control.

Know How to Start (and Finish) a Lift

You won't always be able to lift from a perfect position—maybe it's on a rack or off to the side. That's okay, as long as you brace yourself. Engage your core by imagining cinching a wide belt tightly around your torso before lifting.

- **Stand directly over the kettlebells** and use a deadlift pattern to raise & lower.
- **To swing it, take a squat position** 1-2 feet behind the kettlebell. With straight arms, hike the bell like a football snap into a backswing. When finished, reverse the hike by dropping your hips and guiding the swing to the floor in front of you, keeping your back neutral throughout.

How to Hold a Kettlebell in the Rack Position and Overhead

For safety, comfort, and control, employ a proper kettlebell grip (also called a "false grip" or "olympic grip:" fingers relaxed, handle at a diagonal across your palm, wrist neutral.

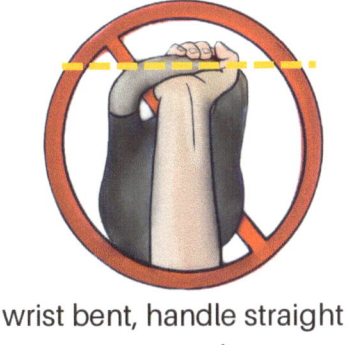

wrist bent, handle straight across palm

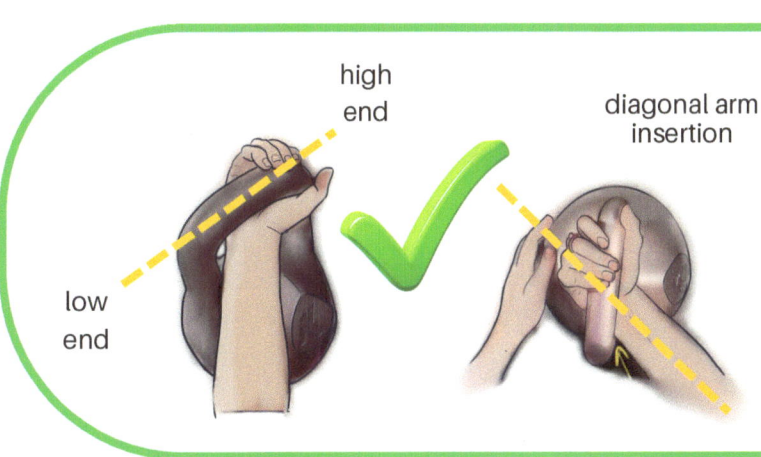

high end / low end / diagonal arm insertion

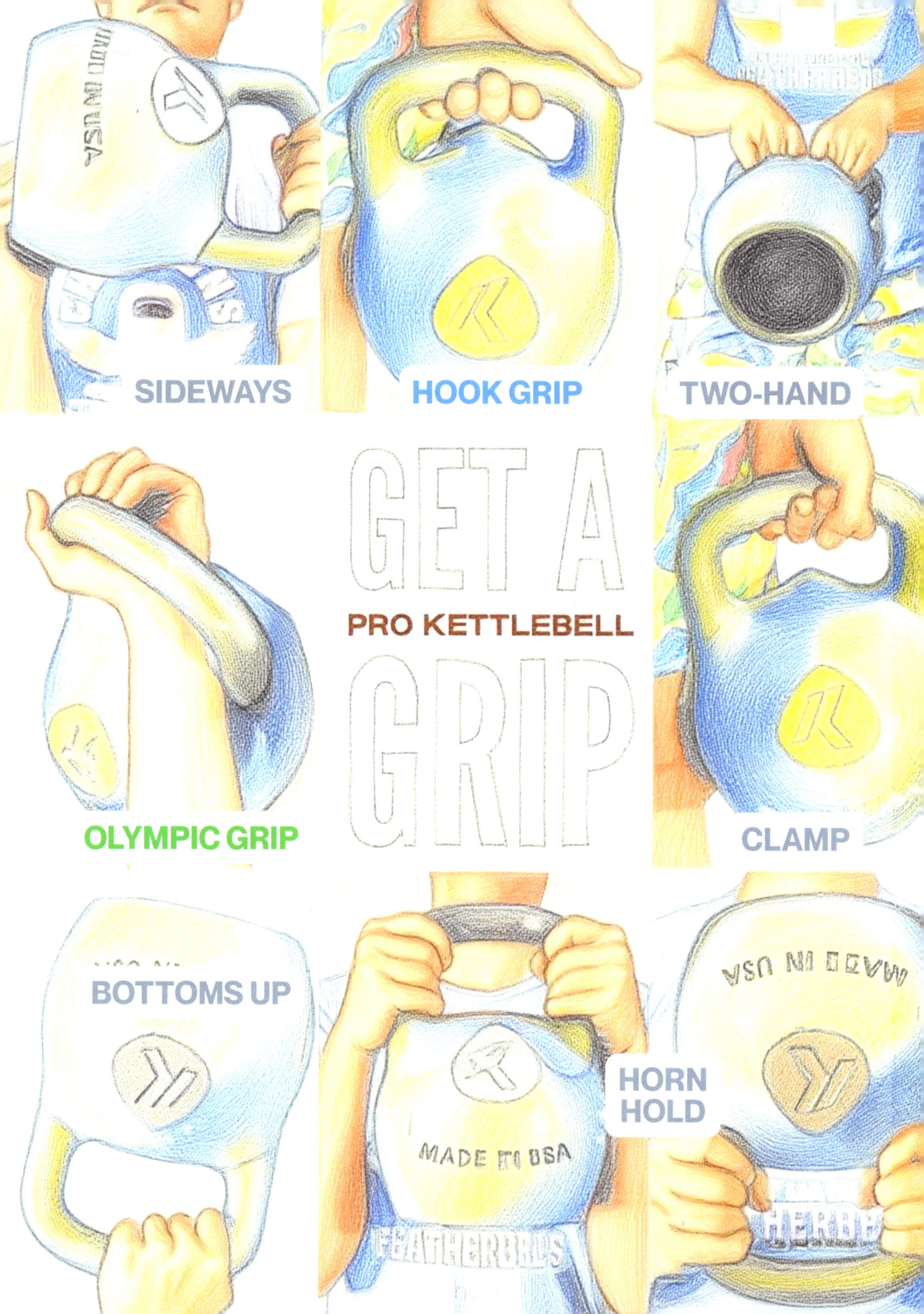

Upper-Body

———————— Section One ————————

The Rack Position
Presses
Push-Ups
Rows
Curls & Miscellaneous

Upper Body

1. Presses

Rack Position	15
Alternating Press	16
Bottoms-Up Floor Press	16
Bottoms-Up Press	16
Bridge Crush Press	17
Double Bridge Press	17
Double Seated Press	17
Double Step-Thru Press	18
Floor Press	18
Front Press	18
Kneeling Press	19
Military Press (Strict Press)	19
Palm Press	19
Seated Twister Press	20
Standing Chest Press	20
Straddle Press, Two-Hand	20
Strict Press (Two-Hand Side Hold)	21
Superman Press	21
Wiper Press	21
Push Press	22
See Saw Press	22
Kneeling Crab Press	22
Racked Circle Press	23
Shinbox Press	23
Slingshot Curtsy Press	23
Warrior Press	24
Iron Cross Circle Press	24

2. Push-Ups

Diamond Cutter Push-Ups	25
Narrow Kettlebell Push-Ups	25
Offset (Uneven Push-Ups)	25
Steam Rollers	26
Decline Kettlebell Push-Ups	26
KB Kick Thru Push-Ups	26
Plyo Push-Up	27
Rolling Push-Ups	27
Slider Push-Ups	27

3. Rows

Alternating Stop Row	28
Ballistic Row	28
Bent Over Gurney Row	28
One-Arm Row	29
Renegade Row	29
Upright Row	29

4. Miscellaneous & Compounds

21-Curls	30
Axe Chops	30
Barn Door Fly	30
Bridge Pull Over	31
Cheat Curls	31
Concentration Curls	31
Cross Curl Press	32
Cross Curls (High Fives)	32
Flat Kettlebell Fly	32
Floor Pullover	33
Front Raise	33
Front Raise Rotations	33
Halos	34
Kettlebell Dips	34
Kettlebell Skull Crushers	34
Kneeling Curl + Press	35
Reverse Curls	35
Ribbon	35
Seated Ribbons	36
Seated Woodchopper	36
Shrugs	36
Tricep Extension	37
Two-Hand Sprays	37
Vertical Halos	37
Wheel Turns	38
Double Reverse Fly	38
Dynamic Ribbons	38
Flat Lat Pullover	39
Lawn Mower Pull	39
Single Leg Ribbons	39

First Things First!

We begin our kettlebell exercise library with the rack position because you must learn it before performing many of the exercises in this book. Learning how to properly hold and rest the kettlebell at your chest ensures safety, efficiency, and balance, and teaches you how to align your body under load for long-term success with more dynamic lifts. Your rack position may look different based on your anatomy, but the rules are simple: keep the bells in alignment with your joints, and your upper arm in contact with your body.

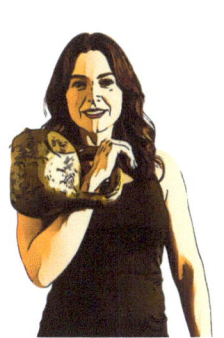 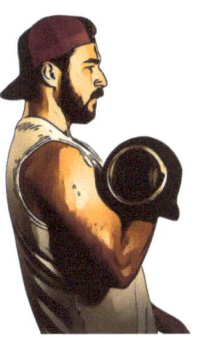 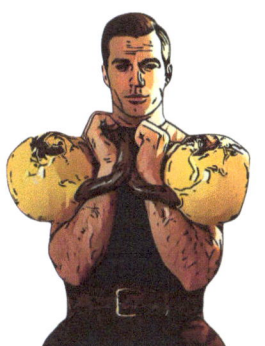 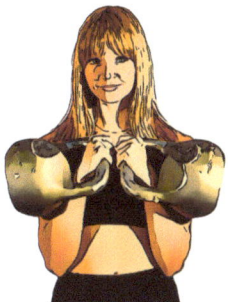 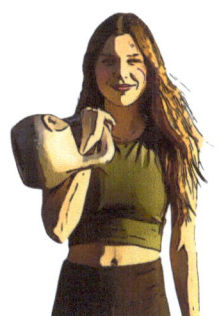

The Rack Position

	Single Bell	Double Bell
	✓	✓

Technical Difficulty	Movement Pattern	Recommended Load
2	Hold	Light, Medium, and Heavy Weights

PRIMARY BENEFIT	UPPER BODY STRENGTH
TARGET MUSCLES	ERECTORS, FRONT DELTS, TRAPS, BICEPS, FOREARMS, ABS

What it is:
The rack position is a foundational hold where the kettlebell rests above your waist, supported by your upper body. Think of the "racking" the kettlebell as putting it on a shelf. This is a position to rest, recover, and launch solid reps from.

How to get there:
Kettlebells are typically moved into the rack position by performing a "clean." A "clean" is a swing you catch in the rack. Before you learn the swing and clean, lift the kettlebell into position using your free hand to assist.

Lower Body:
Begin with a shoulder-width stance. Squeeze your glutes to protect your lower back and shift your hips slightly forward. Stack the kettlebell's center of mass over your hips, between your heels and toes. You may feel a slight groin stretch but no tension in your lower back.

Upper Body / Positioning:
Relax your shoulders slightly forward to allow natural spinal flexion so your elbow(s) rest on your hip. If your arms are shorter or your belly limits this, the forearm can rest along your abdomen.

Bring your hands toward your center so the kettlebell's center of mass, cradled by your bicep and forearm, stays within your frame.

Tips:
It's personal preference whether you stack the handles, lightly touch them, or keep them separated during double-bell work. In all cases, keep your fingers open so they don't get caught between the handles.

With two bells, your body becomes—and should remain—symmetrical, but during single bell work you will feel asymmetrical, which is normal and okay.

PRO KETTLEBELL

1. Alternating Press

	Single Bell	Double Bell
SLOW	✗	✓

🔧 Technical Difficulty	💪 Movement Pattern	⚖️ Recommended Load
1	Push	Medium Weight

PRIMARY BENEFIT	UPPER BODY STRENGTH
TARGET MUSCLES	LATS, DELTOIDS, TRICEPS

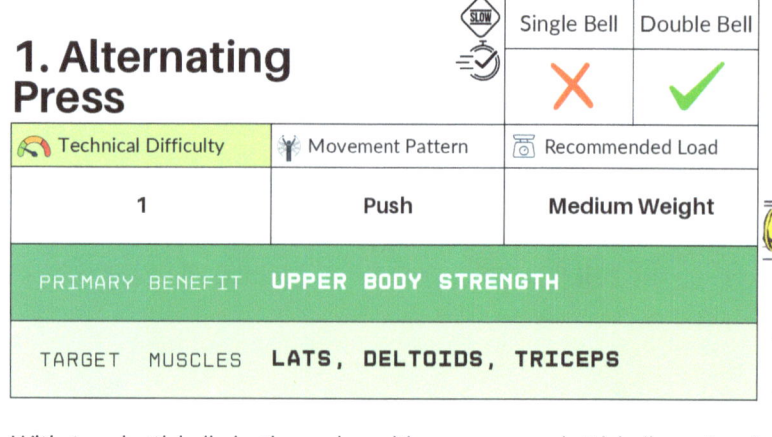

With two kettlebells in the rack position, press one kettlebell overhead while keeping the other in the rack. Lower the bell back to the rack, then switch arms. Keep each press controlled and aligned over the shoulder. Rest between reps in the rack if needed or press one up as the other comes down to increase intensity. ▶ PROKETTLEBELL.COM/1

2. Bottoms-Up Floor Press

	Single Bell	Double Bell
SLOW	✓	✓

🔧 Technical Difficulty	💪 Movement Pattern	⚖️ Recommended Load
1	Push	Light, Medium Weight

PRIMARY BENEFIT	UPPER BODY STRENGTH
TARGET MUSCLES	TRICEPS, PECS, DELTOIDS, LATS

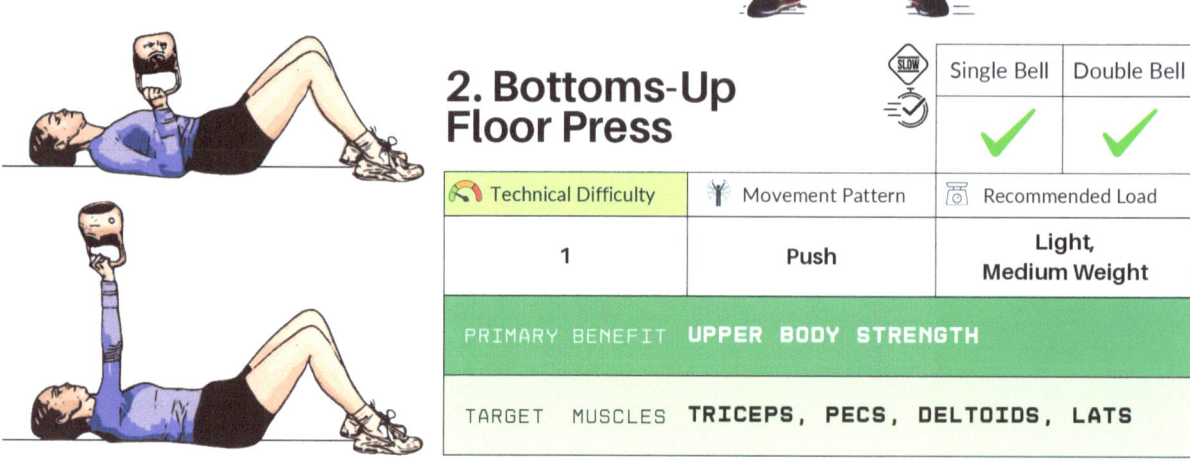

Lie on your back with knees bent and hold a kettlebell by the handle, upside down. Keep the weight balanced over your shoulder and press straight up, then lower under control. For more tricep focus, keep the elbows tight; for more chest involvement, allow them to flare slightly to about 45 degrees. Double bells can be attempted with care or with assistance from a partner. ▶ PROKETTLEBELL.COM/2

3. Bottoms-Up Press

	Single Bell	Double Bell
SLOW	✓	✓

🔧 Technical Difficulty	💪 Movement Pattern	⚖️ Recommended Load
1	Push	Light, Medium Weight

PRIMARY BENEFIT	SHOULDER, ELBOW, WRIST STRENGTH AND STABILITY
TARGET MUSCLES	DELTOIDS, TRICEPS, FOREARMS

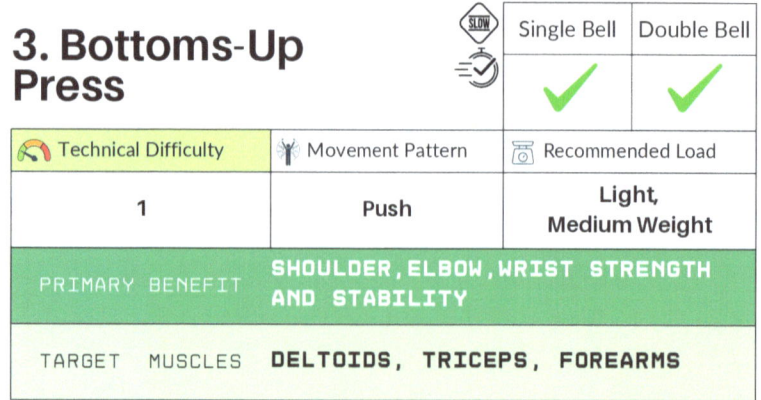
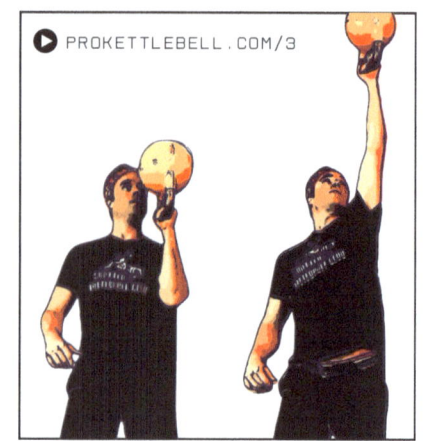

▶ PROKETTLEBELL.COM/3

Hold the kettlebell by the handle in a bottoms-up position, gripping near the corner of the handle for maximum control. Begin with your arm bent and your forearm vertical. Press the kettlebell upward until your arm is fully extended, keeping the bell stacked directly over the shoulder. Lower under control to the starting position. Maintain balance and full-body tension at the top. To increase difficulty, grip closer to the center of the handle to further challenge stability and grip strength.

4. Bridge Crush Press

	Single Bell	Double Bell
	✓	✗

Technical Difficulty	Movement Pattern	Recommended Load
1	Push	Medium, Heavy Weight

PRIMARY BENEFIT	CHEST AND ARM STRENGTH
TARGET MUSCLES	GLUTES, PECS, LATS, DELTOIDS, TRICEPS

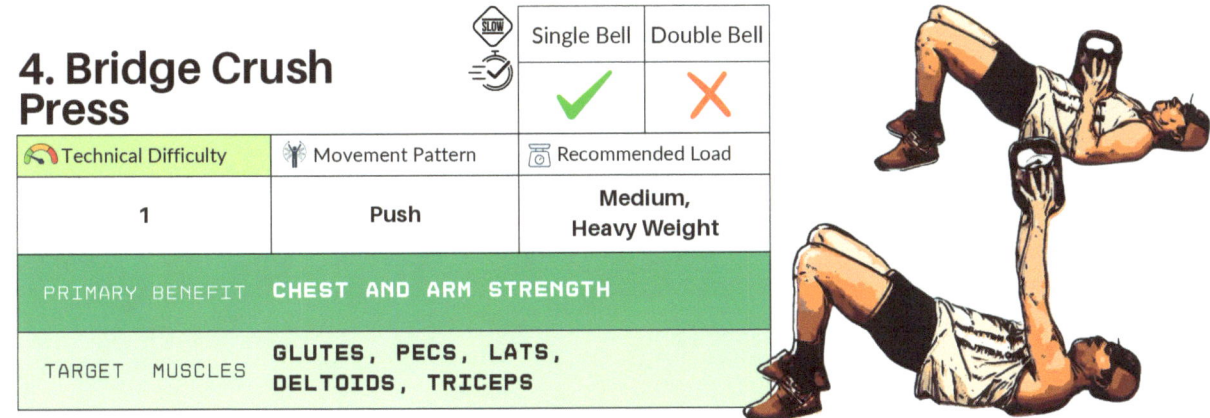

Lie on your back with knees bent and hold a single kettlebell between both palms, base aligned at your chest. Drive through your heels to lift your hips into a bridge. Squeeze the kettlebell as if crushing it, then press it straight up over your chest, aligning wrists, elbows, and shoulders at the top. Control the descent and repeat. Grip style may vary depending on the kettlebell and your comfort.   ▶ PROKETTLEBELL.COM/4

▶ PROKETTLEBELL.COM/5

5. Double Bridge Press

	Single Bell	Double Bell
	✗	✓

Technical Difficulty	Movement Pattern	Recommended Load
1	Push	Medium Weight

PRIMARY BENEFIT	UPPER BODY STRENGTH
TARGET MUSCLES	GLUTES, ERECTORS, LATS, PECS, DELTOIDS, TRICEPS

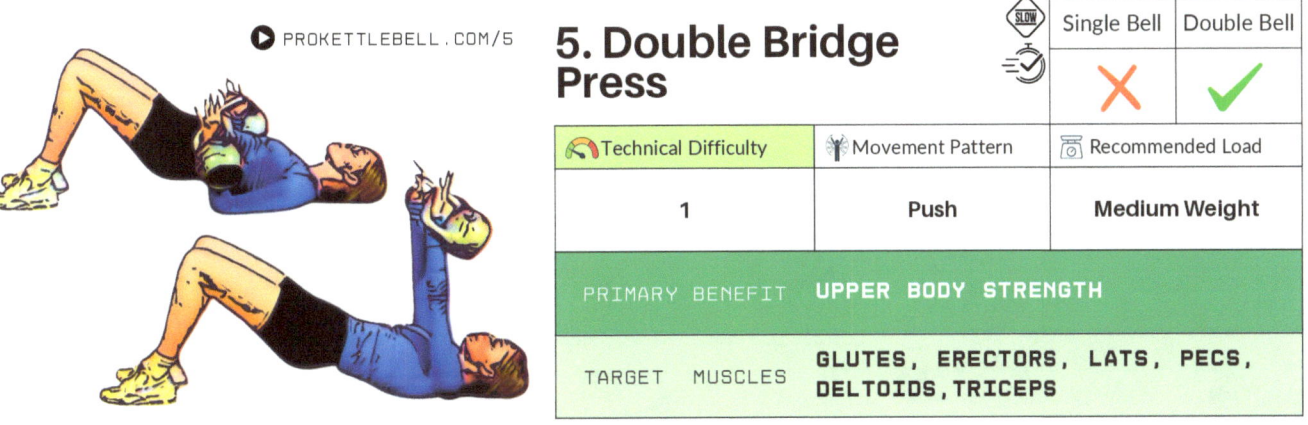

Begin lying on your back with knees and arms bent, forearms perpendicular to the floor. Drive through your heels to lift your hips, forming a straight line from shoulders to knees. From this bridged position, press the kettlebells overhead with control until arms are totally straight. Keep elbows tucked in for more triceps focus or slightly wider for more pec activation, avoiding angles wider than 45 degrees for shoulder safety.

6. Double Seated Press

	Single Bell	Double Bell
	✗	✓

Technical Difficulty	Movement Pattern	Recommended Load
1	Push	Medium Weight

PRIMARY BENEFIT	UPPER BODY STRENGTH AND MOBILITY
TARGET MUSCLES	ABS, ERECTORS, LATS, DELTOIDS, TRICEPS

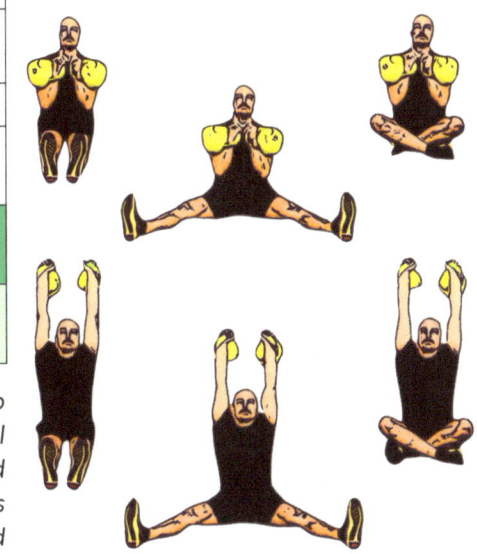

Sit in a straddle, cross-legged, or legs-extended position with two kettlebells held at your chest. Press the kettlebells straight over head until arms are fully extended, then lower back to the rack. Choose a seated posture that supports good form and allows for full overhead range. As you progress, try more difficult positions to improve shoulder mobility and upper-body strength.   ▶ PROKETTLEBELL.COM/6

PRESSES

7. Double Step-Thru Press

		Single Bell	Double Bell
		✗	✓

Technical Difficulty	Movement Pattern	Recommended Load
1	Push	Medium Weight

PRIMARY BENEFIT	FULL-BODY STRENGTH
TARGET MUSCLES	QUADRICEPS, GLUTES, HAMSTRINGS ERECTORS, LATS, DELTOIDS, TRICEPS

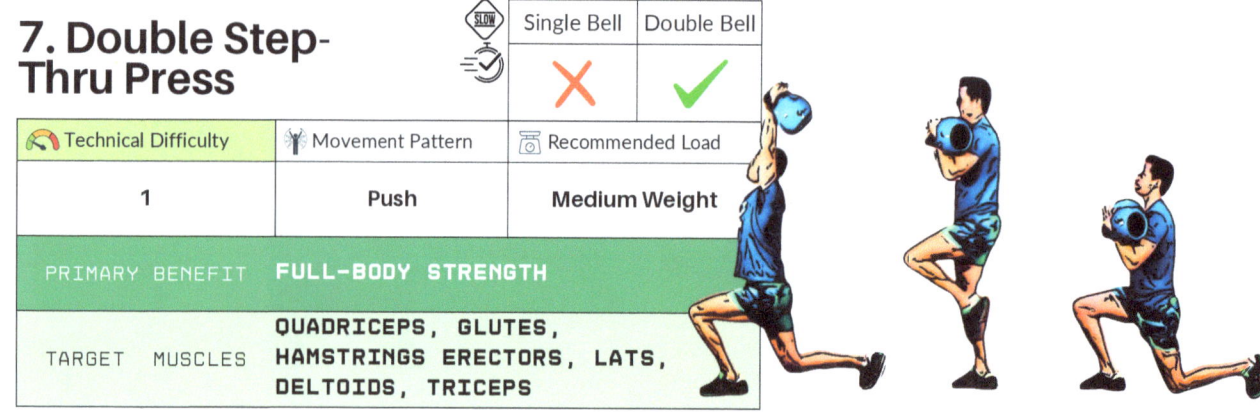

Start with two kettlebells held at the chest. Step into a forward lunge, then perform a strict overhead press. After fixation at the top, return the kettlebells to the chest and take a giant step backward into a reverse lunge position. Complete another press, return the bells to the rack position, and take a giant step into a forward lunge again. Repeat. Work one leg at a time, switching legs after a set period of time or reps. ▶ PROKETTLEBELL.COM/7

8. Floor Press

▶ PROKETTLEBELL.COM/8

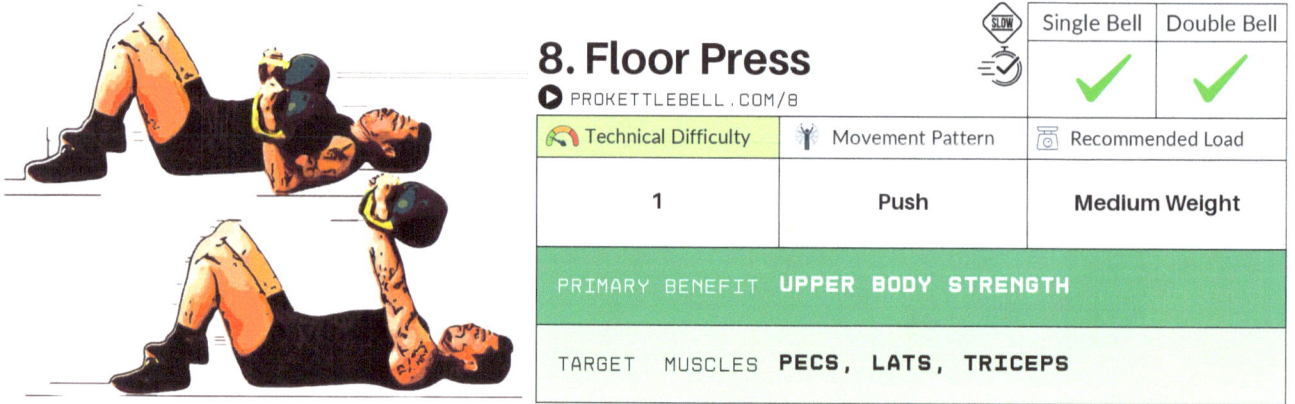

		Single Bell	Double Bell
		✓	✓

Technical Difficulty	Movement Pattern	Recommended Load
1	Push	Medium Weight

PRIMARY BENEFIT	UPPER BODY STRENGTH
TARGET MUSCLES	PECS, LATS, TRICEPS

Lie on your back with knees bent, holding one or two kettlebells with forearms vertical and elbows resting on the floor. Press the kettlebells straight up until your arms are fully extended and the bells are directly over your shoulders, gently squeezing them together at the top. Lower with control until your triceps lightly touch the ground, then repeat. Keep your core engaged, wrists neutral, and elbows at a 45-degree angle or tucked close for more tricep emphasis.

9. Front Press

		Single Bell	Double Bell
		✓	✓

Technical Difficulty	Movement Pattern	Recommended Load
1	Push	Medium Weight

PRIMARY BENEFIT	ARM AND CHEST STRENGTH
TARGET MUSCLES	UPPER PECS, DELTOIDS, TRICEPS

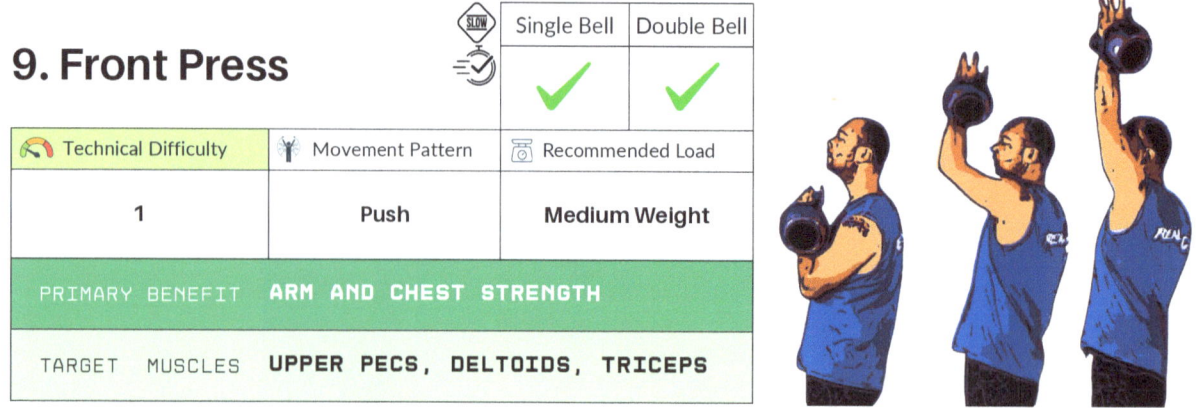

Hold a kettlebell in the rack position with your elbow pointing straight ahead; a 90-degree bend to your arm. **Keep this elbow position throughout the movement.** *Press the kettlebell up as high as you can while keeping your elbows in front of you—some people will be able to fully lock out over their shoulder but some cannot. Return to the starting position and repeat. This variation targets the triceps, front delts, and upper chest while maintaining tension and alignment for isolation.* ▶ PROKETTLEBELL.COM/9

10. Kneeling Press

	Single Bell	Double Bell
	✓	✓

Technical Difficulty	Movement Pattern	Recommended Load
1	Push	Medium Weight

PRIMARY BENEFIT	UPPER BODY STRENGTH
TARGET MUSCLES	DELTOIDS AND TRICEPS

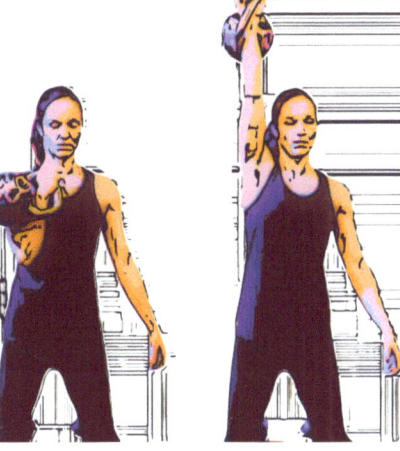

To perform the kneeling press, begin in a kneeling position on the floor with one or both knees down, depending on your preference. Hold the kettlebell in the rack position. From this position, press the kettlebell straight overhead, emphasizing shoulder and triceps engagement. The kneeling stance removes any lower-body assistance, isolating the upper body for a strict press. Use a pad under the knee for comfort. ▶ PROKETTLEBELL.COM/10

11. Military Press

▶ PROKETTLEBELL.COM/11

	Single Bell	Double Bell
	✓	✓

Technical Difficulty	Movement Pattern	Recommended Load
1	Push	Medium Weight

PRIMARY BENEFIT	UPPER BODY STRENGTH
TARGET MUSCLES	DELTOIDS, TRICEPS

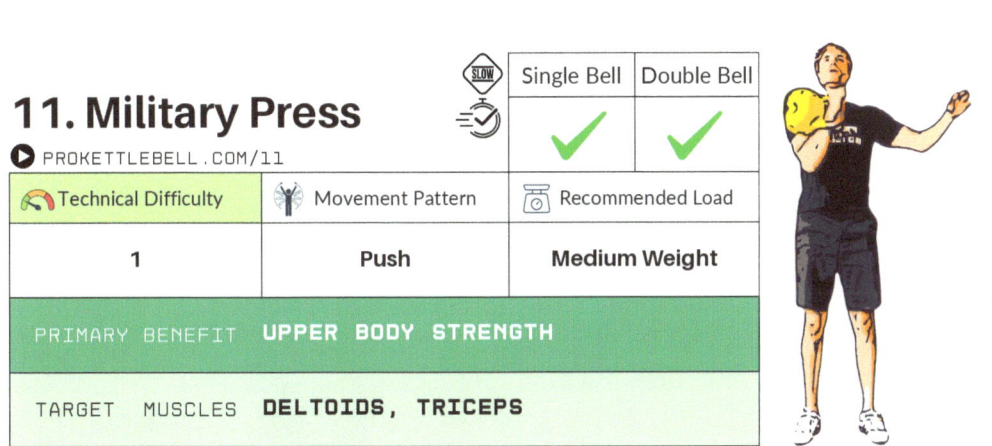

(*"Strict Press"*) Begin standing with a kettlebell in the rack position, legs straight. Keep the kettlebell within your frame, stacked over the hip when viewed from the front and side. Press the kettlebell straight up without using the legs. As the bell passes the shoulder, allow the upper body to shift slightly forward; as it lowers, let the chest and torso move slightly backward to maintain a straight vertical bell path throughout the movement.

12. Palm Press

▶ PROKETTLEBELL.COM/12

	Single Bell	Double Bell
	✓	✓

Technical Difficulty	Movement Pattern	Recommended Load
1	Push	Medium Weight

PRIMARY BENEFIT	UPPER BODY STRENGTH AND STABILITY
TARGET MUSCLES	LATS, DELTOIDS, TRICEPS

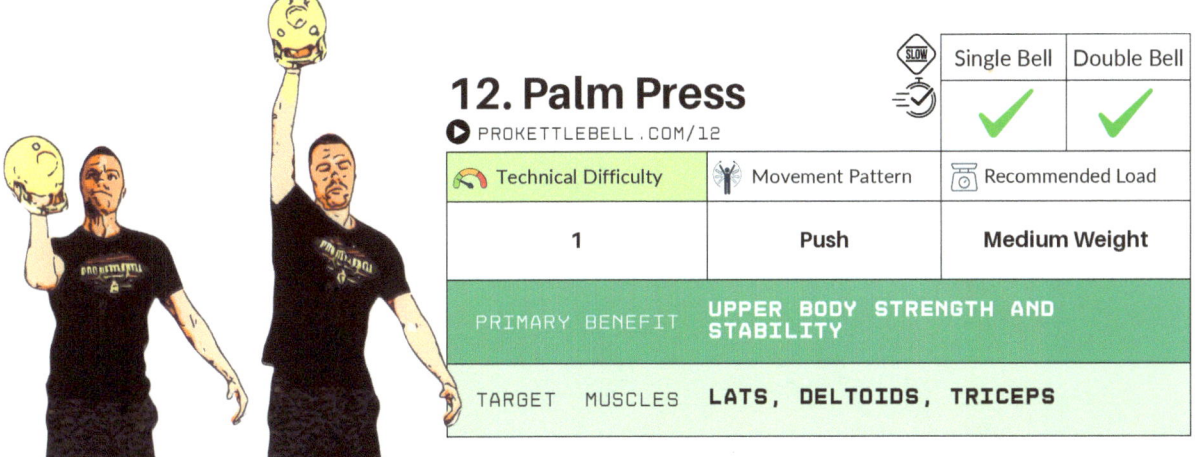

Hold the kettlebell upright with the base resting in the palm and the handle draped over the wrist. This setup places the load directly over the palm, increasing the demand on shoulder stability and pec engagement. Slightly turn the palm outward and align the kettlebell with the shoulder. Press the weight overhead with control, keeping the elbow slightly forward. Lower the kettlebell slowly back to the start, maintaining control and alignment throughout the movement.

PRESSES

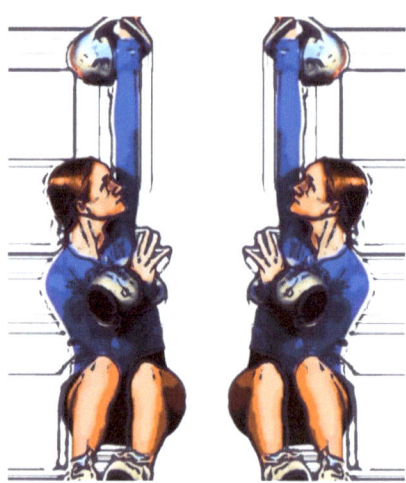

13. Seated Twister Press

	Single Bell	Double Bell
SLOW	✗	✓

Technical Difficulty	Movement Pattern	Recommended Load
1	Push	Light Weight

PRIMARY BENEFIT	UPPER BODY STRENGTH AND MOBILITY
TARGET MUSCLES	ERECTORS, OBLIQUES, LATS, DELTOIDS, TRICEPS

Sit on the ground with your legs extended, splayed, or crossed—whichever position feels the most stable. Hold the kettlebells close to your midline. Rotate your torso to one side and press the kettlebell overhead <u>with the outside arm</u>, then return to center. Repeat on the opposite side, always pressing with the outside arm. This exercise builds shoulder strength and rotational core control. Start with a light weight to emphasize mobility, positioning, and maintaining alignment as close to your center as possible.

▶ PROKETTLEBELL.COM/13

14. Standing Chest Press ▶ PROKETTLEBELL.COM/14

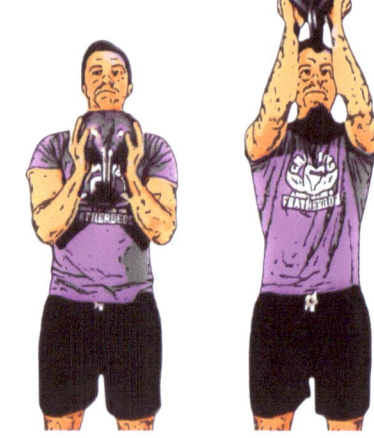

	Single Bell	Double Bell
SLOW	✓	✗

Technical Difficulty	Movement Pattern	Recommended Load
1	Push	Light, Medium Weight

PRIMARY BENEFIT	CHEST STRENGTH AND HYPERTROPHY
TARGET MUSCLES	PEC, DELTOIDS, TRICEPS

Hold a single kettlebell with both hands in a crush grip, positioned directly in front of your chest with forearms parallel. Maintain tension through the pecs as you press the kettlebell slightly forwards and upward, then return to the starting position under control. This movement emphasizes upper chest strength and hypertrophy and is best performed with light to medium weight due to the forward load position. Keep the core braced and posture upright to avoid lower back strain.

15. Two-Hand Straddle Press

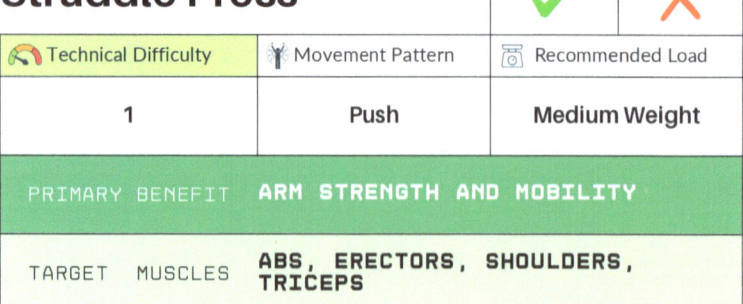

	Single Bell	Double Bell
SLOW	✓	✗

Technical Difficulty	Movement Pattern	Recommended Load
1	Push	Medium Weight

PRIMARY BENEFIT	ARM STRENGTH AND MOBILITY
TARGET MUSCLES	ABS, ERECTORS, SHOULDERS, TRICEPS

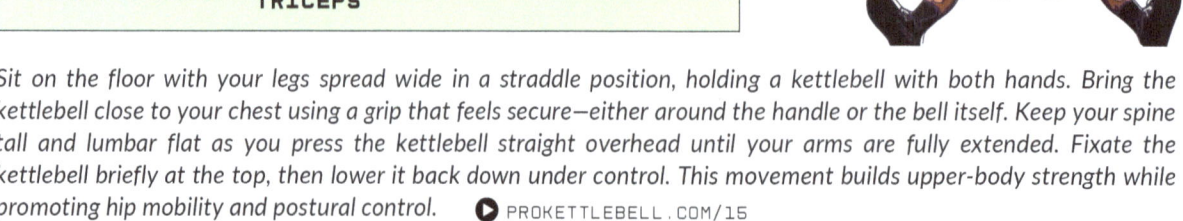

Sit on the floor with your legs spread wide in a straddle position, holding a kettlebell with both hands. Bring the kettlebell close to your chest using a grip that feels secure—either around the handle or the bell itself. Keep your spine tall and lumbar flat as you press the kettlebell straight overhead until your arms are fully extended. Fixate the kettlebell briefly at the top, then lower it back down under control. This movement builds upper-body strength while promoting hip mobility and postural control. ▶ PROKETTLEBELL.COM/15

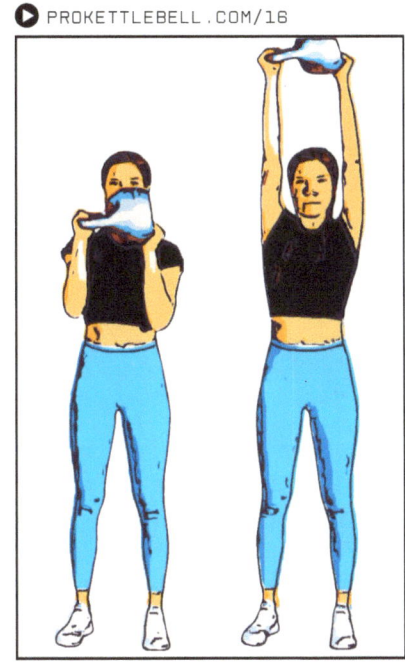

16. Side-Hold Strict Press

PROKETTLEBELL.COM/16

	Single Bell	Double Bell
SLOW	✗	✓

Technical Difficulty	Movement Pattern	Recommended Load
1	Push	Medium Weight

PRIMARY BENEFIT	SHOULDER STRENGTH
TARGET MUSCLES	SHOULDERS, TRICEPS

Hold the kettlebell with one hand on the handle and the other on the base, keeping the forearms parallel. Without using the legs, press the kettlebell straight overhead in line with your center of mass until it is directly above the head. Focus on controlled movement and a stable lockout, avoiding shoulder shrugging. Lower the kettlebell back to the chest under control and repeat. This two-hand variation promotes even force distribution and reinforces proper overhead alignment and fixation.

17. Superman Press

PROKETTLEBELL.COM/17

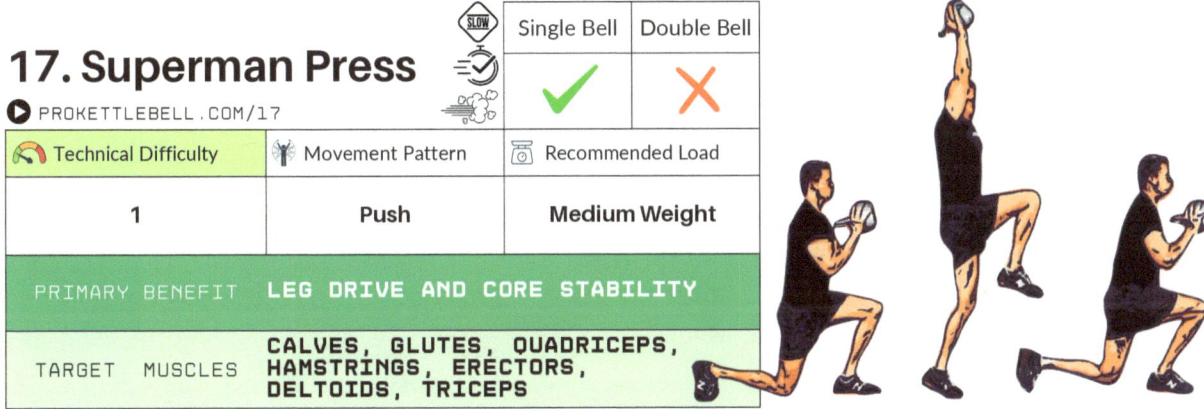

	Single Bell	Double Bell
SLOW	✓	✗

Technical Difficulty	Movement Pattern	Recommended Load
1	Push	Medium Weight

PRIMARY BENEFIT	LEG DRIVE AND CORE STABILITY
TARGET MUSCLES	CALVES, GLUTES, QUADRICEPS, HAMSTRINGS, ERECTORS, DELTOIDS, TRICEPS

Begin the Superman press holding the kettlebell between your palms at chest height, with thumbs positioned between the horns for balance. Step back into a controlled reverse lunge. From there, explosively drive forward and upward, bringing your knee to chest-height while simultaneously pressing the kettlebell overhead. Finish by landing the "up" leg in a forward lunge position as you lower the kettlebell back to your chest. Start with a light load to build coordination before progressing.

18. Wiper Press

PROKETTLEBELL.COM/18

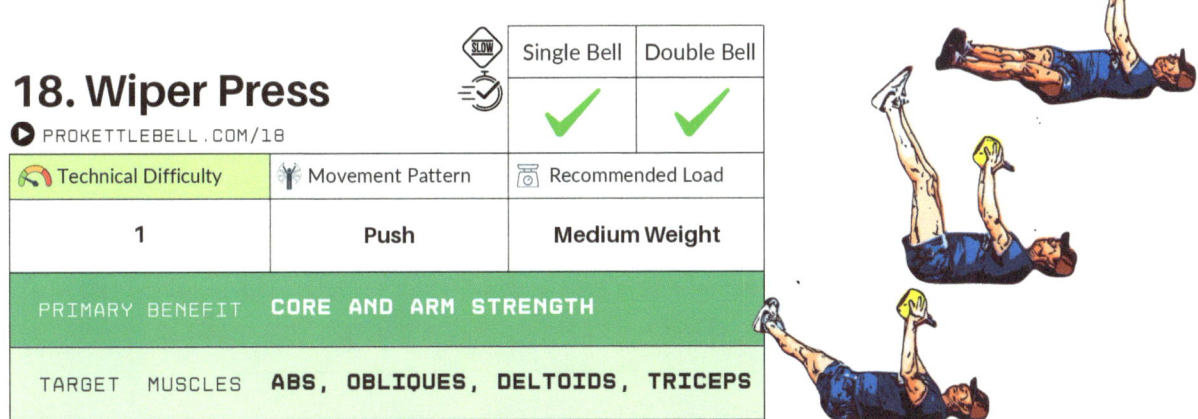

	Single Bell	Double Bell
SLOW	✓	✓

Technical Difficulty	Movement Pattern	Recommended Load
1	Push	Medium Weight

PRIMARY BENEFIT	CORE AND ARM STRENGTH
TARGET MUSCLES	ABS, OBLIQUES, DELTOIDS, TRICEPS

Lie on your back and press one or two kettlebells into position; straight arms, stacked above your shoulders. Extend your legs straight up and move them side to side in a controlled windshield-wiper motion. Maintain core tension and steady control of the kettlebell(s) throughout. To reduce difficulty, slightly bend the knees while keeping the press strong and stable.

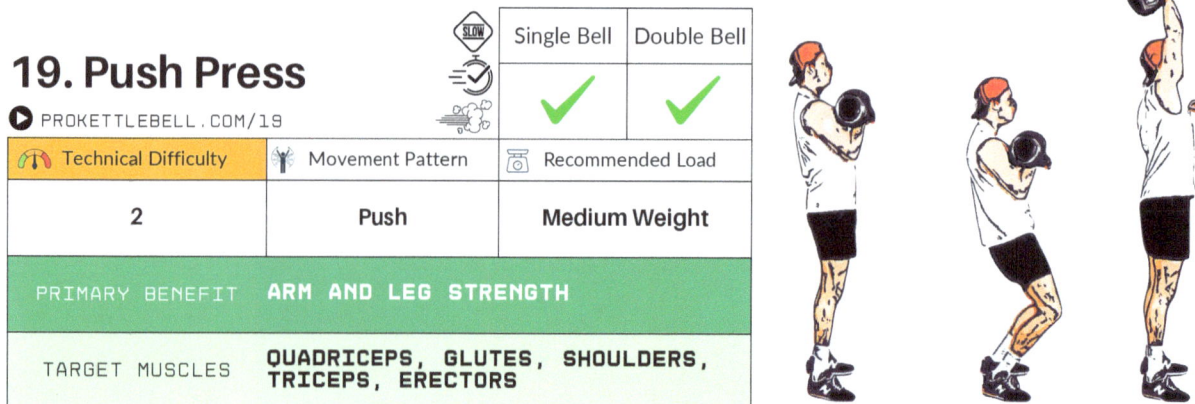

19. Push Press

▶ PROKETTLEBELL.COM/19

	Single Bell	Double Bell
	✓	✓

Technical Difficulty	Movement Pattern	Recommended Load
2	Push	Medium Weight

PRIMARY BENEFIT	ARM AND LEG STRENGTH
TARGET MUSCLES	QUADRICEPS, GLUTES, SHOULDERS, TRICEPS, ERECTORS

Begin the push press by holding the kettlebell in the rack position. While maintaining arm-to-body connection, initiate the movement with a short, controlled dip by slightly bending the knees and keeping the hips forward. Drive upward powerfully using your legs, transferring that momentum into your arm to press the kettlebell overhead. Allow the bell to fixate briefly before lowering it back to the rack position. Arm-to-body contact and proper alignment are key to safe and effective execution.

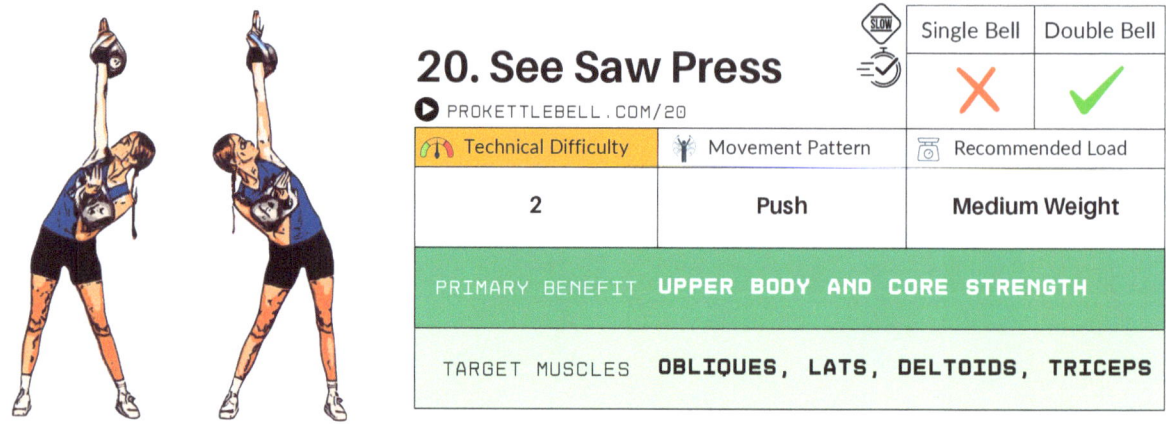

20. See Saw Press

▶ PROKETTLEBELL.COM/20

	Single Bell	Double Bell
	✗	✓

Technical Difficulty	Movement Pattern	Recommended Load
2	Push	Medium Weight

PRIMARY BENEFIT	UPPER BODY AND CORE STRENGTH
TARGET MUSCLES	OBLIQUES, LATS, DELTOIDS, TRICEPS

With a kettlebell in each hand at the rack position, stand with a wide, stable base. Press one kettlebell overhead while keeping the other in the rack, driving that elbow into the torso as the hip shifts underneath the pressing bell. As the raised kettlebell lowers, guide the elbow back into the hip and initiate the weight shift and press on the opposite side, creating a smooth, seesaw-like rhythm. This movement is similar to an alternating press but adds a sliding hip shift under the working bell—essentially a blend of a windmill and an alternating press. It challenges mobility, core control, coordination, and balanced shoulder strength.

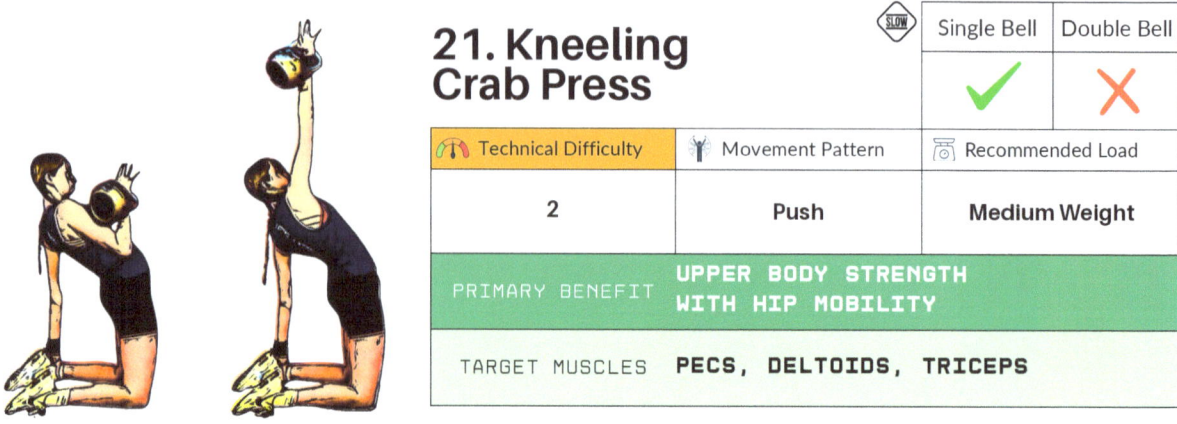

21. Kneeling Crab Press

	Single Bell	Double Bell
	✓	✗

Technical Difficulty	Movement Pattern	Recommended Load
2	Push	Medium Weight

PRIMARY BENEFIT	UPPER BODY STRENGTH WITH HIP MOBILITY
TARGET MUSCLES	PECS, DELTOIDS, TRICEPS

Start in a kneeling position with a single kettlebell in the rack position. Place one hand on your ankle or heel for support, then drive your hips forward until they are stacked over your knees. Press the kettlebell upward, keeping the elbow within your frame and locking out fully at the top. Lower the bell back to the chest and repeat for reps, or hold the top position and relax into the stretch before switching sides. This movement targets the delts, pecs, and upper chest while also developing hip flexor, quad, and core strength and mobility. ▶ PROKETTLEBELL.COM/21

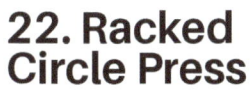 PROKETTLEBELL.COM/22

22. Racked Circle Press

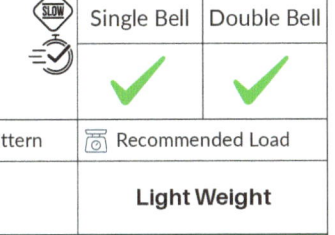

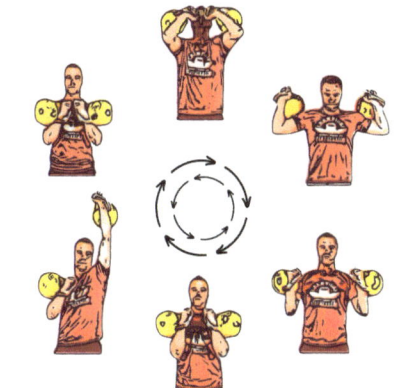

Technical Difficulty	Movement Pattern	Recommended Load
2	Push	Light Weight
PRIMARY BENEFIT	SHOULDER MOBILITY AND CONTROL	
TARGET MUSCLES	PECS, DELTOIDS, LATS, TRICEPS, BICEPS	

Begin with two matching kettlebells held at your chest, hands held close together. Shrug your shoulders and rest the kettlebells on them as you separate your hands and perform a circular motion, drawing the shoulder blades together before returning to the start—think "shoulder circles." As the circle finishes, return one arm to the rack position while pressing the other arm overhead to complete the rep. Lower the pressed bell back to the rack and repeat, beginning again with the shoulder circles. Alternate which side is pressing with each repetition.

23. Shinbox Press

PROKETTLEBELL.COM/23

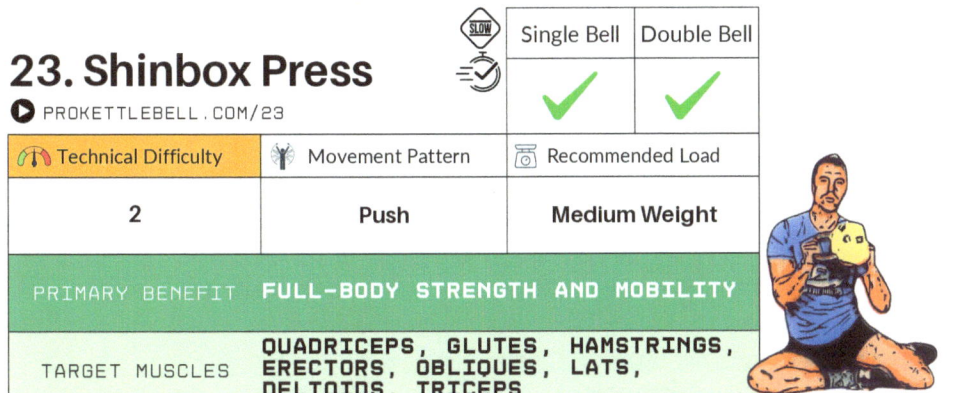

Technical Difficulty	Movement Pattern	Recommended Load
2	Push	Medium Weight
PRIMARY BENEFIT	FULL-BODY STRENGTH AND MOBILITY	
TARGET MUSCLES	QUADRICEPS, GLUTES, HAMSTRINGS, ERECTORS, OBLIQUES, LATS, DELTOIDS, TRICEPS	

Start seated in the shinbox position, with both legs bent at 90 degrees—one leg in front, the other to the side. Hold the kettlebell with both hands, ideally at the handle and base for control. From here, rise up onto both knees and simultaneously press the kettlebell overhead. Lower it back down and return to the seated position. This press builds hip mobility, core stability, and upper body strength. You can increase the challenge by progressing to a double kettlebell rack position once the base movement is mastered.

24. Slingshot Curtsy Press

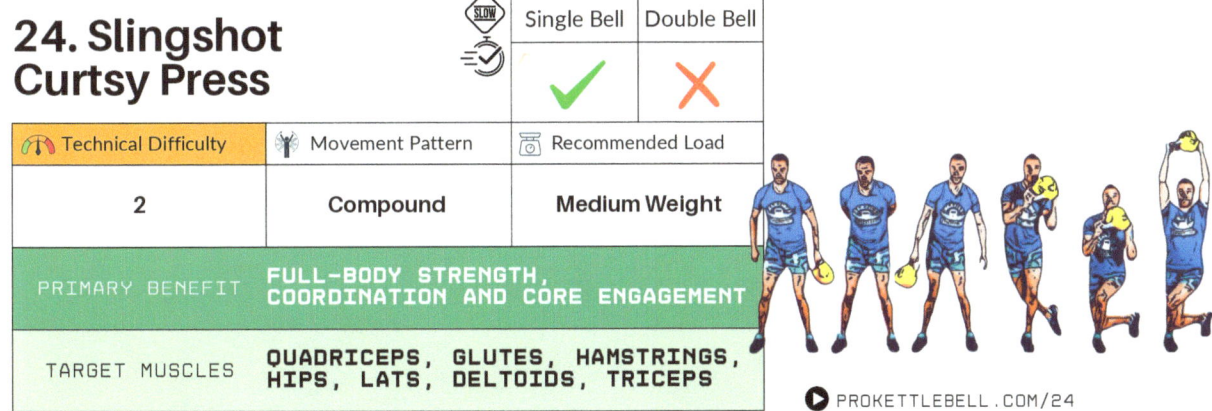

Technical Difficulty	Movement Pattern	Recommended Load
2	Compound	Medium Weight
PRIMARY BENEFIT	FULL-BODY STRENGTH, COORDINATION AND CORE ENGAGEMENT	
TARGET MUSCLES	QUADRICEPS, GLUTES, HAMSTRINGS, HIPS, LATS, DELTOIDS, TRICEPS	

PROKETTLEBELL.COM/24

Begin by performing a kettlebell slingshot to the left, catching the bell with one hand on the handle and the other supporting the base. As you catch it, step the left leg behind you at a 45-degree angle and lower into a curtsy squat. Once stable, press the kettlebell overhead, straighten your arms completely, find momentary stillness and return to standing. Lower the bell back to your chest and mirror the movement on the opposite side by initiating a slingshot to the right. Adjust squat depth based on your mobility and control.

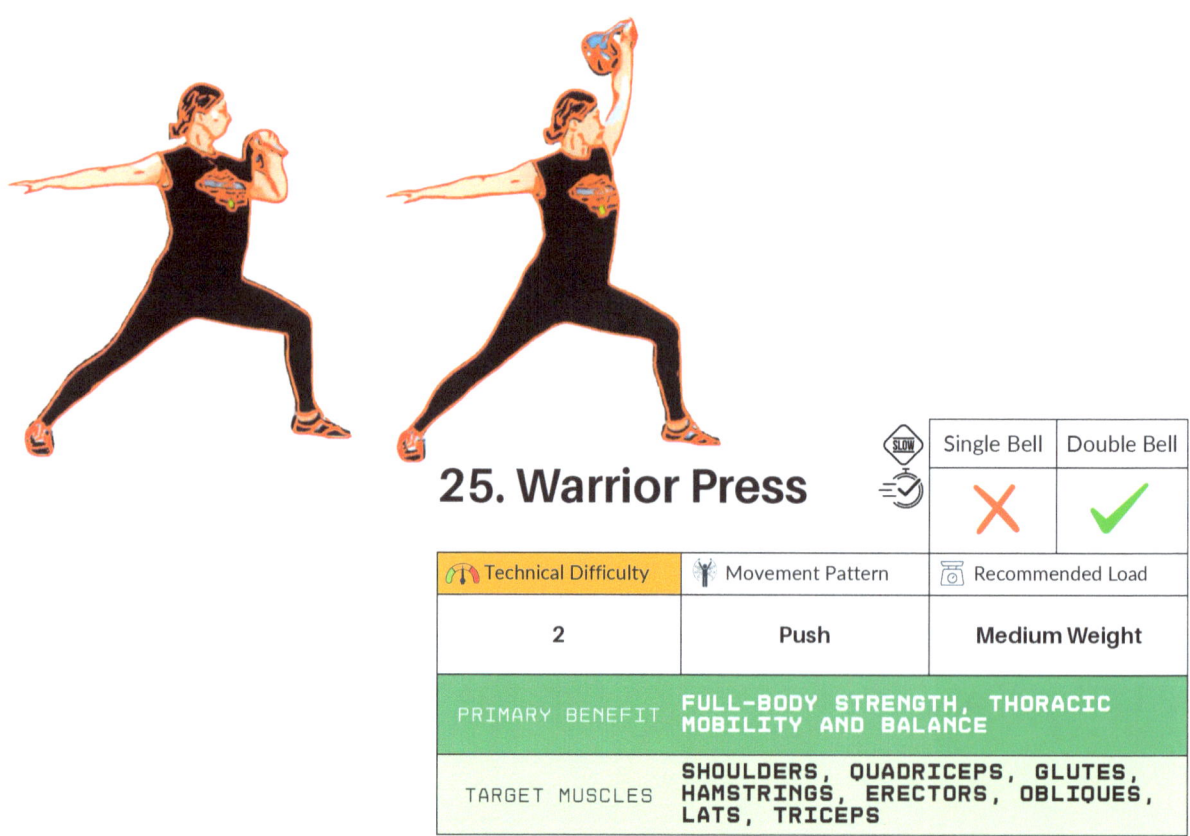

25. Warrior Press

	Single Bell	Double Bell
SLOW	✗	✓

Technical Difficulty	Movement Pattern	Recommended Load
2	Push	Medium Weight

PRIMARY BENEFIT	FULL-BODY STRENGTH, THORACIC MOBILITY AND BALANCE
TARGET MUSCLES	SHOULDERS, QUADRICEPS, GLUTES, HAMSTRINGS, ERECTORS, OBLIQUES, LATS, TRICEPS

Begin by holding a single kettlebell at the chest. Step forward with the kettlebell-side leg into a wide lunge, front foot facing forward and turn out the back foot ~90 degrees. Lift the front elbow and raise your back arm so both arms are parallel to the floor, tracking over the legs. From here, press the kettlebell overhead while facing forward and maintaining an upright posture. Keeping the rest of the body static, return the bell to the starting position and repeat before mirroring the same number of repetitions on the opposite side. ▶ PROKETTLEBELL.COM/25

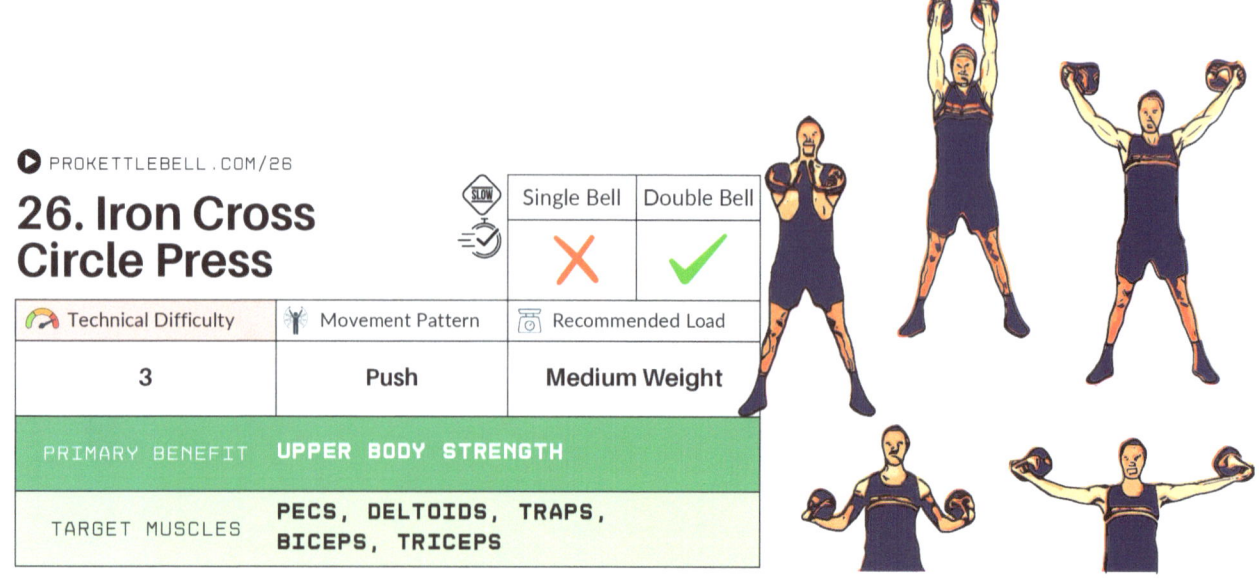

▶ PROKETTLEBELL.COM/26

26. Iron Cross Circle Press

	Single Bell	Double Bell
SLOW	✗	✓

Technical Difficulty	Movement Pattern	Recommended Load
3	Push	Medium Weight

PRIMARY BENEFIT	UPPER BODY STRENGTH
TARGET MUSCLES	PECS, DELTOIDS, TRAPS, BICEPS, TRICEPS

Begin with two kettlebells in the rack position. Press both overhead until arms are fully extended, then turn your palms outward. Keeping your arms straight, slowly lower them in a wide arc, letting the kettlebells balance on your forearms as you go. When the bells reach approximately shoulder height (arms parallel to the floor) or become too heavy to control, bend the arms and draw the elbows toward the ribs to circle the kettlebells back into the rack position to begin the next repetition. Maintain control and constant tension throughout.

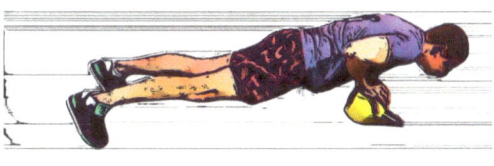

27. Diamond Cutter Push-Ups

	Single Bell	Double Bell
SLOW	✓	✗

Technical Difficulty	Movement Pattern	Recommended Load
1	Push	Heavy Weight

PRIMARY BENEFIT	UPPER BODY STRENGTH
TARGET MUSCLES	LATS, DELTOIDS, PECS, TRICEPS

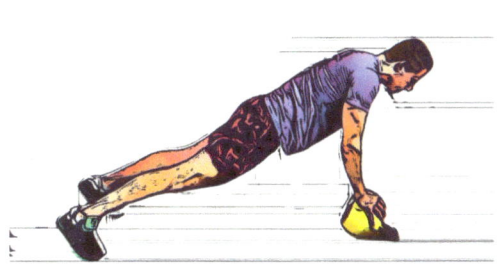

▶ PROKETTLEBELL.COM/27

Place a kettlebell on its side, handle pointing away from you. Take a plank position with both hands coming together to form a diamond shape on the kettlebell. Lower your chest to the kettlebell while keeping your elbows angled back at about 45 degrees. Squeeze your core, avoid shoulder shrugging, and keep a straight back throughout. Perform from your knees if planking from your toes is too challenging.

28. Narrow Kettlebell Push-Ups

	Single Bell	Double Bell
SLOW	✗	✓

▶ PROKETTLEBELL.COM/28

Technical Difficulty	Movement Pattern	Recommended Load
1	Push	Medium Weight

PRIMARY BENEFIT	UPPER BODY STRENGTH
TARGET MUSCLES	ABS, ERECTORS, LATS, DELTOIDS, PECS, TRICEPS

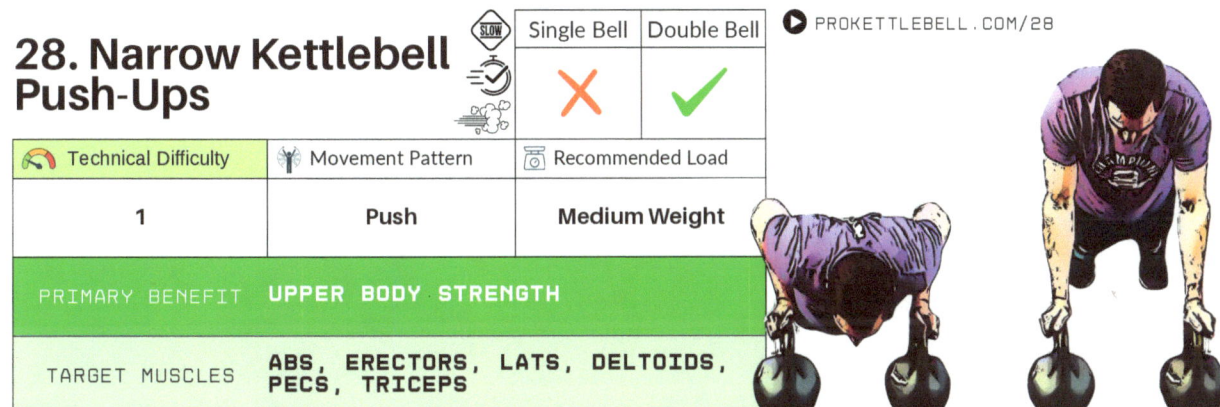

Place two kettlebells on the floor with handles aligned vertically and set slightly narrower than shoulder width. Grip the handles and assume a strong plank position with a neutral spine and engaged core. Lower your chest between the bells while keeping the elbows close to the ribs. Press back to the top, emphasizing triceps engagement. This variation enhances overhead strength and can be performed on knees for an easier option.

29. Off-Set Push-Ups

	Single Bell	Double Bell
SLOW	✓	✗

Technical Difficulty	Movement Pattern	Recommended Load
1	Push	Heavy Weight

PRIMARY BENEFIT	UPPER BODY STRENGTH
TARGET MUSCLES	LATS, PECS, DELTOIDS, TRICEPS

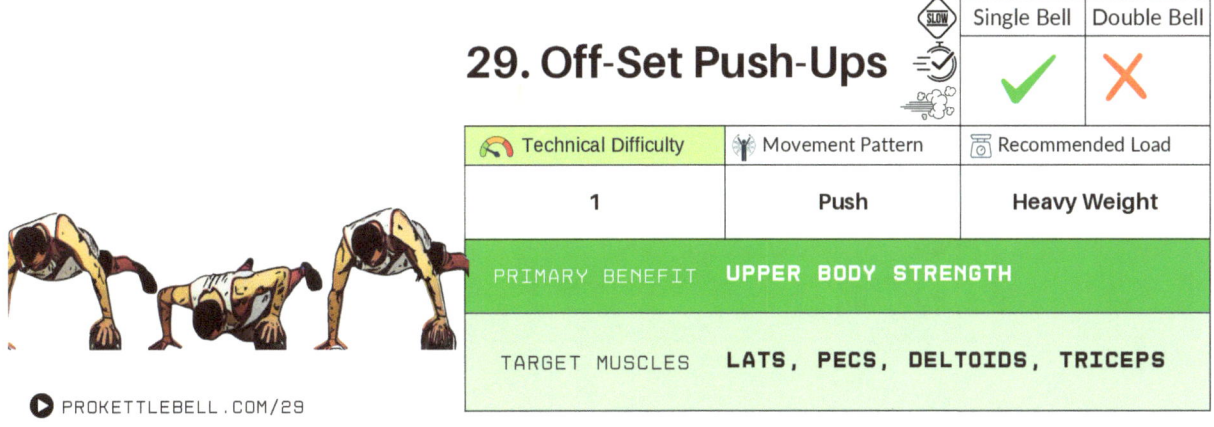

▶ PROKETTLEBELL.COM/29

("Uneven Push-Ups") Place one hand on a kettlebell and the other directly on the ground to create an uneven setup. Lower your chest, increasing the stretch and demand on one arm and pectoral muscle. Push-up, keeping your body straight, elbows angled back about 45 degrees, and core tight throughout. Switch sides after a set to train both arms evenly. This move is a great precursor to more advanced single-arm push-up variations.

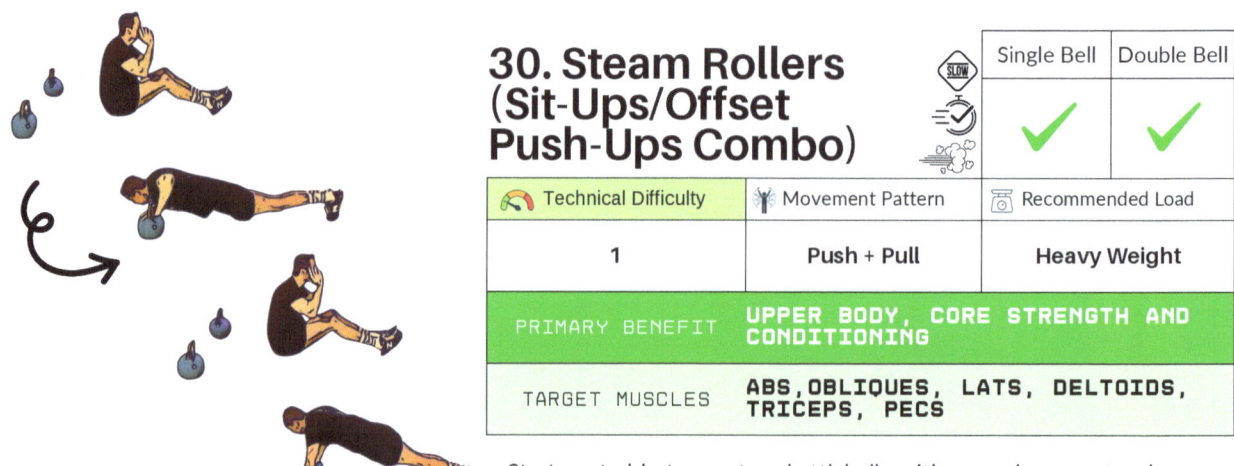

30. Steam Rollers (Sit-Ups/Offset Push-Ups Combo)

	Single Bell	Double Bell
SLOW	✓	✓

Technical Difficulty	Movement Pattern	Recommended Load
1	Push + Pull	Heavy Weight

PRIMARY BENEFIT	UPPER BODY, CORE STRENGTH AND CONDITIONING
TARGET MUSCLES	ABS, OBLIQUES, LATS, DELTOIDS, TRICEPS, PECS

Start seated between two kettlebells with enough space to place one hand on a bell and the other on the floor. Perform three sit-ups, then roll to one side and complete three offset push-ups with one hand on a kettlebell. Roll back, perform three more sit-ups, then roll to the opposite side for three push-ups on the other arm. This fun combination challenges your chest, shoulders, triceps, abs, and obliques all in one sequence. ▶ PROKETTLEBELL.COM/30

31. Decline Kettlebell Push-Ups

	Single Bell	Double Bell
SLOW	✗	✓

Technical Difficulty	Movement Pattern	Recommended Load
2	Push	Heavy Weight

PRIMARY BENEFIT	UPPER BODY STRENGTH
TARGET MUSCLES	PECS, DELTOIDS, TRICEPS, LATS

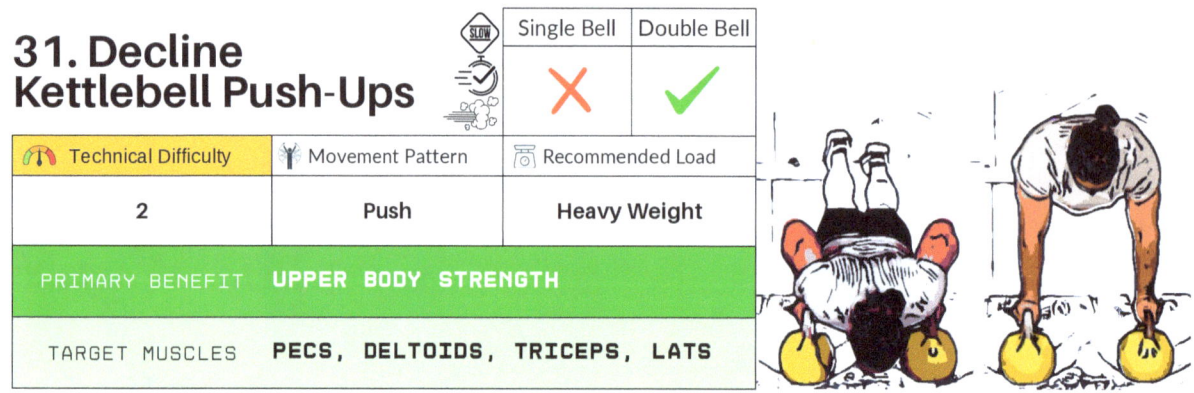

Place two kettlebells directly under your shoulders and elevate your feet on a bench or box. Grip the handles and assume a strong plank position with an engaged core. Lower your chest between the bells, keeping the elbows tucked close to the body for triceps emphasis or slightly flared to increase chest involvement. Press back up to full arm extension while maintaining a straight body line. If the decline position is too advanced, perform from a pike position for added stability (hips up high, like a yoga "down-dog"). It's safest to use wide-base and heavy kettlebells to increase stability. ▶ PROKETTLEBELL.COM/31

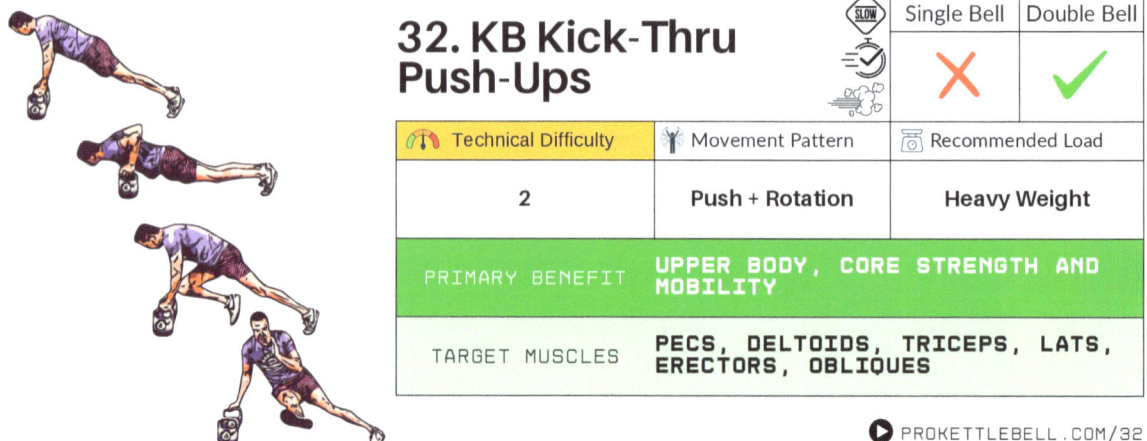

32. KB Kick-Thru Push-Ups

	Single Bell	Double Bell
SLOW	✗	✓

Technical Difficulty	Movement Pattern	Recommended Load
2	Push + Rotation	Heavy Weight

PRIMARY BENEFIT	UPPER BODY, CORE STRENGTH AND MOBILITY
TARGET MUSCLES	PECS, DELTOIDS, TRICEPS, LATS, ERECTORS, OBLIQUES

▶ PROKETTLEBELL.COM/32

Set two wide-based kettlebells at a comfortable width for a stable push-up position. Perform a controlled push-up, then drive one knee toward the chest before kicking it laterally across the body, extending through the hip as you straighten the leg. Return to a plank position and repeat on the opposite side. Keep the core braced and the movement smooth throughout. Balance on one kettlebell for increased rotational demand if desired.

33. Plyo Push-Up

PROKETTLEBELL.COM/33

	Single Bell	Double Bell
	✓	✗

Technical Difficulty	Movement Pattern	Recommended Load
2	Push	Heavy Weight

PRIMARY BENEFIT	UPPER BODY STRENGTH AND POWER
TARGET MUSCLES	LATS, PECS, DELTOIDS, TRICEPS

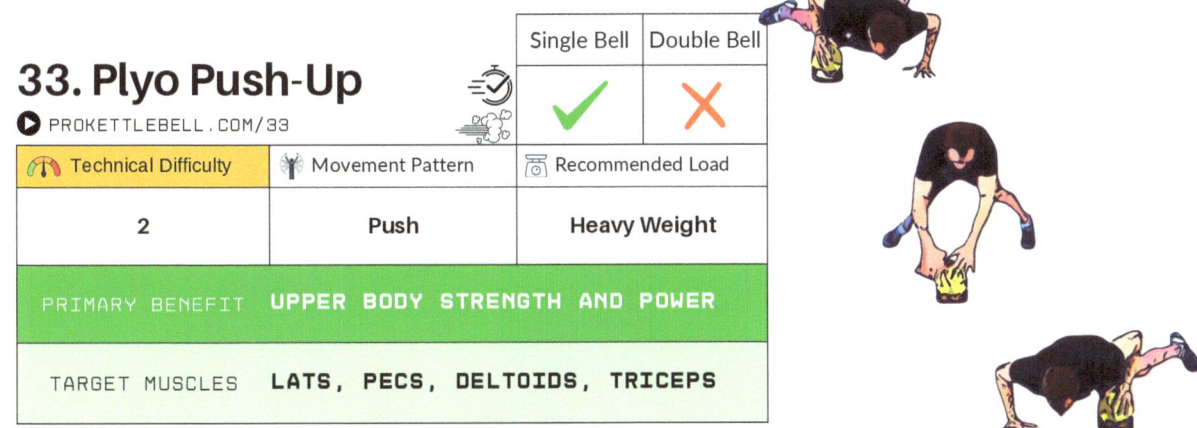

Place the kettlebell on its side with the handle pointing away from you. Set up in a strong plank position with one hand on the kettlebell and the other on the floor. Lower your chest with control, then explosively press up and switch hand positions so the opposite hand lands on the kettlebell. Repeat, mirroring the move. Maintain a tight core and neutral spine throughout. If switching hands in the air is too challenging, step the hands over instead. This exercise can also be performed from the knees for a regression.

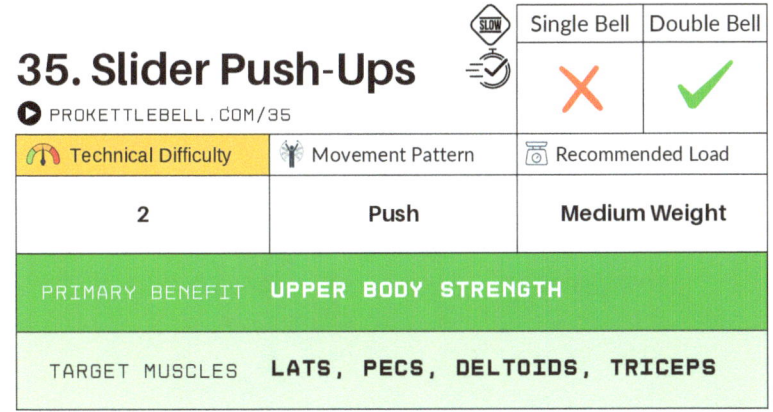

34. Rolling Push-Ups

PROKETTLEBELL.COM/34

Begin seated, holding a kettlebell. Roll back onto your shoulder blades (not your neck). Using as little momentum as possible, 1) roll up, 2) place your feet on the ground shoulder-width apart or wider, 3) place the kettlebell between your feet, 4), walk your hands out to a push-up position, 5) perform a push-up, and then 6) walk your hands back to your feet to return to seated. Repeat. This fluid move trains core control, mobility, and upper body strength.

	Single Bell	Double Bell
	✓	✗

Technical Difficulty	Movement Pattern	Recommended Load
2	Push + Rotation	Light, Medium, Heavy Weight

PRIMARY BENEFIT	UPPER BODY, CORE STRENGTH AND MOBILITY
TARGET MUSCLES	ABS, PECS, DELTOIDS, LATS, TRICEPS

35. Slider Push-Ups

PROKETTLEBELL.COM/35

	Single Bell	Double Bell
	✗	✓

Technical Difficulty	Movement Pattern	Recommended Load
2	Push	Medium Weight

PRIMARY BENEFIT	UPPER BODY STRENGTH
TARGET MUSCLES	LATS, PECS, DELTOIDS, TRICEPS

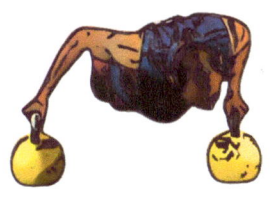
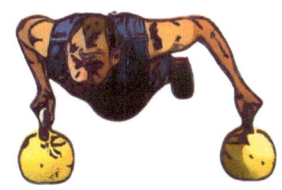

Set two kettlebells just outside of shoulder-width. Assume a plank with each hand on a kettlebell. Lower your chest to one side. Slide across toward the other kettlebell, then press up. Reverse the motion on the next rep. This demanding variation mimics a blend of single-arm, wide, and standard push-ups, offering enhanced chest activation, unilateral strength, and mobility. Beginners can start on their knees to learn the movement safely.

PUSH-UPS

36. Alternating Stop Row

	Single Bell	Double Bell
	✓	✗

Technical Difficulty	Movement Pattern	Recommended Load
1	Pull	Medium Weight

PRIMARY BENEFIT	BACK AND BICEP STRENGTH
TARGET MUSCLES	LATS, REAR DELTOIDS, BICEPS

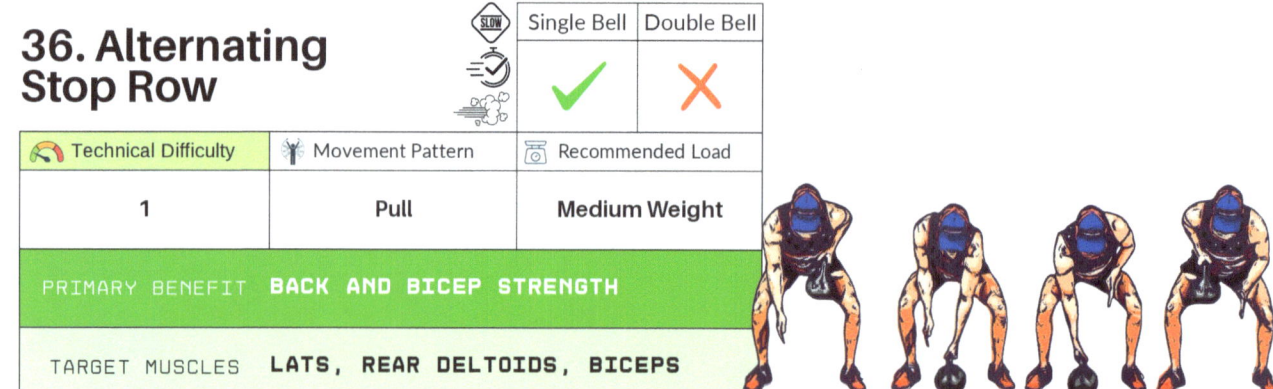

Begin with a kettlebell positioned on the floor between your feet. Hinge at the hips into an athletic stance with a flat back and chest tall. Row the kettlebell with one arm, driving the elbow tightly alongside the ribcage. Lower the bell back to the floor and switch hands. Repeat. Keep the torso steady and spine neutral throughout, engaging both the legs and upper back. ▶ PROKETTLEBELL.COM/36

37. Ballistic Row

▶ PROKETTLEBELL.COM/37

	Single Bell	Double Bell
	✓	✗

Technical Difficulty	Movement Pattern	Recommended Load
1	Compound	Medium Weight

PRIMARY BENEFIT	POWER FOR LEGS, CORE AND ARMS
TARGET MUSCLES	QUADRICEPS, GLUTES, HAMSTRING, CORE, BICEPS

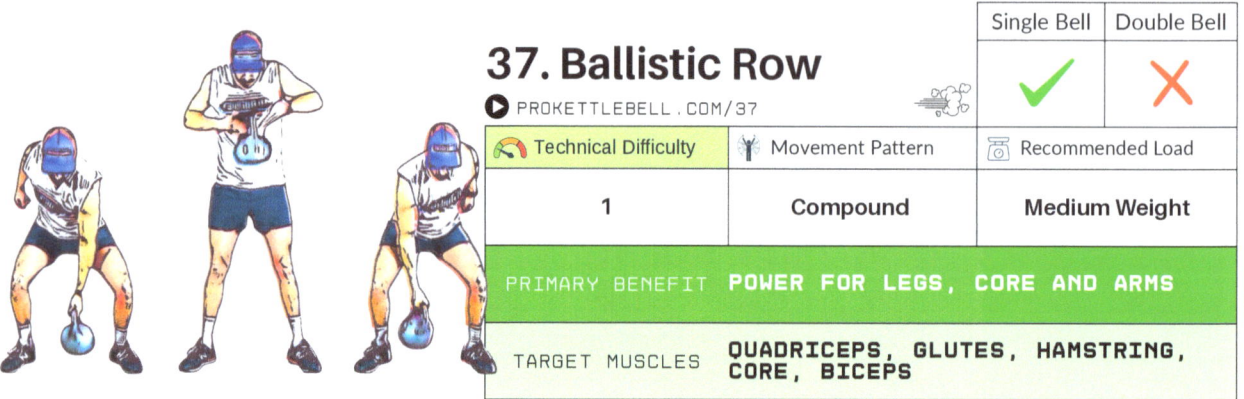

Set the kettlebell on the floor between your feet and assume a wide, athletic stance. Hook the handle with your fingertips. Drive powerfully through the legs and hips to initiate the pull, keeping the bell close to the body as you stand tall. As the kettlebell reaches chest height, shrug the shoulders and switch hands mid-air. Catch the bell softly, absorbing the load by bending the legs as the arm straightens and the bell lowers. Before the bell reaches the floor, initiate the next repetition with another strong leg drive. Focus on proper sequencing: legs and hips first, followed by the core and arms.

38. Bent-Over Gurney Row

	Single Bell	Double Bell
	✓	✓

▶ PROKETTLEBELL.COM/38

Technical Difficulty	Movement Pattern	Recommended Load
1	Pull	Medium Weight

PRIMARY BENEFIT	UPPER BODY STRENGTH
TARGET MUSCLES	ERECTORS, LATS, BICEPS

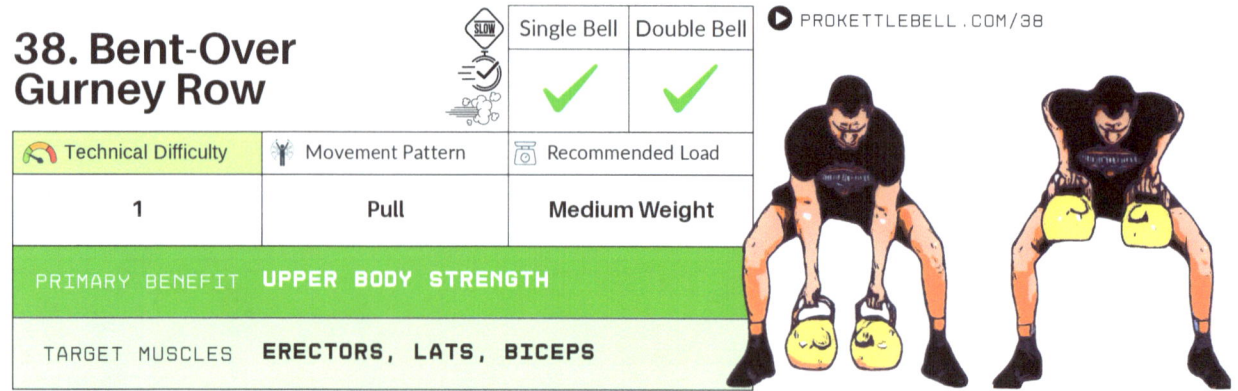

Stand over two kettlebells with a wide stance and hinge at the hips. Grip the bells with palms facing forward in a "gurney grip," arms extended straight. Pull both elbows back, dragging your arms along your ribs and lats to emphasize the biceps. Keep your back flat and the motion tight and controlled. This variation places greater stress on the biceps and forearm tendons while still engaging the back, offering a unique twist on the classic bent-over row.

39. One-Arm Row

	Single Bell	Double Bell
	✓	✗

Technical Difficulty	Movement Pattern	Recommended Load
1	Pull	Medium Weight

PRIMARY BENEFIT	BACK AND ARM STRENGTH
TARGET MUSCLES	LATS, REAR DELTOIDS, BICEPS

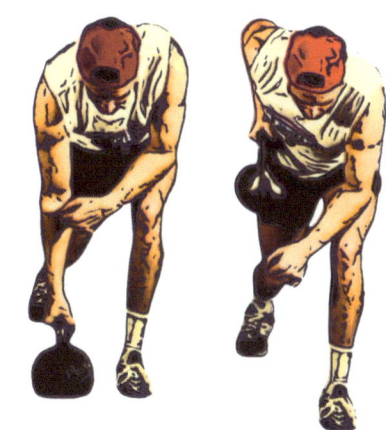

▶ PROKETTLEBELL.COM/39

From a low lunge stance, rest your non-working arm on the front thigh for support. With the working hand, grab the kettlebell positioned directly beneath the shoulder. Maintain a flat back and square shoulders as you row the bell upward, keeping the elbow tucked close so it lightly grazes the ribs. Lower the kettlebell under control and repeat. Resist torso rotation throughout; slow tempo and a brief pause at the top can be used to increase time under tension.

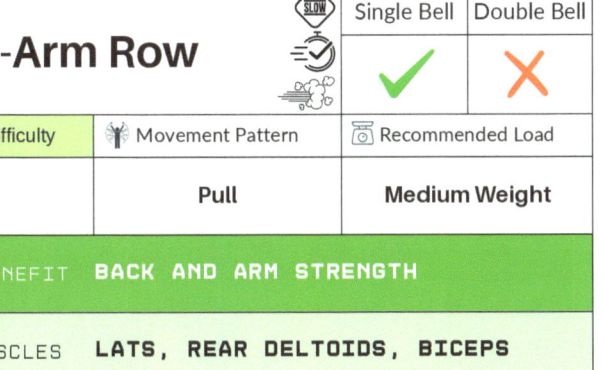

40. Renegade Row

▶ PROKETTLEBELL.COM/40

	Single Bell	Double Bell
	✗	✓

Technical Difficulty	Movement Pattern	Recommended Load
1	Pull	Medium Weight

PRIMARY BENEFIT	CORE AND UPPER BODY STRENGTH
TARGET MUSCLES	ABS, ERECTORS, OBLIQUES, LATS, DELTOIDS, TRICEPS, BICEPS

Start in a strong plank position with hands gripping kettlebells placed directly under the shoulders and feet set wide for stability. Keeping the hips and torso as still as possible, row one kettlebell toward the ribs while maintaining core tension. Lower with control and alternate sides each repetition. Add a brief pause at the top for increased difficulty or narrow the stance to increase anti-rotation demand.

41. Upright Row

	Single Bell	Double Bell
	✓	✗

Technical Difficulty	Movement Pattern	Recommended Load
1	Pull	Medium Weight

PRIMARY BENEFIT	UPPER BACK AND TRAP STRENGTH
TARGET MUSCLES	TRAPS, DELTOIDS, RHOMBOIDS, BICEPS

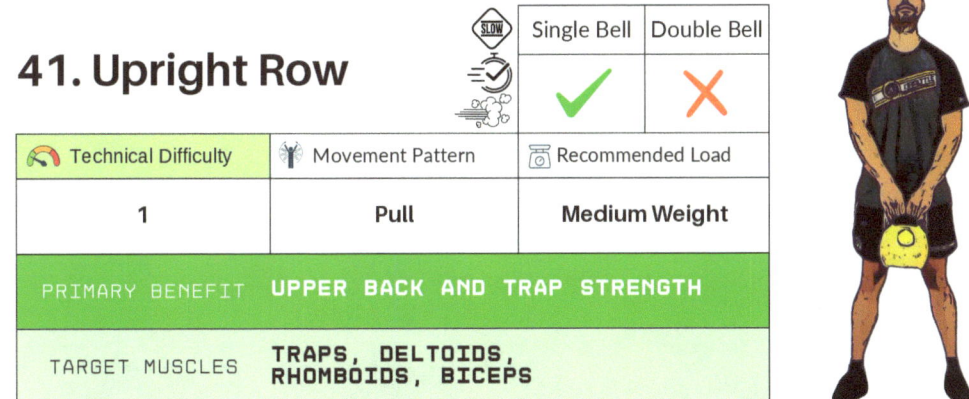

Hold a kettlebell with both hands and let it rest below your center of mass, arms close to your body. From a standing position, row the bell upward toward your chin, leading with your elbows and keeping the handle close to your body. Control the motion both up and down, keeping constant tension for muscle engagement. This movement isolates the upper traps and rhomboids and is great for improving posture and counteracting forward shoulder slouch from prolonged desk work. ▶ PROKETTLEBELL.COM/41

ROWS

42. 21-Curls

PROKETTLEBELL.COM/42

	Single Bell	Double Bell
	✓	✗

Technical Difficulty	Movement Pattern	Recommended Load
1	Pull	Medium Weight

PRIMARY BENEFIT	BICEPS STRENGTH AND HYPERTROPHY
TARGET MUSCLES	BICEPS, FOREARMS

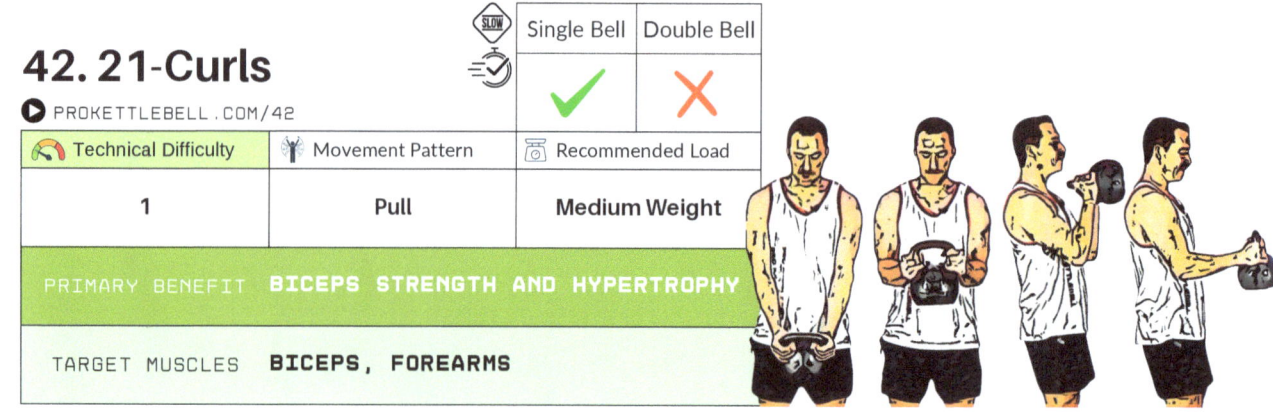

This bicep-focused movement involves three segments: seven curls from the bottom to halfway up, seven from the top to halfway down, and seven full-range curls. You can use a standard grip, horns up or down, or even a towel for added instability. Keep elbows tight to your sides throughout and choose a light enough weight to maintain form across all reps. Full range of motion is essential for optimal hypertrophy.

43. Axe Chops

PROKETTLEBELL.COM/43

	Single Bell	Double Bell
	✓	✗

Technical Difficulty	Movement Pattern	Recommended Load
1	Compound + Rotation	Light, Medium Weight

PRIMARY BENEFIT	UPPER BODY STRENGTH
TARGET MUSCLES	OBLIQUES, ERECTORS, LATS, DELTOIDS, TRICEPS, BICEPS

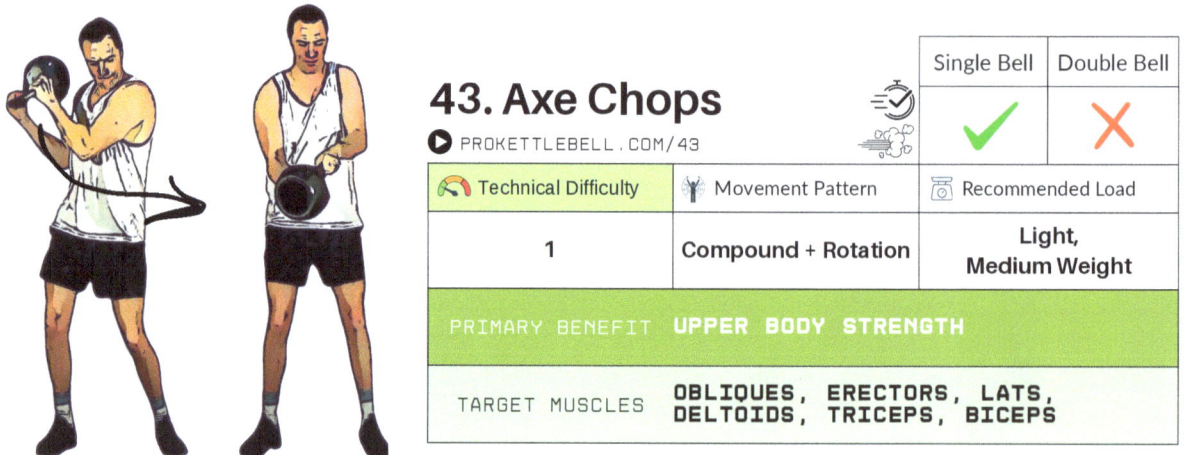

Hold the kettlebell by the horns with the base facing down. Stand in a stable stance and brace the core. Rotate and drive the kettlebell diagonally across the body from shoulder height down toward the opposite hip, mimicking a chopping motion. Keep the forearms parallel and elbows close to the torso. Control the return and repeat for all reps before switching sides.

44. Barn Door Fly

PROKETTLEBELL.COM/44

	Single Bell	Double Bell
	✗	✓

Technical Difficulty	Movement Pattern	Recommended Load
1	Push	Light Weight

PRIMARY BENEFIT	UPPER BODY STRENGTH AND HYPERTROPY
TARGET MUSCLES	DELTOIDS, TRAPS, ROTATOR CUFF

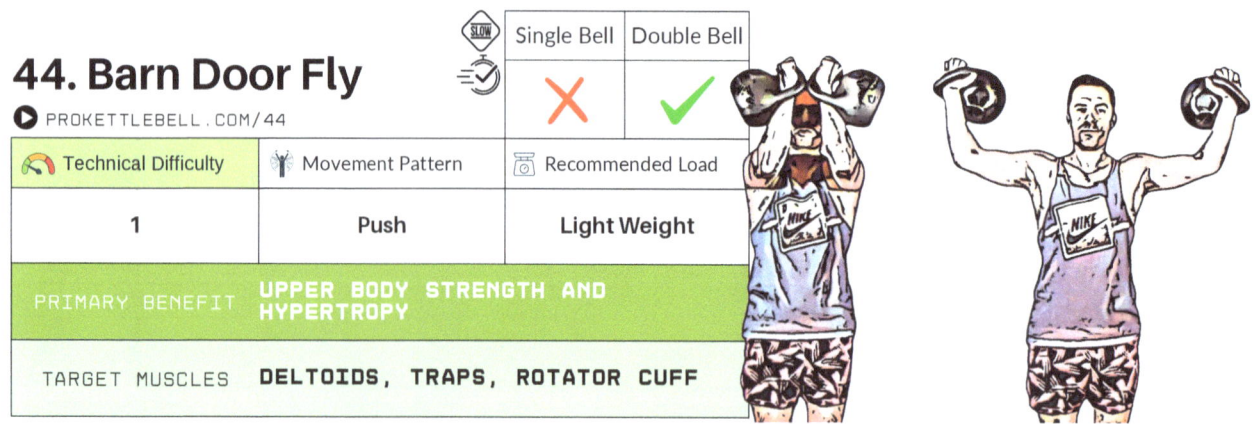

Bring two kettlebells to the rack position. Raise the elbows so the arms are bent at 90 degrees, with forearms vertical and palms facing inward. Open the arms outward, moving the kettlebells laterally away from the body while keeping the elbows lifted and fixed in position. Reverse the motion to bring the bells back toward the front, maintaining elbow height throughout, and repeat. Maintain constant shoulder tension throughout the exercise.

45. Bridge Pull-Over

PROKETTLEBELL.COM/45

Technical Difficulty	Movement Pattern	Recommended Load
1	Pull	Medium, Heavy Weight

PRIMARY BENEFIT	CORE AND UPPER BODY STRENGTH
TARGET MUSCLES	GLUTES, HAMSTRINGS, ERECTORS, LATS, PECS

Single Bell ✓ / Double Bell ✗

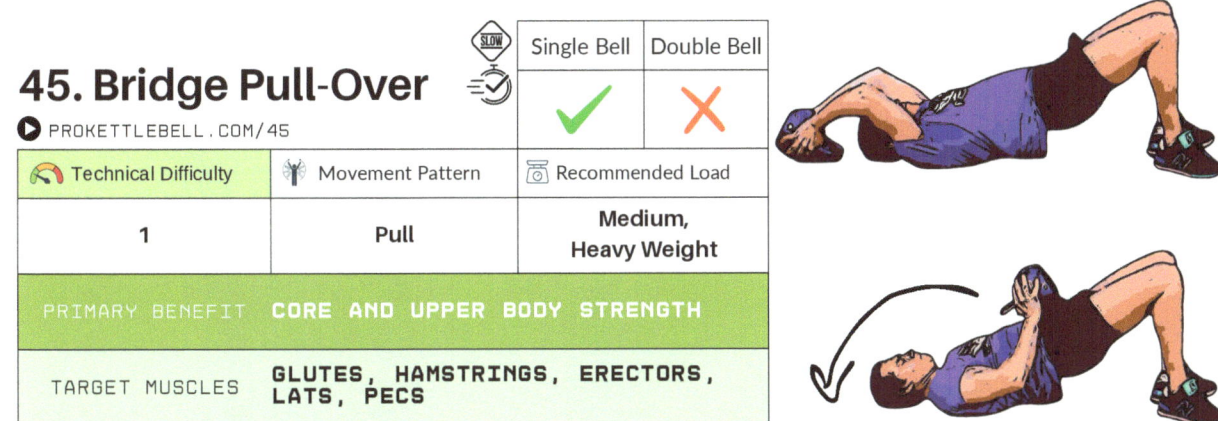

Lie on your back with feet planted and perform a strong glute bridge, forming a straight line from shoulders to knees. Hold the kettlebell with a firm grip and bring it overhead in a controlled arc, tapping the floor behind you before returning to your pelvis. Maintain tension, parallel forearms, and squeezed glutes throughout. This combines lat, core, and posterior chain activation.

46. Cheat Curls

PROKETTLEBELL.COM/46

Technical Difficulty	Movement Pattern	Recommended Load
1	Pull	Medium Weight

PRIMARY BENEFIT	ARM AND CORE STRENGTH
TARGET MUSCLES	BICEPS

Single Bell ✓ / Double Bell ✗

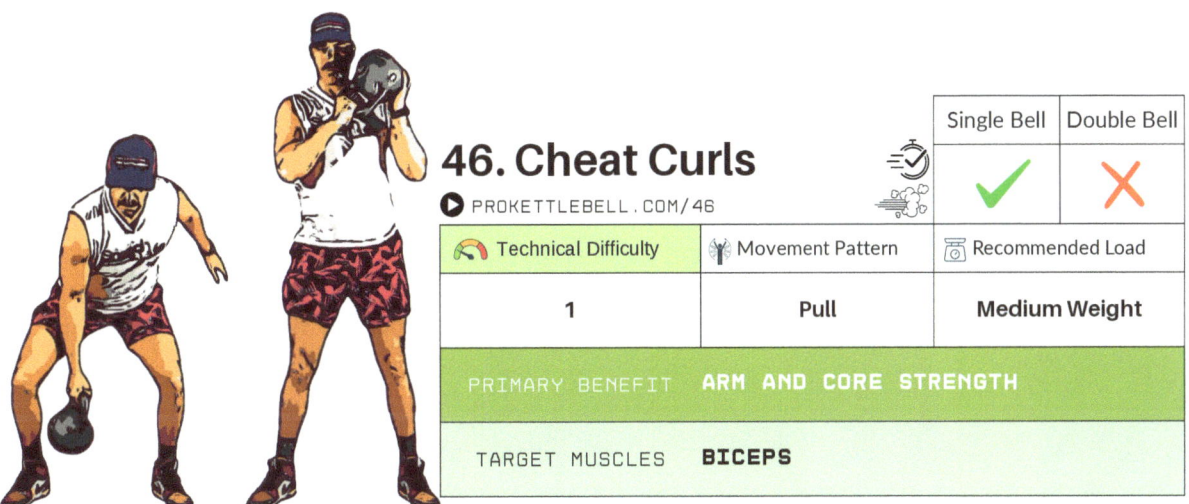

Take an athletic stance and hold the kettlebell with the handle perpendicular to your body (thumb pointing away). Using minimal leg and hip drive, curl the weight up toward your opposite shoulder, relying primarily on biceps. Let the kettlebell drop vertically between your legs on the descent. Avoid swinging and flaring the elbow. This ballistic curl variation allows a heavier load but still emphasizes bicep isolation when done with proper form.

47. Concentration Curls

PROKETTLEBELL.COM/47

Technical Difficulty	Movement Pattern	Recommended Load
1	Pull	Medium Weight

PRIMARY BENEFIT	ARM STRENGTH
TARGET MUSCLES	BICEPS

Single Bell ✓ / Double Bell ✗

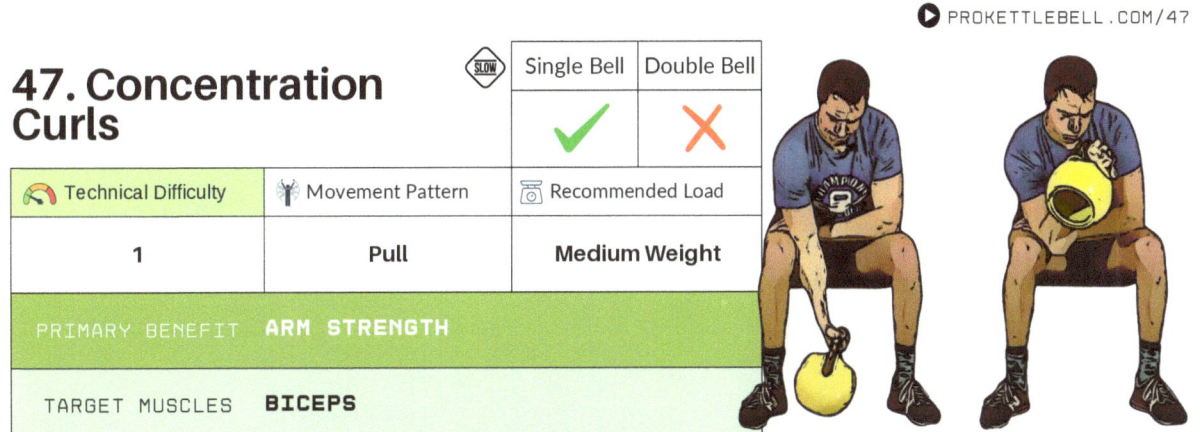

Seated with legs apart, rest one elbow on your inner thigh and hold a kettlebell securely. Curl the weight slowly through a full range of motion and lower it in control. You may stabilize the elbow with your free hand. Use lighter weight if needed, as this isolation movement is all about time under tension and clean execution for bicep growth.

CURLS & MISC UPPER BODY

48. Cross Curl Press

PROKETTLEBELL.COM/48

	Single Bell	Double Bell
	✓	✗

Technical Difficulty	Movement Pattern	Recommended Load
1	Compound	Medium Weight

PRIMARY BENEFIT UPPER BODY STRENGTH

TARGET MUSCLES LATS, OBLIQUES, SHOULDERS, BICEPS

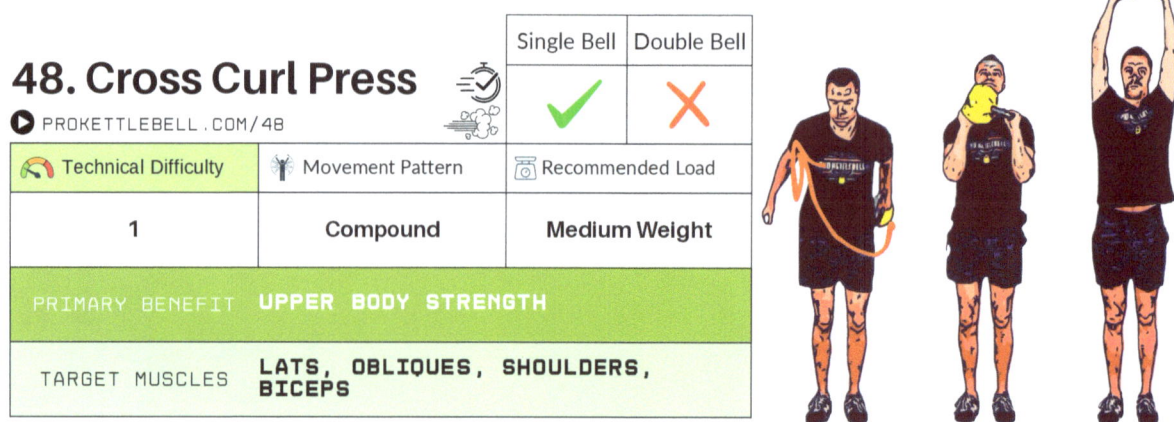

Start with the kettlebell at the outside of your hip and swing it toward your opposite shoulder, catching it with your opposite hand. From there, press it directly overhead, straightening your arms completely. Adjust your grip as necessary, depending on kettlebell type, and use minimal leg involvement during the press.

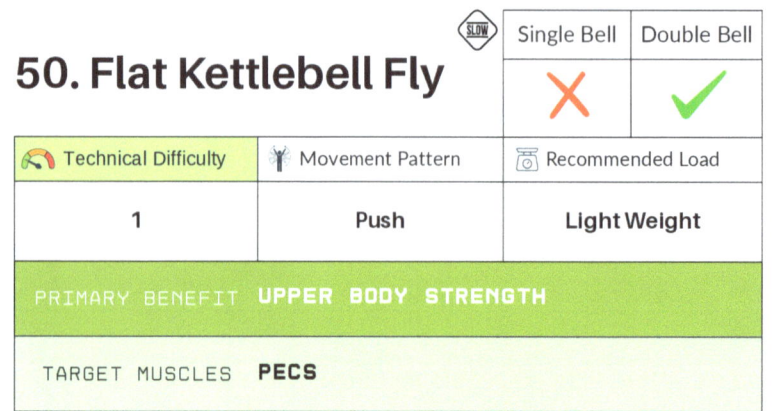

49. Cross Curls

PROKETTLEBELL.COM/49

	Single Bell	Double Bell
	✓	✗

Technical Difficulty	Movement Pattern	Recommended Load
1	Pull	Medium Weight

PRIMARY BENEFIT UPPER BODY STRENGTH

TARGET MUSCLES BICEPS, SHOULDERS, OBLIQUES, FOREARMS

("High-Five's") Swing the kettlebell from your hip upward and across your body, stopping the momentum in front of the opposite shoulder with your free hand, as if giving yourself a high five. Fully extend the working arm at the bottom, then curl the weight back up with controlled movement. Counterbalance naturally with your body and maintain tight elbow positioning to emphasize diagonal biceps engagement.

50. Flat Kettlebell Fly

	Single Bell	Double Bell
	✗	✓

Technical Difficulty	Movement Pattern	Recommended Load
1	Push	Light Weight

PRIMARY BENEFIT UPPER BODY STRENGTH

TARGET MUSCLES PECS

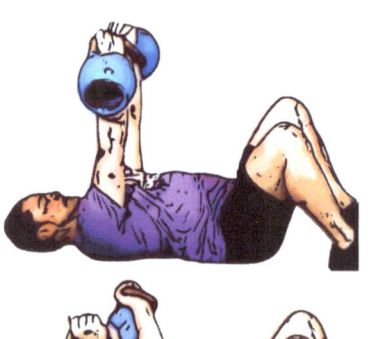
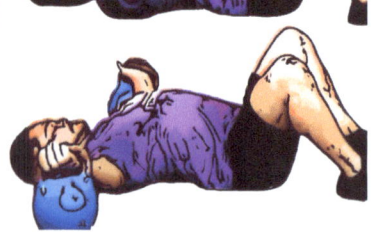

Lie on your back between two kettlebells and press them above your chest. With a slight bend in the elbows, lower your arms out to the sides under control until the weights touch the ground, then squeeze them back together over your chest following the same arc. Move slowly to maximize time under tension. This can also be performed on a bench or stability ball.   PROKETTLEBELL.COM/50

51. Floor Pull-Over

PROKETTLEBELL.COM/51

	Single Bell	Double Bell
SLOW	✓	✗

Technical Difficulty	Movement Pattern	Recommended Load
1	Pull	Medium Weight

PRIMARY BENEFIT — CHEST AND BACK STRENGTH

TARGET MUSCLES — CHEST, LATS, TRICEPS

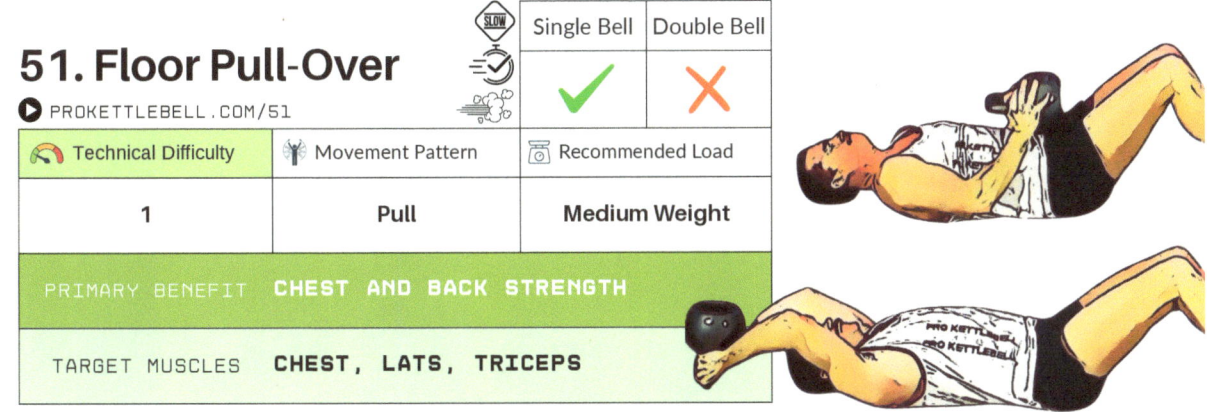

Hold the kettlebell between your palms and lie back with knees bent. Starting at your hips, sweep the bell in a controlled C-shape overhead until it taps the ground behind your head, then return it to your torso. Keep your elbows close and forearms parallel throughout. Use a grip that allows control and stretches the lats without sacrificing form.

52. Front Raise

PROKETTLEBELL.COM/52

	Single Bell	Double Bell
SLOW	✓	✗

Technical Difficulty	Movement Pattern	Recommended Load
1	Compound	Light Weight

PRIMARY BENEFIT — SHOULDER STRENGTH

TARGET MUSCLES — DELTOIDS, TRAPS, CORE

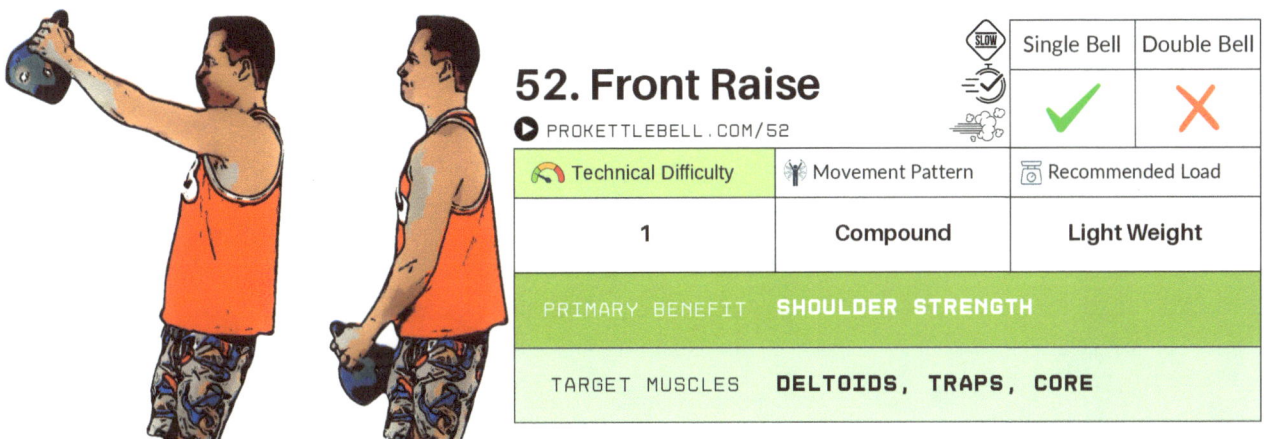

Stand tall with the kettlebell gripped securely in both hands. Keeping your arms straight, raise the bell up to eye level, pause briefly, and then lower it in control. Because the weight is far from your center of mass, this heavily activates the front delts, with support from your core and erectors. Avoid momentum and adjust arm bend to manage leverage.

53. Front Raise Rotations

PROKETTLEBELL.COM/53

	Single Bell	Double Bell
SLOW	✓	✗

Technical Difficulty	Movement Pattern	Recommended Load
1	Rotate	Light Weight

PRIMARY BENEFIT — UPPER BODY AND CORE STRENGTH

TARGET MUSCLES — ERECTORS, OBLIQUES, DELTOIDS

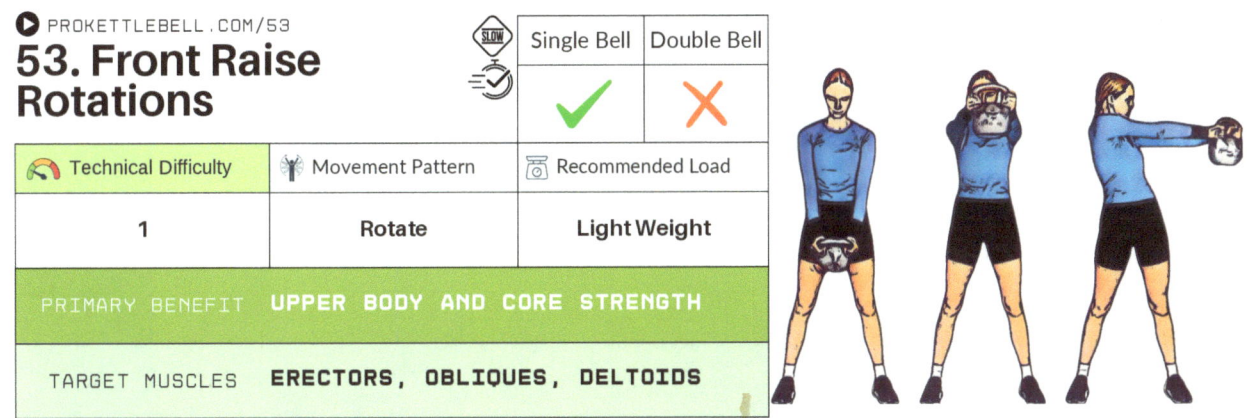

Raise a single kettlebell up to shoulder height with both arms extended. While holding it steady at that height, rotate your upper body to one side, return to center, then rotate to the opposite side. Keep hips and feet facing forward to isolate rotation in the spine and core. This builds delt strength and enhances spinal mobility simultaneously.

CURLS & MISC UPPER BODY

54. Halos

▶ PROKETTLEBELL.COM/54

	Single Bell	Double Bell
	✓	✗

Technical Difficulty	Movement Pattern	Recommended Load
1	Compound	Medium Weight

PRIMARY BENEFIT — SHOULDER MOBILITY AND STABILITY

TARGET MUSCLES — DELTOIDS, UPPER BACK, ROTATOR CUFF, CORE

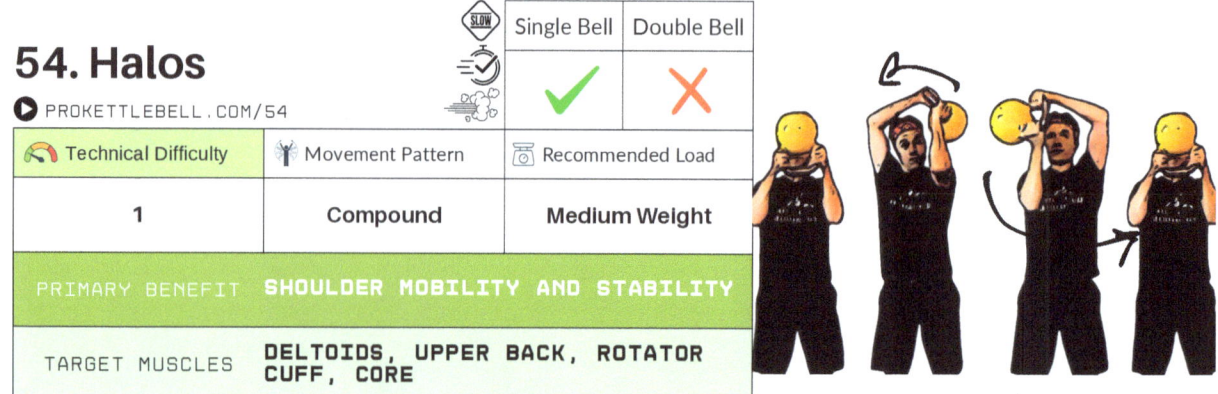

Hold the kettlebell at forehead height with forearms parallel and circle it around your head, lifting the elbows as it passes behind to allow a deep path. Keep the bell above eye level when in front to emphasize shoulder engagement. Hold the bell bottom-up or bottom-down as preferred, performing multiple passes in one direction or alternating each circle.

55. Kettlebell Dips

▶ PROKETTLEBELL.COM/55

	Single Bell	Double Bell
	✗	✓

Technical Difficulty	Movement Pattern	Recommended Load
1	Push	Heavy Weight

PRIMARY BENEFIT — UPPER BODY STRENGTH

TARGET MUSCLES — PECS, TRICEPS

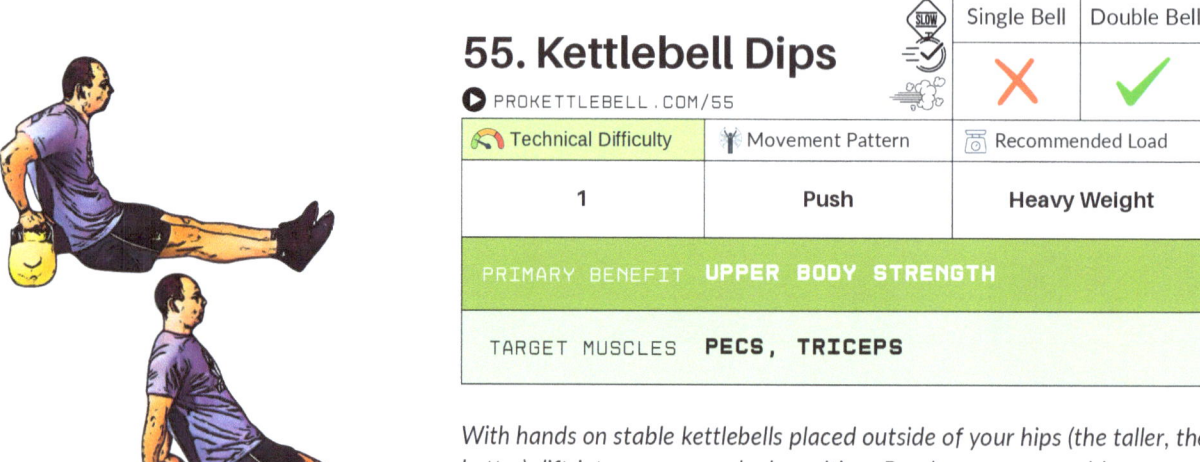

With hands on stable kettlebells placed outside of your hips (the taller, the better), lift into a reverse plank position. Bend your arms and lower your body as close as you can to the ground without touching, then press back up. Keep elbows tight to your ribs and maintain a vertical torso. Adjust leg position to scale difficulty—bent knees make it easier.

56. Kettlebell Skull Crushers

	Single Bell	Double Bell
	✓	✗

Technical Difficulty	Movement Pattern	Recommended Load
1	Push	Light, Medium Weight

PRIMARY BENEFIT — TRICEP STRENGTH

TARGET MUSCLES — TRICEPS

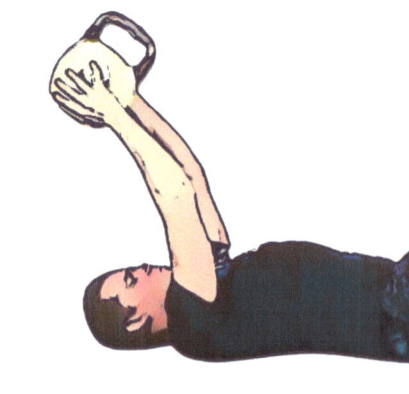
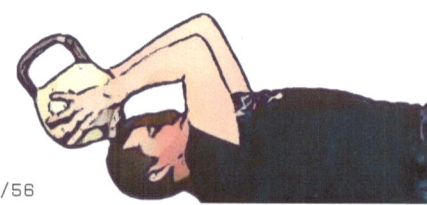

Lie flat while securely holding a kettlebell with two-hands overhead. Lower it by bending your elbows until it nears your forehead, then extend back up. Keep forearms parallel and elbows close together. Use a grip that feels safest based on your kettlebell shape. Control the descent to avoid injury and fully extend to maximize triceps activation. ▶ PROKETTLEBELL.COM/56

57. Kneeling Curl + Press

	Single Bell	Double Bell
	✓	✗

Technical Difficulty	Movement Pattern	Recommended Load
1	Compound	Medium Weight

PRIMARY BENEFIT	ARM STRENGTH
TARGET MUSCLES	BICEPS, DELTOIDS, TRICEPS

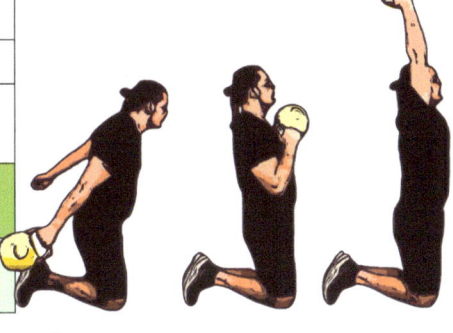

From a kneeling position next to your kettlebell, swing it across your body to chest level, catching it with both hands. Then press it straight overhead, locking out your arms before returning to the starting position. Kneeling removes leg drive, forcing your upper body to carry the workload. Elevate your knees with a mat if needed for clearance.

▶ PROKETTLEBELL.COM/57

58. Reverse Curls

	Single Bell	Double Bell
	✓	✗

Technical Difficulty	Movement Pattern	Recommended Load
1	Pull	Medium Weight

PRIMARY BENEFIT	ARM STRENGTH
TARGET MUSCLES	FOREARMS, BICEPS

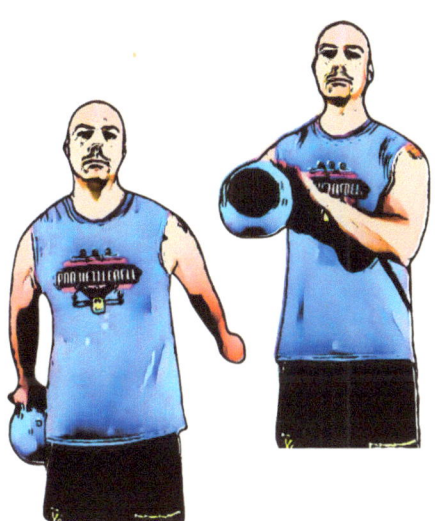

Hold a kettlebell in your fingertips with your palm facing behind and elbow tucked tightly. Curl the weight upward using as little swing assist as possible. Use your free hand as a target at the top to stop the swing. A narrow stance helps avoid hitting your legs. Maintain tension to resist the weight as it returns to the starting position. Repeat and switch sides.

▶ PROKETTLEBELL.COM/58

59. Ribbons

▶ PROKETTLEBELL.COM/59

	Single Bell	Double Bell
	✓	✗

Technical Difficulty	Movement Pattern	Recommended Load
1	Compound	Medium Weight

PRIMARY BENEFIT	SHOULDER AND CORE STRENGTH
TARGET MUSCLES	SHOULDERS, BICEPS, CORE

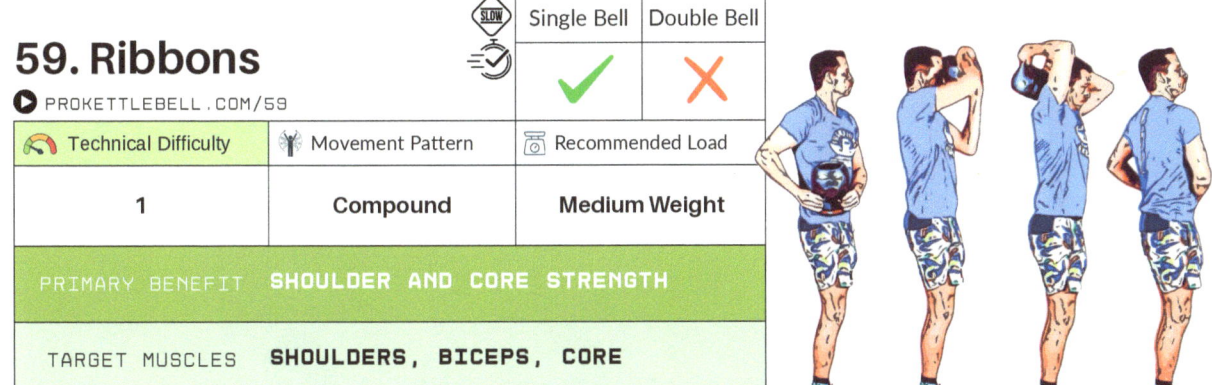

Hold a kettlebell upside-down at your right hip, then move it diagonally across your torso, around the back of your head, and cross your body in front to finish the movement with a return of the kettlebell to your left hip. Repeat by mirroring the movement; starting on your left hip, you'll finish on your right hip. Keep the forearms parallel to maintain joint alignment and maximize stretch through the lats and triceps when moving the bell behind your head.

CURLS & MISC UPPER BODY

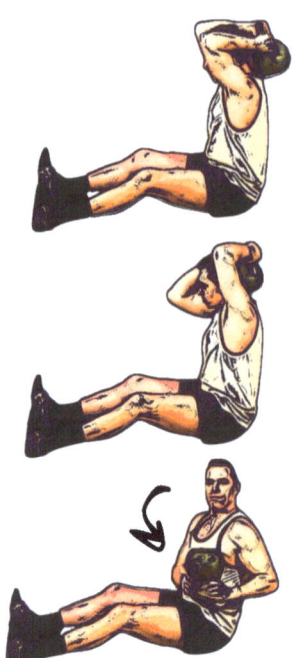

60. Seated Ribbons

	Single Bell	Double Bell
SLOW	✓	✗

Technical Difficulty	Movement Pattern	Recommended Load
1	Compound / Rotation	Medium Weight

PRIMARY BENEFIT	SHOULDER MOBILITY AND CORE STRENGTH
TARGET MUSCLES	DELTOIDS, LATS, TRICEPS, OBLIQUES, CORE

Seated in a straddle, cross-legged, or legs-forward position, hold the kettlebell bottom side up. Bring it diagonally across your body and around your head. Ribbons begin on one hip and conclude on the opposite hip. Keep your chest upright and lumbar flat. Focus on posture to engage your core and protect your back. ▶ PROKETTLEBELL.COM/60

61. Seated Wood Chopper

	Single Bell	Double Bell
SLOW	✓	✗

Technical Difficulty	Movement Pattern	Recommended Load
1	Rotation	Light Weight

PRIMARY BENEFIT	CORE AND ARM STRENGTH
TARGET MUSCLES	OBLIQUES, ABS, ERECTORS, DELTOIDS, FOREARMS

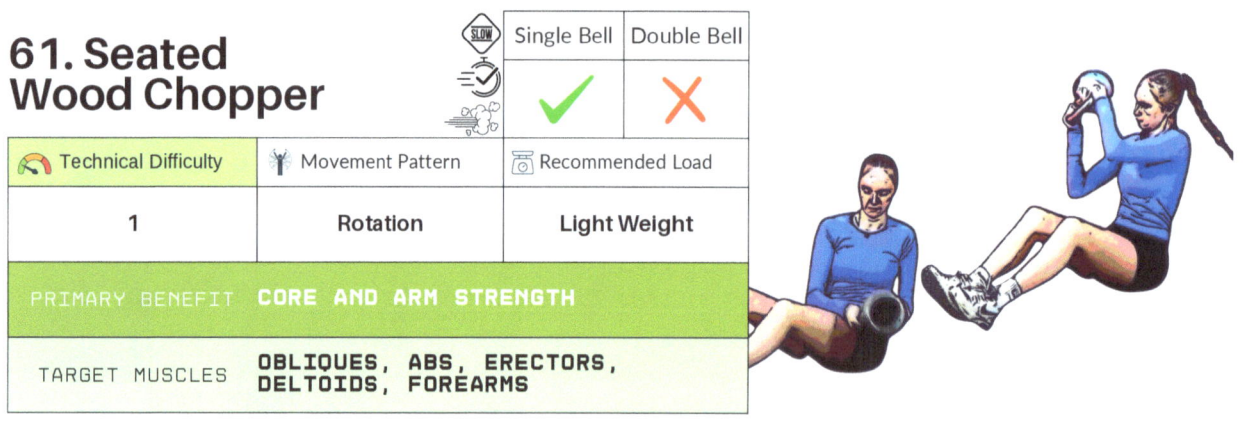

From a seated position, grip the kettlebell bottom side up and move it diagonally from above one shoulder down across your trunk toward the opposite hip as if chopping wood. Repeat equally on both sides. Adjust grip or swing arc depending on the kettlebell's weight. Maintain an upright posture to protect your spine and ensure proper core engagement during each rep. ▶ PROKETTLEBELL.COM/61

62. Shrugs

	Single Bell	Double Bell
SLOW	✗	✓

Technical Difficulty	Movement Pattern	Recommended Load
1	Pull	Medium Weight

PRIMARY BENEFIT	UPPER TRAP STRENGTH
TARGET MUSCLES	TRAPS, RHOMBOIDS, ERECTORS

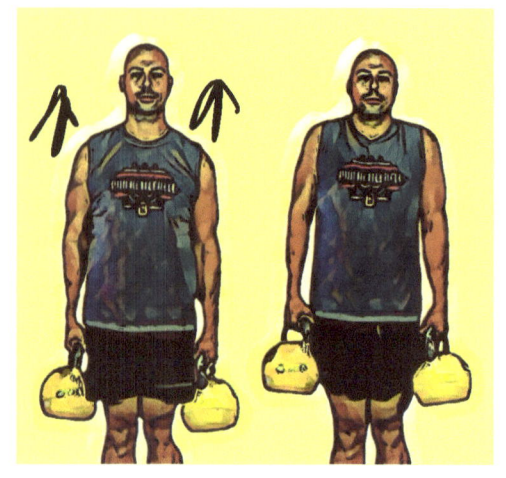

Holding a kettlebell in each hand, roll your shoulders up toward your ears in a front-to-back motion, squeezing your shoulder blades at the top. Use a weight that allows full range without bending the elbows. This exercise strengthens the traps and upper back, key for shoulder stability in overhead lifts. ▶ PROKETTLEBELL.COM/62

63. Tricep Extensions

	Single Bell	Double Bell
SLOW	✓	✗

Technical Difficulty	Movement Pattern	Recommended Load
1	Push	Light Weight

PRIMARY BENEFIT	TRICEP STRENGTH
TARGET MUSCLES	TRICEPS

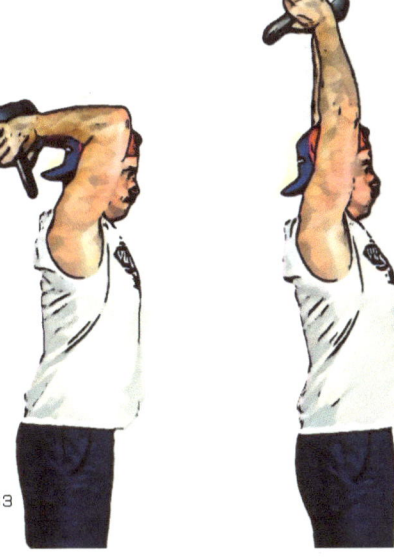

Hold the kettlebell by sandwiching its base between your palms with thumbs between the horns. Raise it overhead with elbows tucked in, then lower it behind your head to at least 90 degrees before extending fully. Maintain parallel forearms and avoid elbow flare. This isolates the triceps and should be done in control to protect the joints. ▶ PROKETTLEBELL.COM/63

64. Two-Hand Sprays

	Single Bell	Double Bell
SLOW	✗	✓

Technical Difficulty	Movement Pattern	Recommended Load
1	Compound / Rotation	Medium Weight

PRIMARY BENEFIT	SHOULDER AND CORE STRENGTH
TARGET MUSCLES	DELTOIDS, OBLIQUES, CORE, UPPER BACK

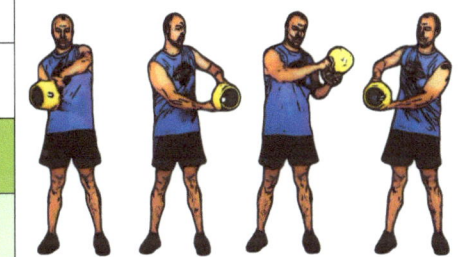

Hold the kettlebell bottom side up by the horns and move it side to side in a slight figure-8 pattern as if spraying a large area with water from a hose. Keep your elbows pointed downward and core tight. You can bring your arms in closer if the weight is too heavy. This full-body movement builds shoulder, arm, and core strength with dynamic motion. ▶ PROKETTLEBELL.COM/64

65. Vertical Halos

▶ PROKETTLEBELL.COM/65

	Single Bell	Double Bell
SLOW	✓	✗

Technical Difficulty	Movement Pattern	Recommended Load
1	Compound	Medium Weight

PRIMARY BENEFIT	SHOULDER MOBILITY AND CORE STABILITY
TARGET MUSCLES	ABS, OBLIQUES, LATS, DELTOIDS, BICEPS

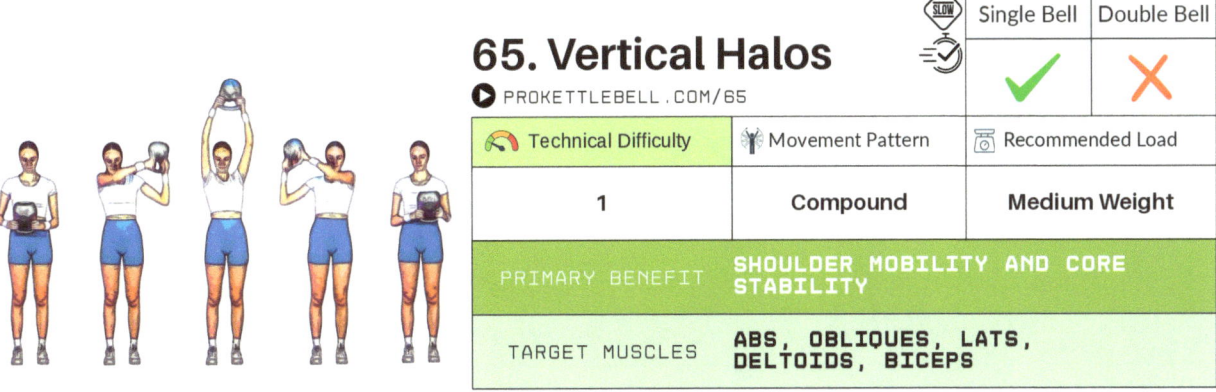

Using a bottoms-up horn grip, move the kettlebell in a vertical circular motion from waist to above your head and back down, alternating directions. Maintain tension throughout and avoid swinging. This works your shoulders, arms, and especially your core, demanding control and stability as the bell moves through its arc.

CURLS & MISC UPPER BODY

66. Wheel Turns

	Single Bell	Double Bell
SLOW	✓	✗

Technical Difficulty	Movement Pattern	Recommended Load
1	Rotation	Light Weight

PRIMARY BENEFIT GRIP AND SHOULDER STRENGTH

TARGET MUSCLES FOREARMS, SHOULDERS, TRICEPS

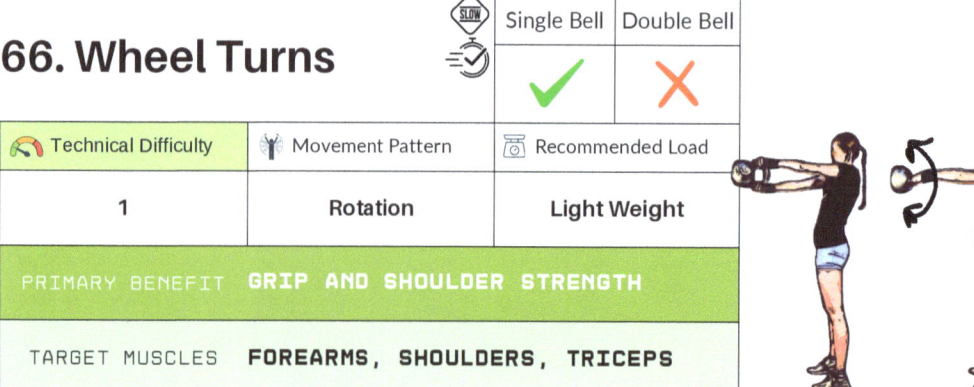

Hold the kettlebell by the horns with the bottom facing away. Twist it side to side like turning a steering wheel. Elbows can be pulled in to make the movement easier with heavier bells. This exercise improves grip, wrist, and shoulder mobility while also challenging arm endurance and control. ▶ PROKETTLEBELL.COM/66

67. Double Reverse Fly

	Single Bell	Double Bell
SLOW	✗	✓

Technical Difficulty	Movement Pattern	Recommended Load
2	Pull	Light Weight

PRIMARY BENEFIT UPPER BACK AND SHOULDER STRENGTH

TARGET MUSCLES RHOMBOIDS, REAR DELTS, TRAPS

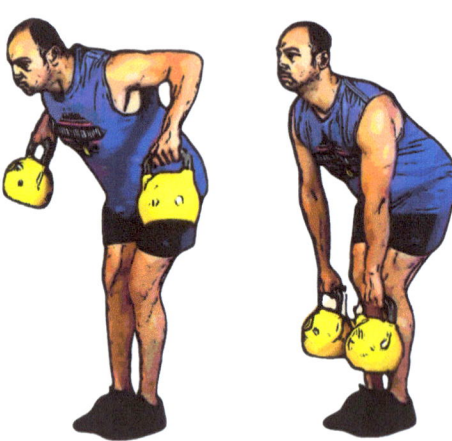

Fold at the hips with a kettlebell in each hand while keeping a flat back. Pull the weights out to the sides in a reverse fly motion, squeezing your shoulder blades together. You can slightly vary your thumb position to adjust muscle activation. This exercise targets the rear delts, rhomboids, and traps with old-school bodybuilding style. ▶ PROKETTLEBELL.COM/67

68. Dynamic Ribbons

	Single Bell	Double Bell
SLOW	✓	✗

Technical Difficulty	Movement Pattern	Recommended Load
2	Compound + Rotation	Medium Weight

PRIMARY BENEFIT COORDINATION AND CORE STRENGTH

TARGET MUSCLES GLUTES, QUADS, ERECTORS, SHOULDERS, LATS, CORE

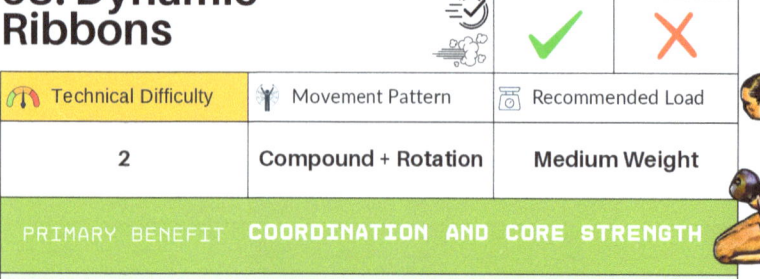

From a kneeling position with the kettlebell held upside-down at your right hip, raise the bell diagonally across your body and around your head as you rise up onto your knees, squeezing your glutes. Sit back down as it moves front and returns to the hip. The rise and fall matches the bell's arc, making this a full-body flow with emphasis on core and upper body. ▶ PROKETTLEBELL.COM/68

69. Flat Lat Pull-Over

	Single Bell	Double Bell
	✓	✓

Technical Difficulty	Movement Pattern	Recommended Load
2	Pull	Light Weight

PRIMARY BENEFIT	LAT STRENGTH
TARGET MUSCLES	LATS, LOWER PECS, TRICEPS

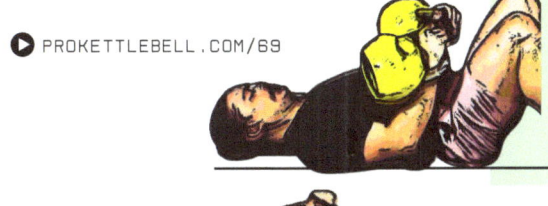
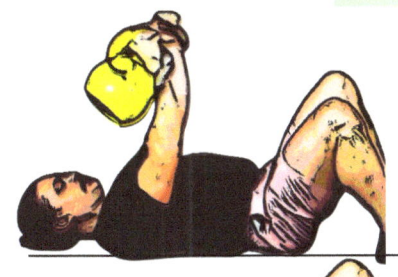
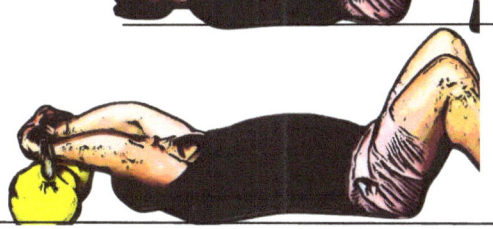

PROKETTLEBELL.COM/69

Lie flat between two kettlebells with both hands fully inserted into the windows, bells resting on the floor behind your head. With straight arms, bring the bells overhead, then slightly bend the elbows and lower them slowly to your low belly. Keep elbows angled down to maximize lat engagement and maintain control through the back and shoulders.

70. Lawn Mower Pull

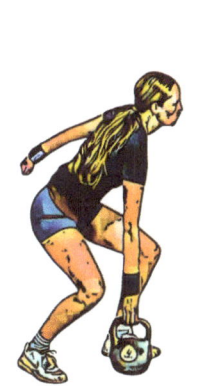
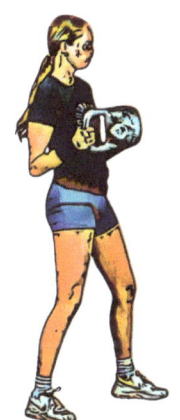

	Single Bell	Double Bell
	✓	✗

Technical Difficulty	Movement Pattern	Recommended Load
2	Pull	Medium Weight

PRIMARY BENEFIT	UPPER BACK AND POWER DEVELOPMENT
TARGET MUSCLES	LATS, REAR DELTOIDS, RHOMBOIDS, BICEPS

Take a split stance over the kettlebell with it centered between your feet. Using the arm on the rear leg side, squat down and hook the handle. Drive through your legs to stand, pulling the kettlebell up along your side like starting a lawnmower. Keep the back flat and path of motion tight to your body. Catch the kettlebell with the opposite hand at the top before carefully returning it to the ground for the next rep. PROKETTLEBELL.COM/70

71. Single Leg Ribbons

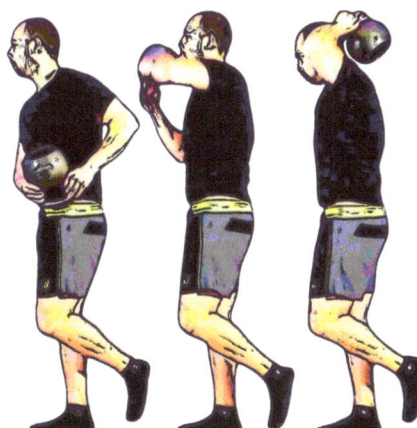
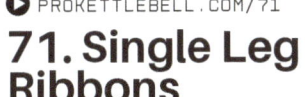

PROKETTLEBELL.COM/71

	Single Bell	Double Bell
	✓	✗

Technical Difficulty	Movement Pattern	Recommended Load
2	Compound + Rotation	Medium Weight

PRIMARY BENEFIT	SHOULDER, CORE STRENGTH AND STABILITY
TARGET MUSCLES	OBLIQUES, ABS, DELTOIDS, LATS, CORE STABILIZERS

Balance on one leg and perform a ribbon by moving the kettlebell diagonally across your body from one hip to the opposite shoulder, around your head, and finishing at the opposite hip. Lift the back leg fully or use the toe as a kickstand for support. Keep elbows tight and the movement controlled to increase core activation, balance, and stability.

CURLS & MISC UPPER BODY

Lower-Body

———————— Section Two ————————

Squats
Lunges
Miscellaneous/Compound

Lower Body

Squats	
Deadlift + Jump Squat	43
Double Rack Squat	43
Double Tip Toe Rack Squat	43
Fireman Squats	44
Front Raise Squat	44
Goblet Squat	44
Loaded Stop Squat	45
Overhead Squat, Two-Hand	45
Pull Over Squats	45
Rack Squat, One-Arm	46
Single Back Squat	46
Squat Curl	46
Ab Squat	47
Bottoms-Up Squat	47
Bulgarian Back Squat	47
Cossack Squat	48
Cross Squat	48
Curtsy Squat	48
Deck Squat	49
Double Overhead Squat	49
Double Rack Curtsy Squat	49
Double Rack Squat Slider	50
Figure-4 Chair Squat	50
Figure-4 Squat	50
Goblet Toss	51
Lateral Frog Squats	51
Loaded Jump Squat	51
Narrow/Wide Goblet Squats	52
Overhead Curtsy Squat	52
Peekaboo Squats	52
Press + Overhead Squat	53
Reverse Jump Squat	53
Semi Squat	53
Slingshot Squat Variations	54
Squat Sliders	54
Curtsy Toss	54
Pistol Squat	55
Speed-Switch Front Squat	55

Lunges	
Clock Lunges	56
Horn Hold Reverse Lunge	56
Hug Lunges	56
Lateral Lunges (Goblet Hold)	57
Loaded Stationary Lunge	57
Lunge Pulse	57
Overhead Lunge	58
Side Lunge Twist	58
Stationary Lunge Press, Two-Hand	58
Bottoms-Up Side Lunge	59
Deep Lunge Press	59
Kettlebell Lunge Jumps	59
Kettlebell Lunge Unders	60
Lateral Lunge Row	60
Lateral Lunge Slingers	60
Lunge Twist	61
Lunge Twist, Reverse, Hammer Grip	61
Lunging Halo	61
Overhead Walking Lunge	62
Rack Step-Thru Lunge	62
Shuffle Lunge	62
Side Lunge Ribbons	63
Side Lunge Toss	63
Slingshot Reverse Lunge	63
Split Lunge Jumps	64
Squat Pulse Lunge Jumps	64
Step-Thru Sumo Turns	64
Tactical Lunge	65
Walking Lunge Row	65
Walking Lunges (Horn Hold)	65
Diagonal Lunge Pull	66
Double Lunge Jump Rows	66
Figure-8 Reverse Lunge	66
Racked Lunge Hops	67
Shotgun Reverse Lunge	67
Slingshot Side Lunge	67

Miscellaneous / Compound	
Figure-4 Glute Bridge	68
Marching Glute Bridge	68
Kettlebell Leg Extensions	68
Step Ups	69
Toe Lifts	69
Weighted Wall Sit	69

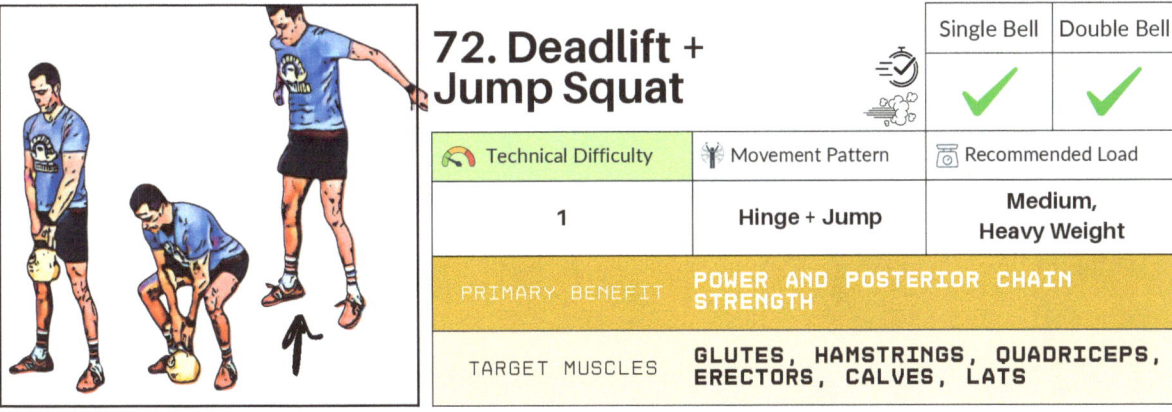

72. Deadlift + Jump Squat

	Single Bell	Double Bell
	✓	✓

Technical Difficulty	Movement Pattern	Recommended Load
1	Hinge + Jump	Medium, Heavy Weight

PRIMARY BENEFIT	POWER AND POSTERIOR CHAIN STRENGTH
TARGET MUSCLES	GLUTES, HAMSTRINGS, QUADRICEPS, ERECTORS, CALVES, LATS

Start by performing a kettlebell deadlift with proper form: hips back, flat lumbar, and weight centered under you. After the lift, set the kettlebell down, let go of the bell and perform a bodyweight jump squat. Land softly with your hips back and heels down. Repeat. This combination improves power, coordination, and leg strength by alternating between controlled lifting and explosive jumping. ▶ PROKETTLEBELL.COM/72

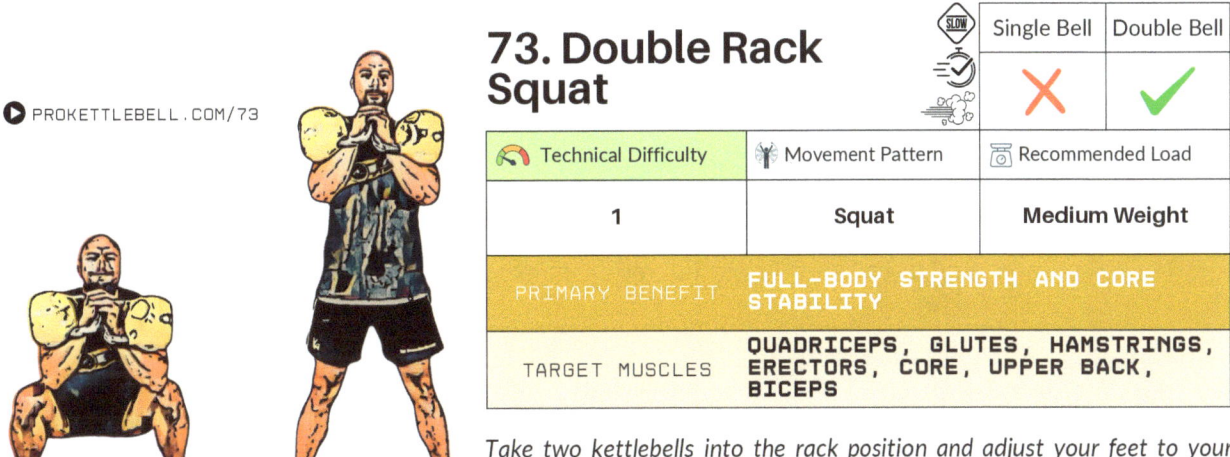

▶ PROKETTLEBELL.COM/73

73. Double Rack Squat

	Single Bell	Double Bell
	✗	✓

Technical Difficulty	Movement Pattern	Recommended Load
1	Squat	Medium Weight

PRIMARY BENEFIT	FULL-BODY STRENGTH AND CORE STABILITY
TARGET MUSCLES	QUADRICEPS, GLUTES, HAMSTRINGS, ERECTORS, CORE, UPPER BACK, BICEPS

Take two kettlebells into the rack position and adjust your feet to your ideal squat width. With chest up and lumbar flat, lower into a squat, while slightly lifting your elbows. Drive through the heels to return to standing. The rack position forces you to engage your core and upper back while building lower-body strength. Rest in the rack as needed between reps.

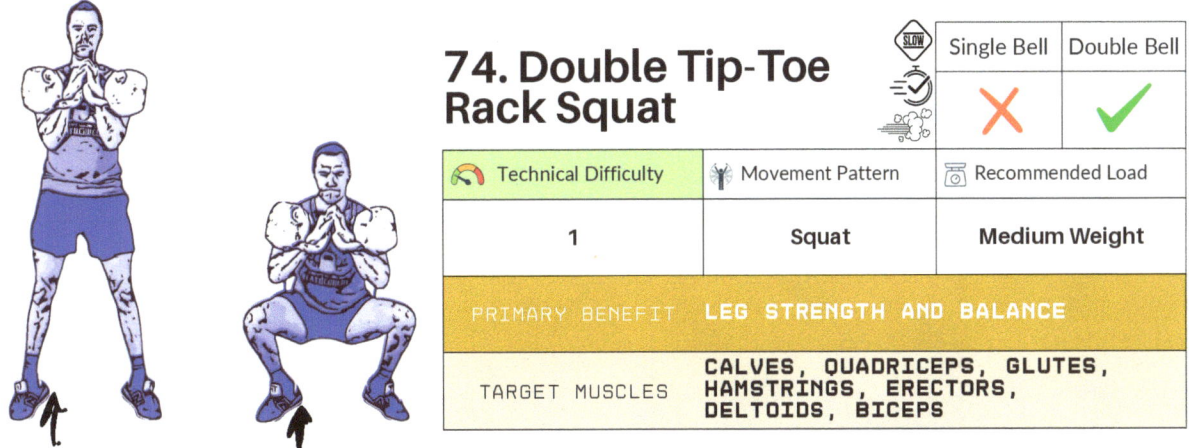

74. Double Tip-Toe Rack Squat

	Single Bell	Double Bell
	✗	✓

Technical Difficulty	Movement Pattern	Recommended Load
1	Squat	Medium Weight

PRIMARY BENEFIT	LEG STRENGTH AND BALANCE
TARGET MUSCLES	CALVES, QUADRICEPS, GLUTES, HAMSTRINGS, ERECTORS, DELTOIDS, BICEPS

Hold two kettlebells in the rack position and rise onto your tiptoes. From this elevated stance, perform a squat, keeping your balance and form intact. Lower with control, maintaining upright posture and flat lumbar. This variation targets lower leg muscles like the calves and feet, in addition to strengthening your core and quads due to the balance challenge. ▶ PROKETTLEBELL.COM/74

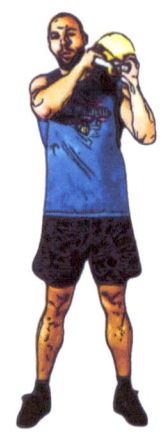
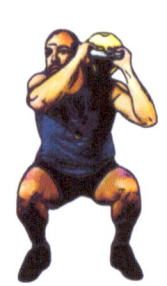

75. Fireman Carry Squats

	Single Bell	Double Bell
	✓	✗

Technical Difficulty	Movement Pattern	Recommended Load
1	Squat	Medium Weight

PRIMARY BENEFIT — LOWER BODY AND CORE STRENGTH

TARGET MUSCLES — QUADRICEPS, GLUTES, HAMSTRINGS, ERECTORS, OBLIQUES, UPPER BACK

Begin by holding the kettlebell by the horns, between your legs, with your elbows and upper arms pressed tightly against your ribs. Generate momentum with a hip thrust, swinging the kettlebell up and over one shoulder as if lifting a heavy object or person. Let the kettlebell rest securely on your trap muscle, not your clavicle. From here, perform a squat while maintaining symmetry, even though the load is asymmetrical. Keep your hips back, lumbar spine flat, heels grounded, and knees tracking your toes. ▶ PROKETTLEBELL.COM/75

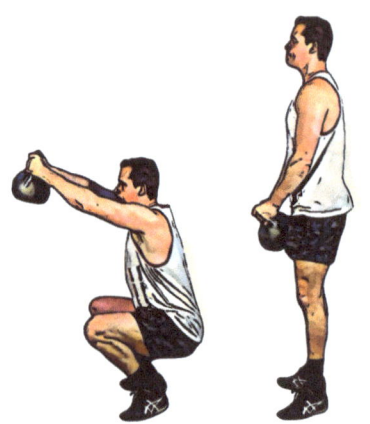

76. Front Raise Squat

	Single Bell	Double Bell
	✗	✓

Technical Difficulty	Movement Pattern	Recommended Load
1	Squat	Medium Weight

PRIMARY BENEFIT — LEG AND ANTERIOR CORE STRENGTH

TARGET MUSCLES — QUADRICEPS, GLUTES, HAMSTRINGS, DELTOIDS, CORE

Start by holding the kettlebell at rest using your preferred grip—horns, side, or crush grip. As you descend into a squat, with arms straight, raise the kettlebell in front of you until you can look straight through the window of the handle. Maintain a flat lumbar and strong posture throughout. ▶ PROKETTLEBELL.COM/76

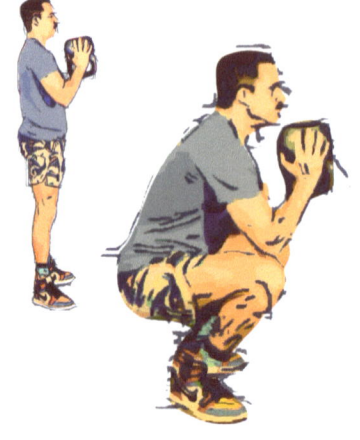

77. Goblet Squat

	Single Bell	Double Bell
	✓	✗

Technical Difficulty	Movement Pattern	Recommended Load
1	Squat	Medium Weight

PRIMARY BENEFIT — LEG AND CORE STRENGTH

TARGET MUSCLES — QUADRICEPS, GLUTES, HAMSTRINGS, CORE, UPPER BACK, BICEPS

▶ PROKETTLEBELL.COM/77

Hold the kettlebell bottom-side up and sandwiched between your palms with forearms parallel (the "goblet" position). Lower into a squat; hips back, heels down, and chest up. Ensure the knees track the toes and maintain a flat lumbar spine. This foundational movement builds lower body and core strength, especially due to the front-loaded weight.

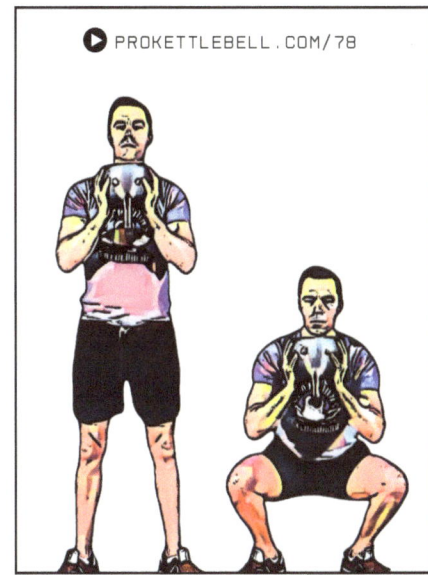

PROKETTLEBELL.COM/78

78. Loaded Stop Squat

	Single Bell	Double Bell
SLOW	✓	✗

Technical Difficulty	Movement Pattern	Recommended Load
1	Squat	Medium Weight

PRIMARY BENEFIT: ISOMETRIC SQUAT STRENGTH AND CORE STABILITY

TARGET MUSCLES: QUADRICEPS, GLUTES, HAMSTRINGS, ERECTORS, CORE

Hold the kettlebell in a goblet or preferred grip and descend into a squat, stopping at the point of maximum tension—typically just above parallel. Hold this position for a few seconds, then return to standing. Ensure your heels stay down, lumbar is flat, and chest is upright. This isometric hold builds static strength and reinforces proper squat posture under tension.

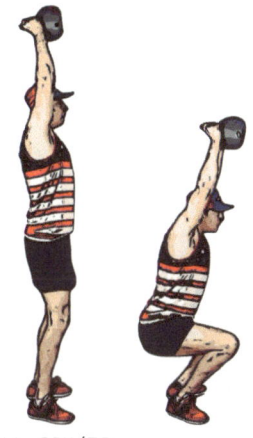

79. Overhead Squat, Two-Hand

	Single Bell	Double Bell
SLOW	✓	✗

Technical Difficulty	Movement Pattern	Recommended Load
1	Squat	Medium Weight

PRIMARY BENEFIT: LEG, CORE STRENGTH AND MOBILITY

TARGET MUSCLES: GLUTES, QUADRICEPS, HAMSTRINGS, ERECTORS, DELTOIDS, UPPER BACK, CORE

PROKETTLEBELL.COM/79

With arms locked out and shoulders actively engaged, the athlete descends into a deep squat, keeping the torso upright and the kettlebells stacked over the midfoot. This exercise builds strength and endurance in the shoulders and upper back while improving hip, ankle, and thoracic mobility. It's a total-body movement that demands focus, balance, and coordination from start to finish.

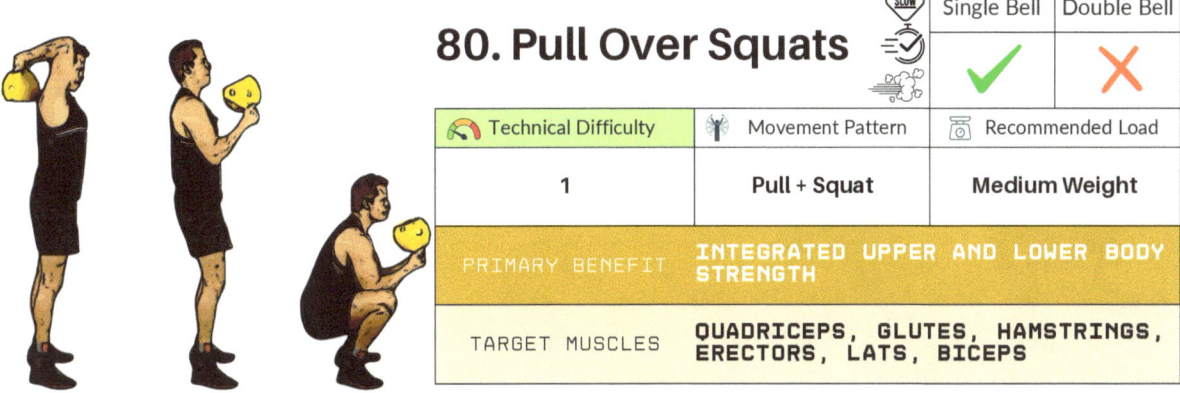

80. Pull Over Squats

	Single Bell	Double Bell
SLOW	✓	✗

Technical Difficulty	Movement Pattern	Recommended Load
1	Pull + Squat	Medium Weight

PRIMARY BENEFIT: INTEGRATED UPPER AND LOWER BODY STRENGTH

TARGET MUSCLES: QUADRICEPS, GLUTES, HAMSTRINGS, ERECTORS, LATS, BICEPS

Hold the kettlebell upside down by the horns at chest level, keeping your forearms parallel. Initiate the movement by performing a pullover—bring the kettlebell behind your head in a controlled arc, maintaining parallel forearms and an upright posture. Once you've reached your max depth behind you, reverse the motion to bring the kettlebell back over your head. As you pull the kettlebell into its forward descent, simultaneously drop into a squat. Stand up to return to the starting position and repeat. This exercise integrates shoulder mobility, upper-body control, and lower-body strength in a fluid, coordinated movement. PROKETTLEBELL.COM/80

PROKETTLEBELL.COM/81

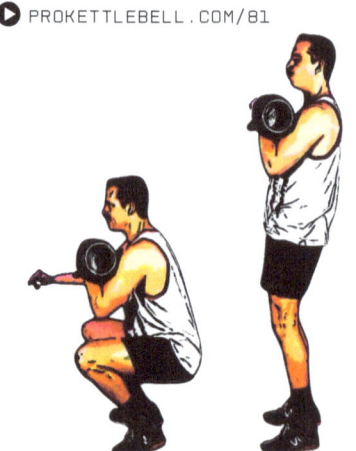

81. Rack Squat, One-Arm

	Single Bell	Double Bell
	✓	✗

Technical Difficulty	Movement Pattern	Recommended Load
1	Squat	Medium Weight

PRIMARY BENEFIT — UNILATERAL LEG AND CORE STRENGTH

TARGET MUSCLES — GLUTES, QUAD, HAMSTRINGS, ERECTORS, DELTOIDS, BICEPS

Begin standing with a kettlebell in the rack position on one side—elbow tucked, wrist straight, and the bell resting on your forearm and bicep. With your feet set at shoulder width or slightly wider, brace your core and descend into a controlled squat, raising your elbow slightly and keeping the kettlebell stable throughout. Maintain an upright torso and even weight distribution through your feet. Push through your heels to return to standing. This exercise builds unilateral strength, core stability, and reinforces proper squat mechanics under asymmetrical load.

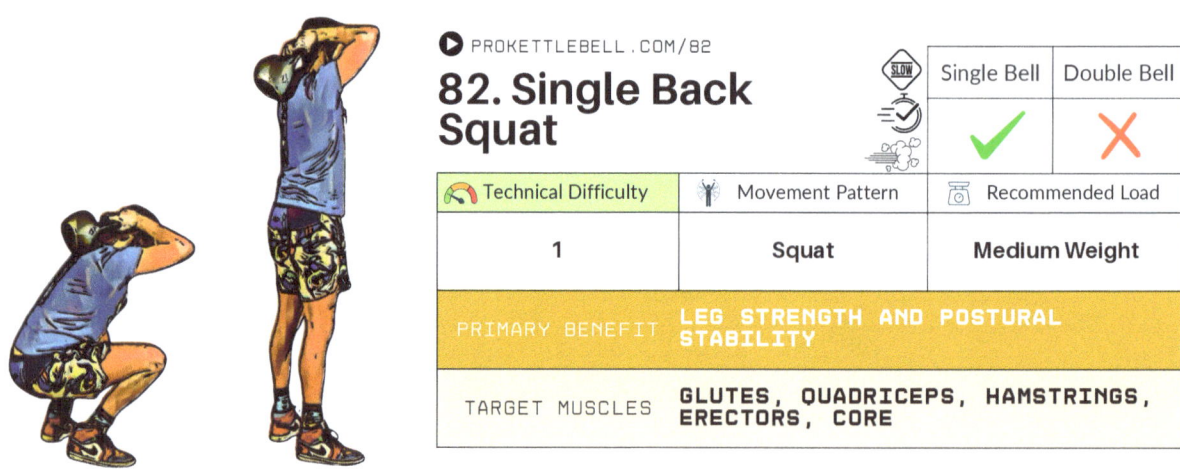

PROKETTLEBELL.COM/82

82. Single Back Squat

	Single Bell	Double Bell
	✓	✗

Technical Difficulty	Movement Pattern	Recommended Load
1	Squat	Medium Weight

PRIMARY BENEFIT — LEG STRENGTH AND POSTURAL STABILITY

TARGET MUSCLES — GLUTES, QUADRICEPS, HAMSTRINGS, ERECTORS, CORE

Position a single kettlebell behind your head, resting across the upper back and shoulders. Stand tall with feet at shoulder-width or more apart. Initiate the squat by driving the hips back and down, keeping the chest lifted and spine neutral. Lower until your hips are at or below parallel, then drive through your heels to return to standing. This variation challenges postural control and core stability while effectively targeting the lower body with minimal equipment.

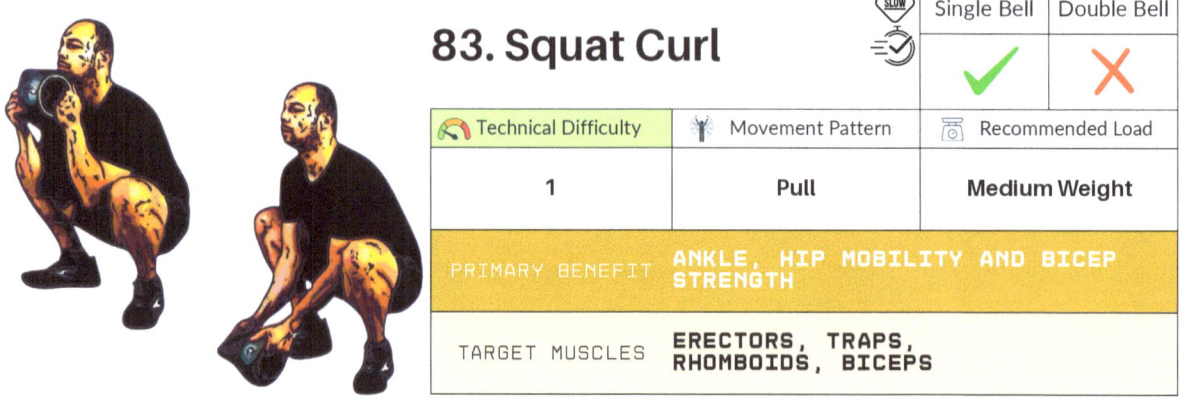

83. Squat Curl

	Single Bell	Double Bell
	✓	✗

Technical Difficulty	Movement Pattern	Recommended Load
1	Pull	Medium Weight

PRIMARY BENEFIT — ANKLE, HIP MOBILITY AND BICEP STRENGTH

TARGET MUSCLES — ERECTORS, TRAPS, RHOMBOIDS, BICEPS

Hold a single kettlebell by the horns at chest height and lower into a deep squat— keeping your heels grounded, chest upright, and elbows inside your knees. While maintaining the squat position, extend your arms fully to lower the kettlebell, then perform a controlled bicep curl to bring it back to your chest. Keep your upper body stable and core engaged throughout. This movement builds lower-body endurance, bicep strength, and postural control, making it an excellent addition to flow or hypertrophy-focused circuits. PROKETTLEBELL.COM/83

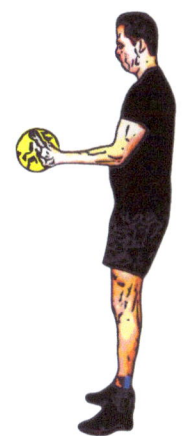

84. Ab Squat
PROKETTLEBELL.COM/84

	Single Bell	Double Bell
	✓	✗

Technical Difficulty	Movement Pattern	Recommended Load
2	Squat	Medium Weight

PRIMARY BENEFIT	ANTERIOR CORE AND LEG STRENGTH
TARGET MUSCLES	QUADRICEPS, GLUTES, HAMSTRINGS, ERECTORS, ABS, DELTOIDS, BICEPS

Hold a kettlebell with both hands and extend it in front of you, with minimal arm bend. The farther the kettlebell is from your body, the more your abs will be engaged. From this position, perform a standard squat with hips back, heels down, and knees tracking the toes. Keep your torso upright and lumbar flat throughout. As your core strength improves, increase the challenge by extending the kettlebell farther during the movement.

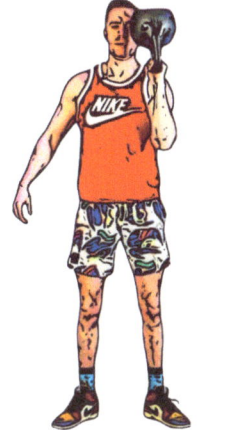
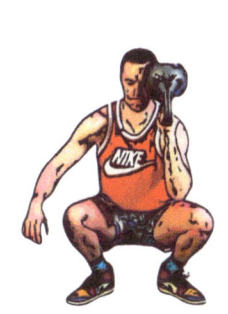

85. Bottoms-Up Squat

	Single Bell	Double Bell
	✓	✗

Technical Difficulty	Movement Pattern	Recommended Load
2	Squat	Medium Weight

PRIMARY BENEFIT	LEG STRENGTH, CORE STABILITY, AND GRIP ENDURANCE
TARGET MUSCLES	QUADRICEPS, GLUTES, HAMSTRINGS, DELTOIDS, CORE, BICEPS, FOREARMS, HANDS

PROKETTLEBELL.COM/85

Begin by holding a kettlebell in a bottoms-up position, with the base facing upward. Grip it in the center of the handle to intensify the challenge, or in the corner for added control. Maintain alignment between the wrist, elbow, and shoulder. Perform a controlled squat, keeping your chest up and back flat.

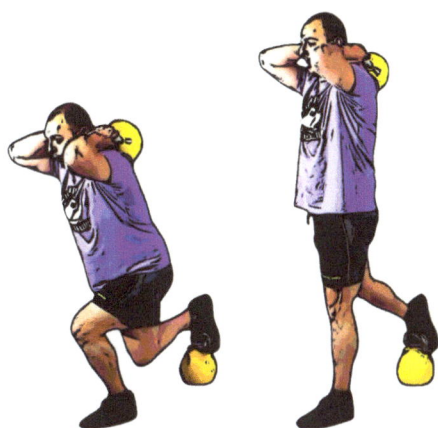

86. Bulgarian Back Squat

	Single Bell	Double Bell
	✓	✗

Technical Difficulty	Movement Pattern	Recommended Load
2	Squat	Medium Weight

PRIMARY BENEFIT	SINGLE-LEG STRENGTH AND STABILITY
TARGET MUSCLES	QUADRICEPS, GLUTES, HAMSTRINGS, ERECTORS, CORE

Hold the kettlebell behind your shoulders. Step one foot forward and the other behind you, placing it on a bench or otherwise elevating it slightly. Lower into a squat, keeping the front knee aligned with the toe and the back knee tracking similarly. Drive through the front heel to return to standing. Maintain an upright torso and flat lumbar throughout the movement to protect your spine. PROKETTLEBELL.COM/86

SQUATS

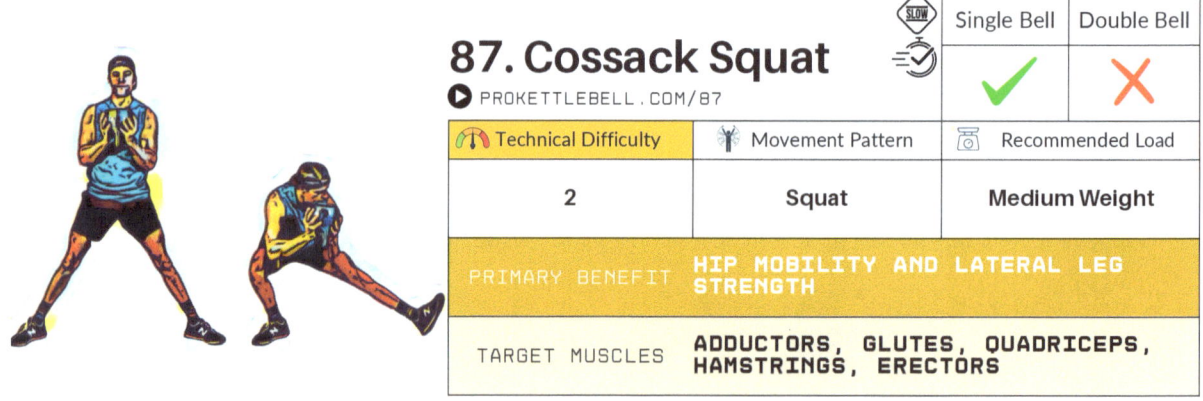

87. Cossack Squat
PROKETTLEBELL.COM/87

	Single Bell	Double Bell
	✓	✗
Technical Difficulty	Movement Pattern	Recommended Load
2	Squat	Medium Weight
PRIMARY BENEFIT	HIP MOBILITY AND LATERAL LEG STRENGTH	
TARGET MUSCLES	ADDUCTORS, GLUTES, QUADRICEPS, HAMSTRINGS, ERECTORS	

Hold the kettlebell in front of your body in a secure grip and take a wide stance. Shift your weight onto one leg, bending it deeply while keeping the opposite leg straight with the toe lifted. Lower under control with the knee tracking the toe and chest upright, then return to center and alternate sides. This movement builds hip mobility, balance, and inner-thigh and glute strength.

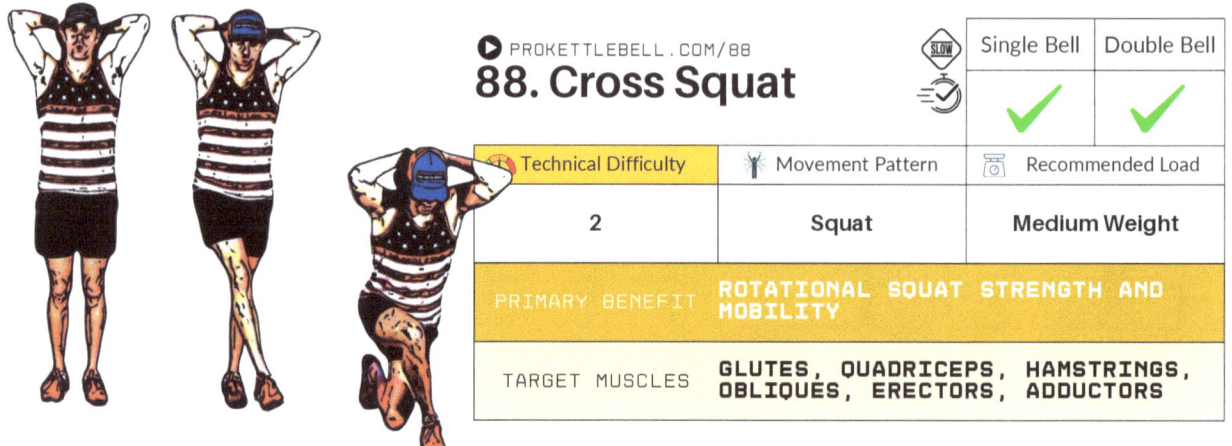

88. Cross Squat
PROKETTLEBELL.COM/88

	Single Bell	Double Bell
	✓	✓
Technical Difficulty	Movement Pattern	Recommended Load
2	Squat	Medium Weight
PRIMARY BENEFIT	ROTATIONAL SQUAT STRENGTH AND MOBILITY	
TARGET MUSCLES	GLUTES, QUADRICEPS, HAMSTRINGS, OBLIQUES, ERECTORS, ADDUCTORS	

With the kettlebell resting behind your shoulders, step forward and diagonally across your body so the lead foot lands clearly in front of the opposite knee, creating an imaginary line from your back foot through the knee to the front foot. Lower into a squat with your knees tracking your toes and torso upright, then drive through the lead foot to return to the start. This is essentially a forward curtsy squat.

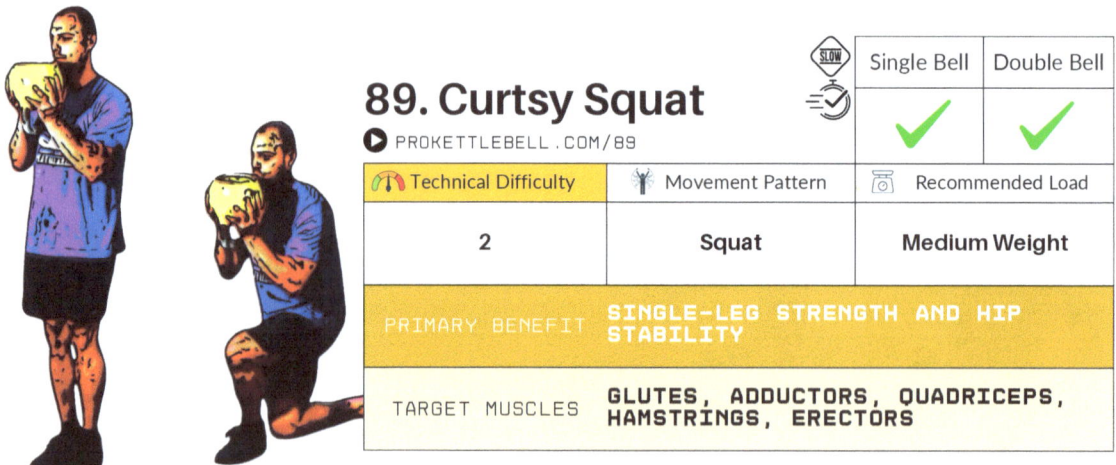

89. Curtsy Squat
PROKETTLEBELL.COM/89

	Single Bell	Double Bell
	✓	✓
Technical Difficulty	Movement Pattern	Recommended Load
2	Squat	Medium Weight
PRIMARY BENEFIT	SINGLE-LEG STRENGTH AND HIP STABILITY	
TARGET MUSCLES	GLUTES, ADDUCTORS, QUADRICEPS, HAMSTRINGS, ERECTORS	

Hold the kettlebell in a goblet position with forearms as parallel as possible. Step one leg back and diagonally to about 45 degrees. Lower the back knee toward the floor while keeping most of your weight on the front leg, aligning the back foot, down knee, and front foot along the same diagonal. Keep your torso upright and the front knee tracking the toes. Drive through the front heel to stand. Repeat for multiple reps on one side or alternate legs.

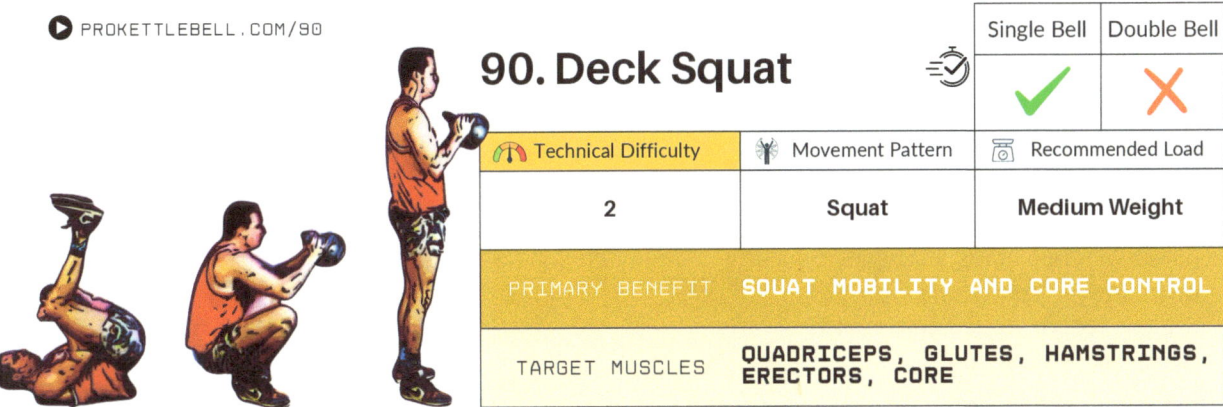

90. Deck Squat

	Single Bell	Double Bell
	✓	✗

Technical Difficulty	Movement Pattern	Recommended Load
2	Squat	Medium Weight

PRIMARY BENEFIT	SQUAT MOBILITY AND CORE CONTROL
TARGET MUSCLES	QUADRICEPS, GLUTES, HAMSTRINGS, ERECTORS, CORE

Begin seated with a kettlebell held securely in both hands. Roll back onto your shoulders—not your neck—then use momentum and core engagement to roll forward into a deep squat. Push through your feet to stand. The kettlebell provides counterbalance, assisting with control. To modify, practice with elevated mats or use assistance like a rope to develop the mobility and strength required.

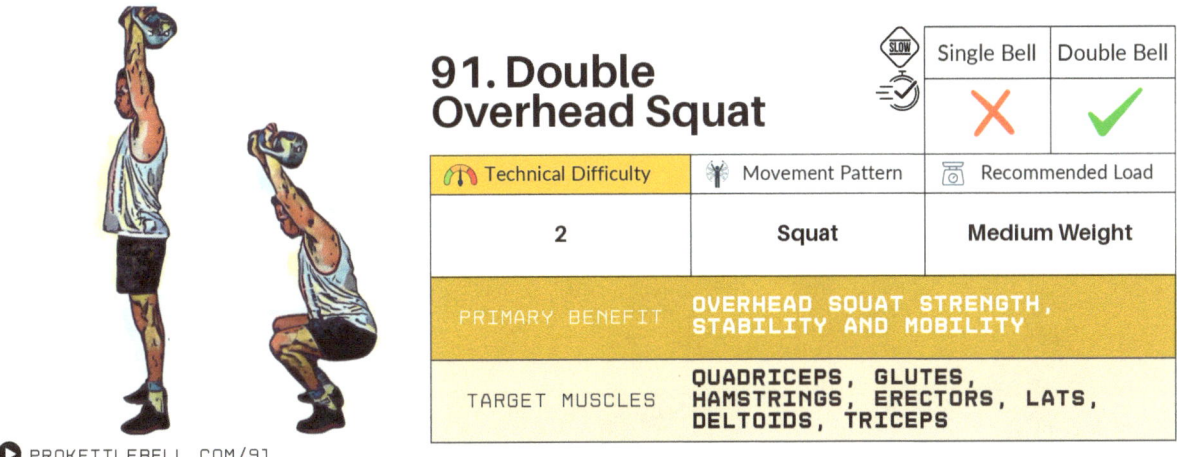

91. Double Overhead Squat

	Single Bell	Double Bell
	✗	✓

Technical Difficulty	Movement Pattern	Recommended Load
2	Squat	Medium Weight

PRIMARY BENEFIT	OVERHEAD SQUAT STRENGTH, STABILITY AND MOBILITY
TARGET MUSCLES	QUADRICEPS, GLUTES, HAMSTRINGS, ERECTORS, LATS, DELTOIDS, TRICEPS

Start with two kettlebells pressed and locked out overhead. Keep the bells stacked directly over your shoulders as you descend. Squat only as deep as you can while maintaining proper alignment—flat lumbar spine, chest up, and knees tracking the toes. Actively engage the upper back by squeezing the shoulder blades together rather than shrugging. This movement challenges thoracic mobility, balance, and total-body control.

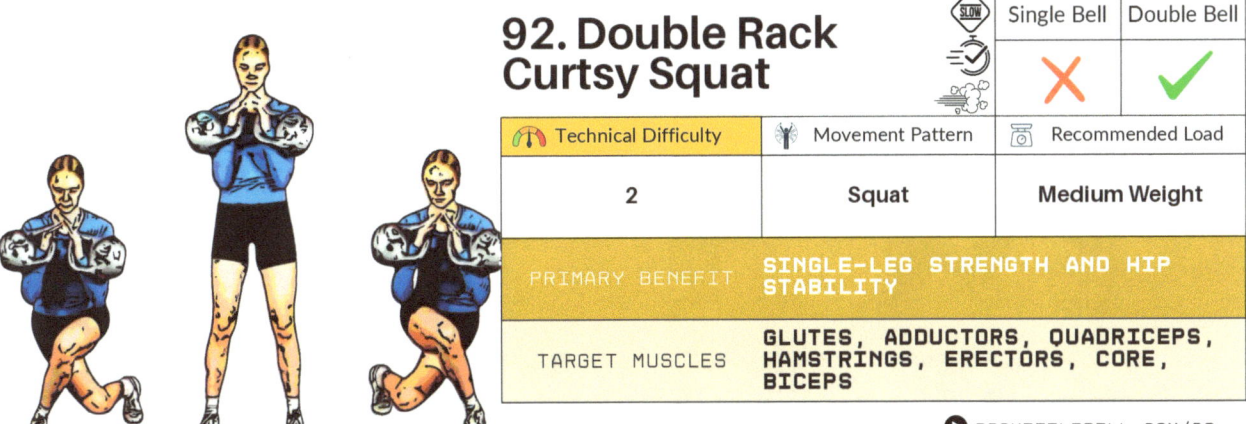

92. Double Rack Curtsy Squat

	Single Bell	Double Bell
	✗	✓

Technical Difficulty	Movement Pattern	Recommended Load
2	Squat	Medium Weight

PRIMARY BENEFIT	SINGLE-LEG STRENGTH AND HIP STABILITY
TARGET MUSCLES	GLUTES, ADDUCTORS, QUADRICEPS, HAMSTRINGS, ERECTORS, CORE, BICEPS

Hold two kettlebells in the rack position. Keeping them within your frame, step one leg back and diagonally behind the front leg. Lower into a squat, ensuring the front knee tracks the toes and the torso stays upright. Drive through the front heel to return. The rear leg acts as a support while the front leg does most of the work. Alternate sides or complete all reps on one side before switching.

SQUATS

▶ PROKETTLEBELL.COM/93

Begin with two kettlebells racked and a wide stance. Shift your weight to one side and squat deeply, then slide in a smooth semi-circle to the opposite side, as if ducking under an imaginary barrier. You may stand and reset at center between reps, or stay low and glide side to side for a deeper stretch and greater challenge. Keep your torso upright and chest lifted throughout.

93. Double Rack Squat Slider

	Single Bell	Double Bell
SLOW	✗	✓

Technical Difficulty	Movement Pattern	Recommended Load
2	Squat	Medium Weight

PRIMARY BENEFIT	LATERAL SQUAT STRENGTH AND HIP MOBILITY
TARGET MUSCLES	QUADRICEPS, GLUTES, HAMSTRINGS, ERECTORS, DELTOIDS, BICEPS

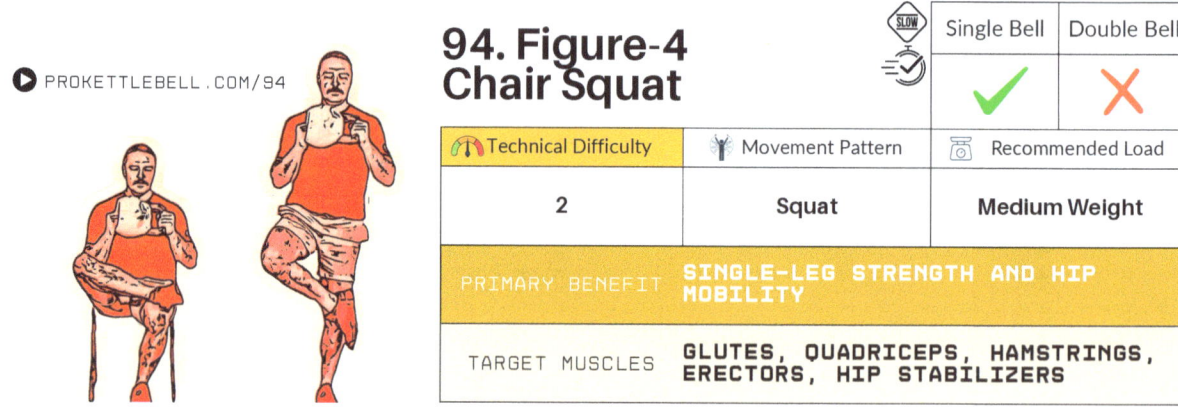

▶ PROKETTLEBELL.COM/94

94. Figure-4 Chair Squat

	Single Bell	Double Bell
SLOW	✓	✗

Technical Difficulty	Movement Pattern	Recommended Load
2	Squat	Medium Weight

PRIMARY BENEFIT	SINGLE-LEG STRENGTH AND HIP MOBILITY
TARGET MUSCLES	GLUTES, QUADRICEPS, HAMSTRINGS, ERECTORS, HIP STABILIZERS

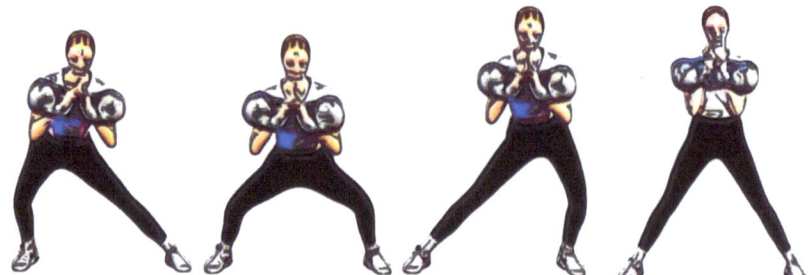

Sit on a chair or bench with a kettlebell in hand. Cross one ankle over the opposite knee to form a figure four. With control, stand up, then sit back down, keeping the raised shin as parallel to the ground as possible. Beginners can extend the kettlebell slightly to assist with balance; holding it close to the chest increases the challenge.

95. Figure-4 Squat

	Single Bell	Double Bell
SLOW	✓	✗

Technical Difficulty	Movement Pattern	Recommended Load
2	Squat	Medium Weight

PRIMARY BENEFIT	SINGLE-LEG STRENGTH AND BALANCE
TARGET MUSCLES	GLUTES, QUADRICEPS, HAMSTRINGS, ERECTORS, HIP STABILIZERS

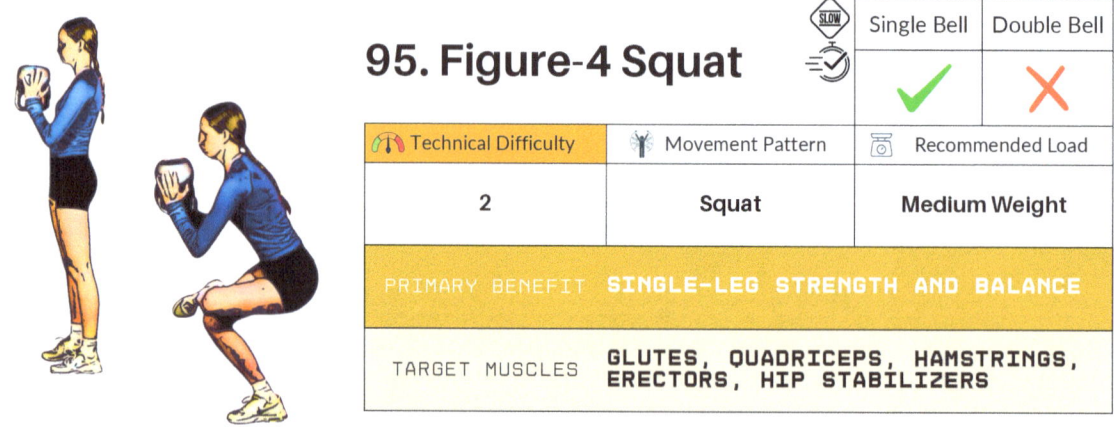

Hold a kettlebell in a secure position at chest height. Cross one ankle over the opposite knee. With the ankle resting just above the knee, lower into a squat while keeping your balance, chest lifted, and lumbar flat. Rise to standing, keeping the kettlebell close to your body. Repeat on both sides. ▶ PROKETTLEBELL.COM/95

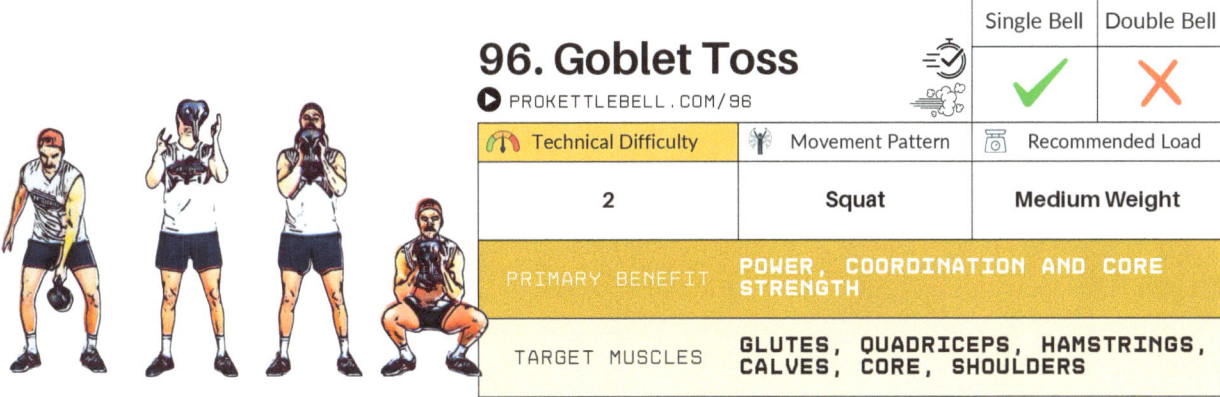

96. Goblet Toss

PROKETTLEBELL.COM/96

	Single Bell	Double Bell
	✓	✗

Technical Difficulty	Movement Pattern	Recommended Load
2	Squat	Medium Weight

PRIMARY BENEFIT	POWER, COORDINATION AND CORE STRENGTH
TARGET MUSCLES	GLUTES, QUADRICEPS, HAMSTRINGS, CALVES, CORE, SHOULDERS

Begin with a goblet squat. Once complete, lightly toss the kettlebell upward and quickly release it, regrasping the handle with one hand. Guide the kettlebell into a swing between your legs as it falls. On the upswing, as the bell reaches the apex, let it rotate upside down, release the handle, and quickly catch the body with both hands to return to the goblet hold. Repeat the goblet squat > toss > swing sequence, alternating hands each swing.

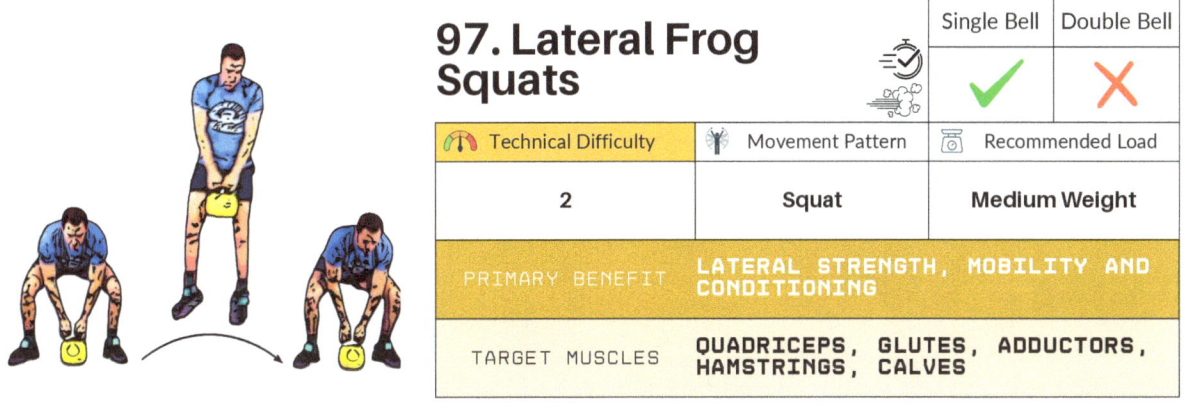

97. Lateral Frog Squats

	Single Bell	Double Bell
	✓	✗

Technical Difficulty	Movement Pattern	Recommended Load
2	Squat	Medium Weight

PRIMARY BENEFIT	LATERAL STRENGTH, MOBILITY AND CONDITIONING
TARGET MUSCLES	QUADRICEPS, GLUTES, ADDUCTORS, HAMSTRINGS, CALVES

Start in a wide stance with the kettlebell on the floor directly under your center of mass. Sit down into a deep frog squat with a flat lumbar spine, chest up, and arms straight and locked, holding the bell. From this low position, hop laterally to one side while keeping the kettlebell low and centered, then continue hopping side to side for distance or single steps. Each rep, bring the kettlebell all the way back to the floor under your body. Keep movement controlled, arms straight, and posture solid throughout. PROKETTLEBELL.COM/97

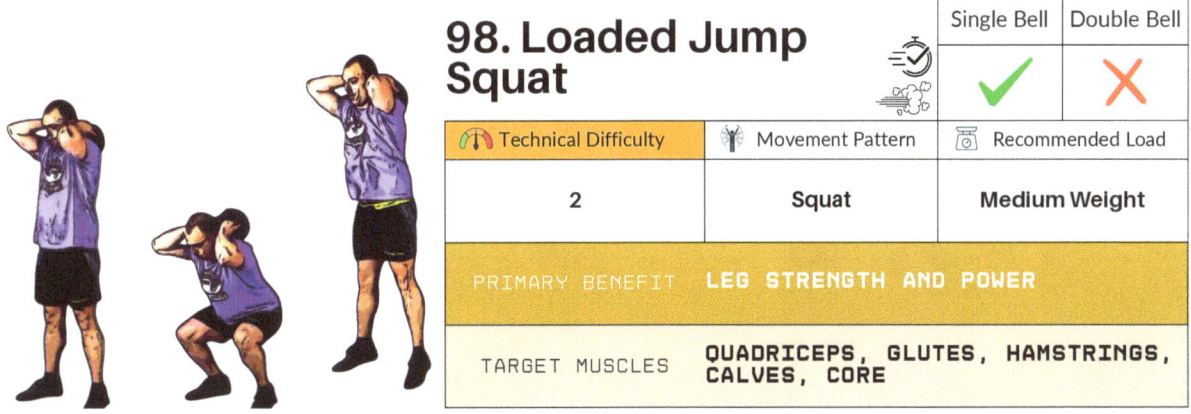

98. Loaded Jump Squat

	Single Bell	Double Bell
	✓	✗

Technical Difficulty	Movement Pattern	Recommended Load
2	Squat	Medium Weight

PRIMARY BENEFIT	LEG STRENGTH AND POWER
TARGET MUSCLES	QUADRICEPS, GLUTES, HAMSTRINGS, CALVES, CORE

Place the kettlebell securely between your shoulder blades by squeezing your shoulder blades together to create a stable shelf. Stand tall, then descend into a squat with good alignment and explode upward into a jump. Land softly on the balls of your feet, absorbing the impact quietly as if landing in a puddle. For a lower-impact option, rise explosively onto your toes instead of jumping. PROKETTLEBELL.COM/98

SQUATS

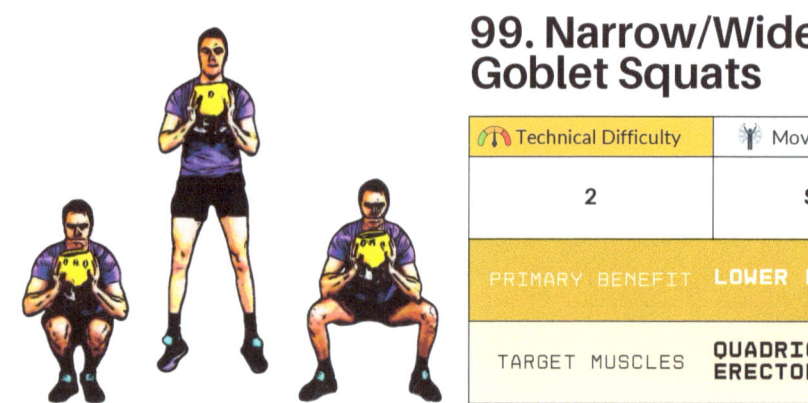

99. Narrow/Wide Goblet Squats

	Single Bell	Double Bell
	✗	✓

Technical Difficulty	Movement Pattern	Recommended Load
2	Squat	Medium Weight

PRIMARY BENEFIT	LOWER BODY

TARGET MUSCLES	QUADRICEPS, GLUTES, HAMSTRINGS, ERECTORS, BICEPS

Begin by holding a kettlebell in the goblet position at chest height. Start with your feet in a narrow stance, perform a squat by sitting back and down, then return to standing. Step one foot out to a wider stance and immediately perform a wide-stance goblet squat. Return to the narrow stance and continue alternating between narrow and wide squats. Keep your chest lifted, core engaged, and heels grounded throughout the movement to ensure proper form and maximize effectiveness. ▶ PROKETTLEBELL.COM/99

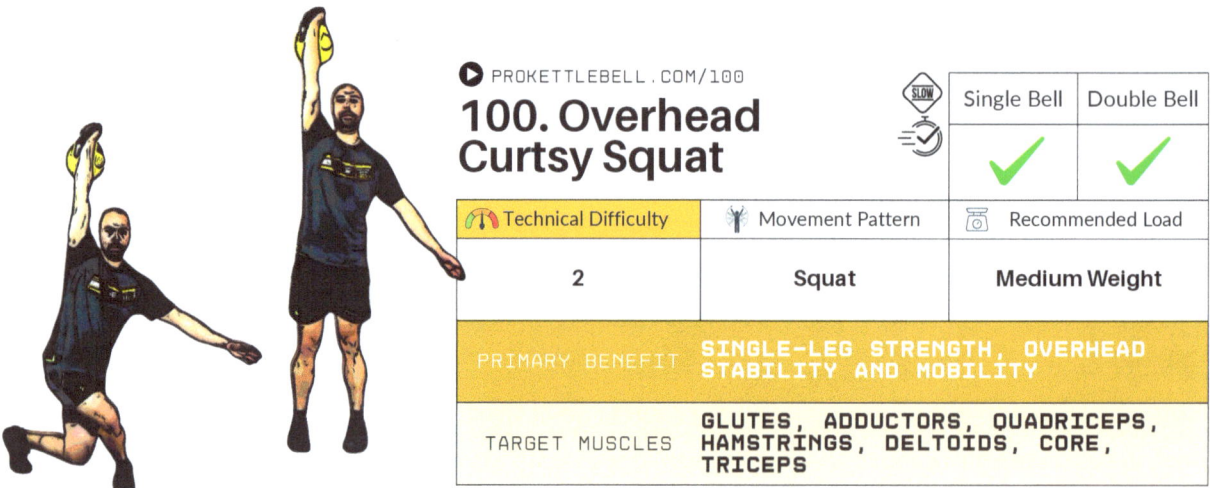

▶ PROKETTLEBELL.COM/100

100. Overhead Curtsy Squat

	Single Bell	Double Bell
	✓	✓

Technical Difficulty	Movement Pattern	Recommended Load
2	Squat	Medium Weight

PRIMARY BENEFIT	SINGLE-LEG STRENGTH, OVERHEAD STABILITY AND MOBILITY

TARGET MUSCLES	GLUTES, ADDUCTORS, QUADRICEPS, HAMSTRINGS, DELTOIDS, CORE, TRICEPS

Starting with a kettlebell pressed overhead, the athlete maintains a strong lockout and braced core while stepping one leg behind and across into a controlled curtsy squat. Keeping as much weight as possible in the front leg, drive through the front heel to return to standing. Repeat on one leg or alternate legs each rep.

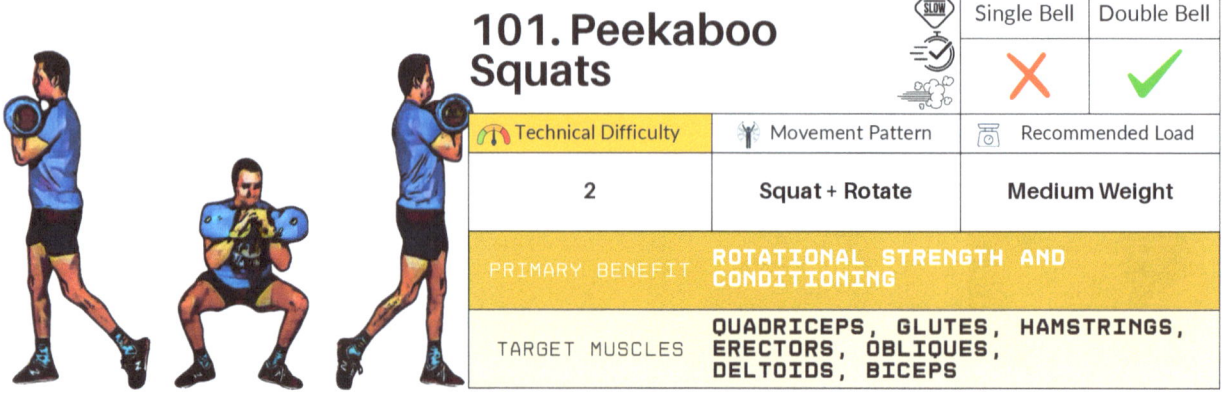

101. Peekaboo Squats

	Single Bell	Double Bell
	✗	✓

Technical Difficulty	Movement Pattern	Recommended Load
2	Squat + Rotate	Medium Weight

PRIMARY BENEFIT	ROTATIONAL STRENGTH AND CONDITIONING

TARGET MUSCLES	QUADRICEPS, GLUTES, HAMSTRINGS, ERECTORS, OBLIQUES, DELTOIDS, BICEPS

Begin in a deep squat with two kettlebells racked at your chest. Keeping your feet in the same place, rotate your torso about 90 degrees to one side and rise to standing, shifting your weight toward the leg on that side. Think of this as an upward punch driven by your legs and core, while the kettlebells stay racked. Lower back into a squat, rotate 180 degrees to the opposite side, and rise again. Continue alternating sides. ▶ PROKETTLEBELL.COM/101

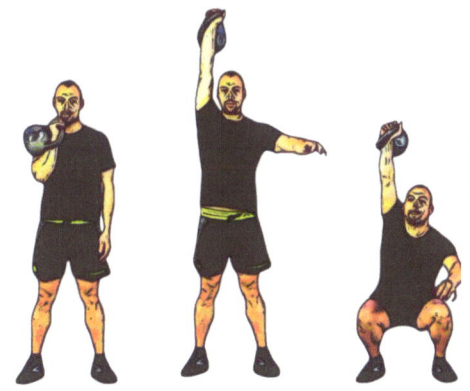

102. Press + Overhead Squat

	Single Bell	Double Bell
SLOW	✓	✓

Technical Difficulty	Movement Pattern	Recommended Load
2	Push	Medium Weight

PRIMARY BENEFIT: INTEGRATED PRESSING STRENGTH AND OVERHEAD SQUAT STABILITY

TARGET MUSCLES: QUADRICEPS, GLUTES, HAMSTRINGS, ERECTORS, LATS, DELTOIDS, TRICEPS

With the kettlebell locked out overhead and your body stabilized, descend into a squat as deeply as you can while keeping the bell stacked over your shoulder. Aim to reach at least parallel, pause briefly at the bottom, then return to standing by driving through your heels. Maintain full-body tension and keep the working arm straight throughout the movement. ▶ PROKETTLEBELL.COM/102

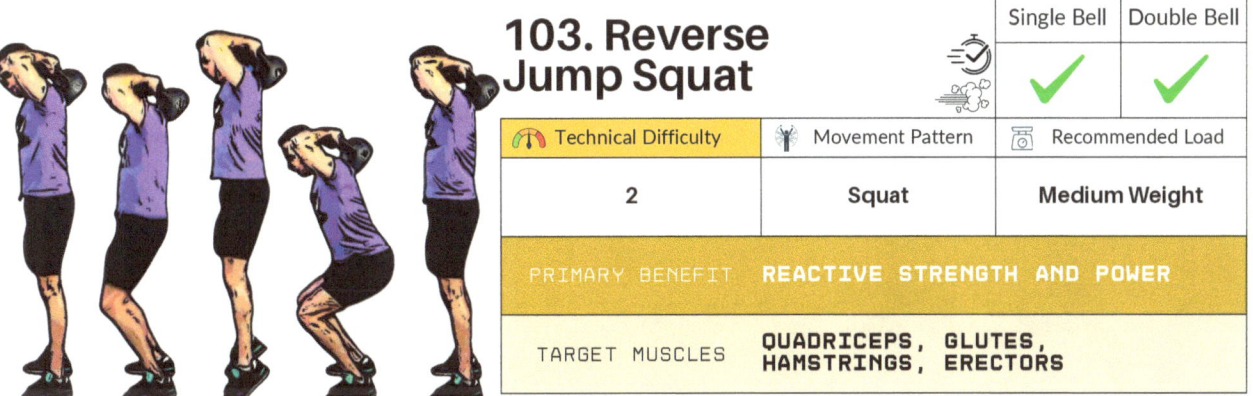

103. Reverse Jump Squat

	Single Bell	Double Bell
	✓	✓

Technical Difficulty	Movement Pattern	Recommended Load
2	Squat	Medium Weight

PRIMARY BENEFIT: REACTIVE STRENGTH AND POWER

TARGET MUSCLES: QUADRICEPS, GLUTES, HAMSTRINGS, ERECTORS

Hold the kettlebell by the horns and rest it securely across your shoulder blades, applying light pressure with your index fingers to prevent bouncing. Initiate a quick hop, lifting your heels off the ground. As you descend, drop smoothly into a squat and catch yourself softly with control. Stand tall to reset, then repeat. This movement trains reactive strength, body control, and lower-body power while challenging your balance under unconventional load placement. ▶ PROKETTLEBELL.COM/103

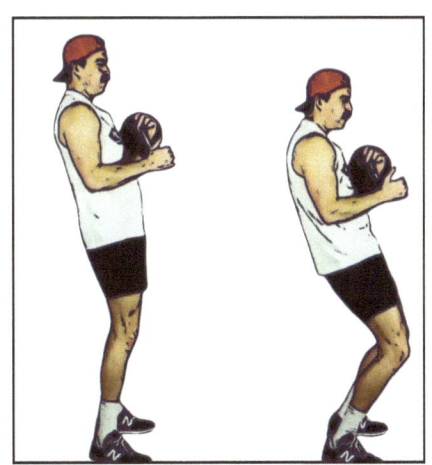

104. Semi-Squat

	Single Bell	Double Bell
SLOW	✓	✓

Technical Difficulty	Movement Pattern	Recommended Load
2	Squat	Medium Weight

PRIMARY BENEFIT: LEG DRIVE AND RACK STABILITY

TARGET MUSCLES: GLUTES, QUADRICEPS, ERECTORS

Hold the kettlebell in the rack position with arm-to-body connection—ideally anchoring the elbow to the hip. Lower into a partial squat while keeping your hips forward to maintain that connection throughout the movement. Stand up quickly to reset and repeat. The semi squat builds leg drive, reinforces rack stability, and primes the body for ballistic lifts like the push press or jerk. ▶ PROKETTLEBELL.COM/104

SQUATS

105. Slingshot Squats

	Single Bell	Double Bell
	✓	✗

Technical Difficulty	Movement Pattern	Recommended Load
2	Squat	Medium Weight

PRIMARY BENEFIT	LOWER BODY STRENGTH AND CORE CONTROL
TARGET MUSCLES	QUADRICEPS, GLUTES, HAMSTRINGS, ERECTORS

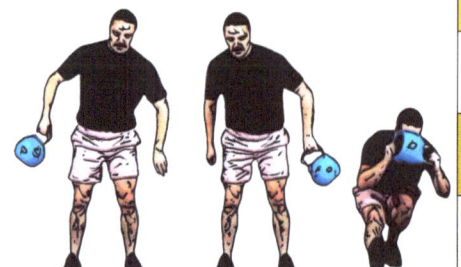

From standing, pass a kettlebell around your waist with momentum, switching hands behind your back. As it comes to the front, grab it with your free hand and drop into a squat, keeping your chest tall and heels grounded. Stand up and repeat, alternating slingshot direction. Variations include adding a pause at the bottom or progressing from slingshot to pistol squat. This movement builds grip strength, core stability, and lower-body control—great for warm-ups, flows, or conditioning. ▶ PROKETTLEBELL.COM/105

106. Squat Sliders

▶ PROKETTLEBELL.COM/106

	Single Bell	Double Bell
	✓	✗

Technical Difficulty	Movement Pattern	Recommended Load
2	Squat	Medium Weight

PRIMARY BENEFIT	LATERAL SQUAT STRENGTH AND CORE STABILITY
TARGET MUSCLES	GLUTES, QUADRICEPS, HAMSTRINGS, ERECTORS, DELTOIDS

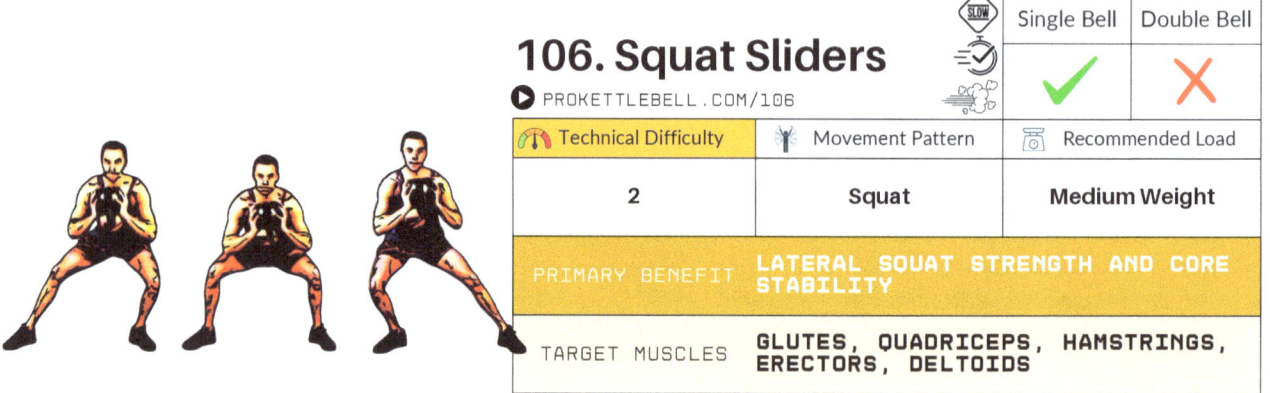

Hold a kettlebell in any secure two-handed grip. Lower into a controlled squat, keeping your chest tall and heels grounded. From the bottom of the squat, shift your hips side to side in a smooth, sliding motion—transferring your weight over one leg while keeping the opposite foot flat and extended. Move slowly and deliberately to maintain balance and tension, then return to center and stand tall to reset.

107. Curtsy Toss

	Single Bell	Double Bell
	✓	✗

Technical Difficulty	Movement Pattern	Recommended Load
2	Lunge	Light, Medium Weight

PRIMARY BENEFIT	COORDINATION, LEG STRENGTH, AND CORE STABILITY
TARGET MUSCLES	QUADRICEPS, GLUTES, ADDUCTORS, HAMSTRINGS, CORE, BICEPS

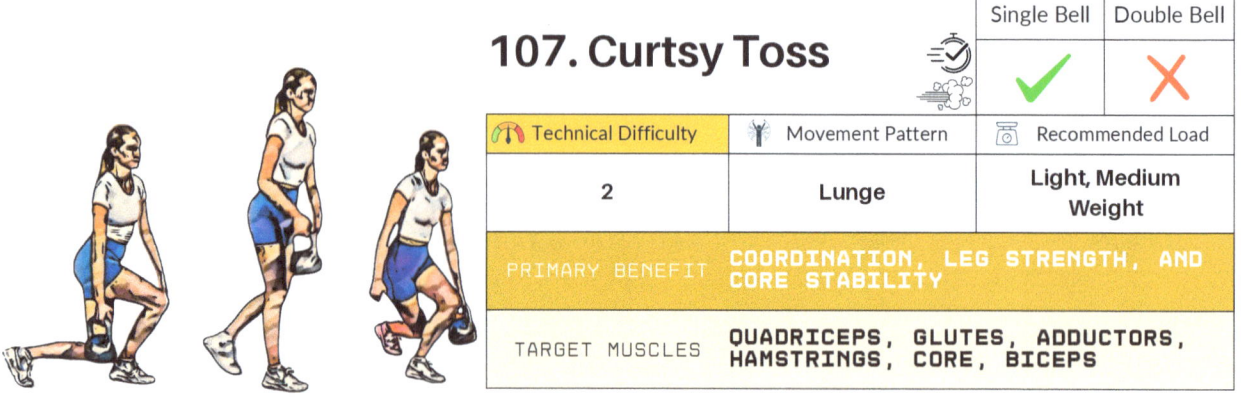

Perform alternating curtsy squats while switching hands each rep: holding a single kettlebell at your side, step the opposite leg back and across into a curtsy lunge with an upright torso. As you stand to switch legs, lightly toss the kettlebell to the opposite hand, creating a smooth "rainbow" arc in front of your body. Continue alternating sides with controlled footwork and clean hand transitions. Timing is everything. ▶ PROKETTLEBELL.COM/107

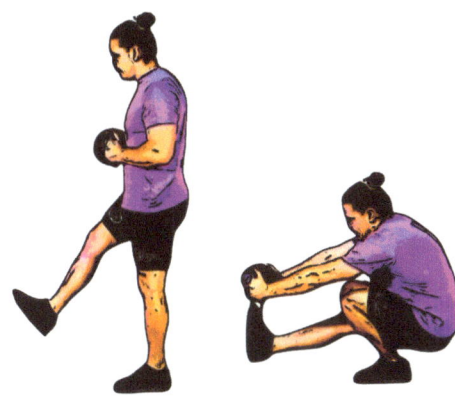

108. Pistol Squat

	Single Bell	Double Bell
	✓	✓

Technical Difficulty	Movement Pattern	Recommended Load
3	Squat	Medium Weight

PRIMARY BENEFIT	SINGLE-LEG STRENGTH AND MOBILITY
TARGET MUSCLES	QUADRICEPS, GLUTES, HAMSTRINGS, ERECTORS

▶ PROKETTLEBELL.COM/108

Holding a kettlebell in any comfortable two-hand grip for counterbalance, extend one leg forward while standing tall on the other. Engage your core and slowly lower into a deep squat on the standing leg, keeping the lifted leg straight and off the ground. Maintain an upright torso and controlled descent. Drive through the heel to return to standing, keeping the kettlebell close to your chest throughout the movement. Alternate sides or complete all reps on one leg before switching, focusing on range of motion.

109. Speed-Switch Front Squat

	Single Bell	Double Bell
	✓	✗

Technical Difficulty	Movement Pattern	Recommended Load
3	Squat	Medium Weight

PRIMARY BENEFIT	LOWER-BODY STRENGTH, COORDINATION AND REACTIVITY
TARGET MUSCLES	QUADRICEPS, GLUTES, HAMSTRINGS, ERECTORS, LATS, BICEPS

▶ PROKETTLEBELL.COM/109

Hold a single kettlebell in the rack position and descend into a front-loaded squat with heels grounded and chest upright. As you stand, initiate a swing and perform a quick "speed switch," tossing the kettlebell to the opposite hand and catching it immediately in the rack. Descend into the next squat without pause. The rapid hand transitions build coordination, rhythm, and reactive strength while developing lower-body power, postural control, and smooth kettlebell handling.

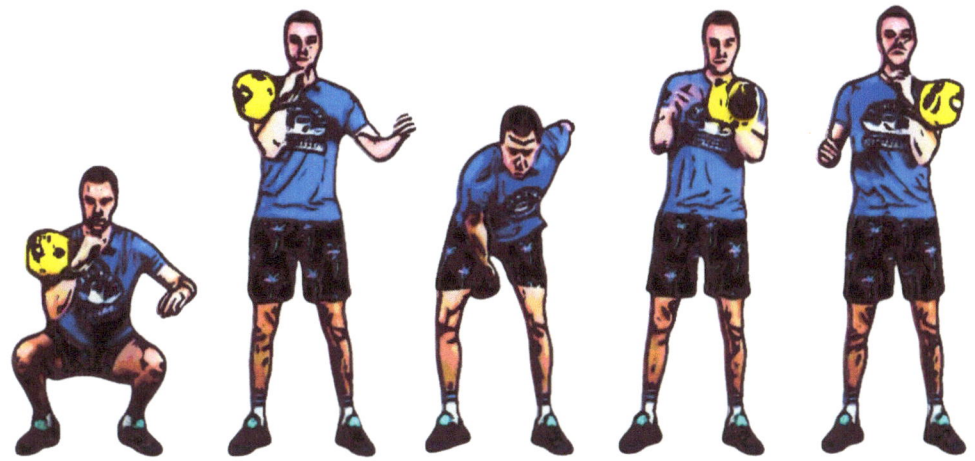

SQUATS

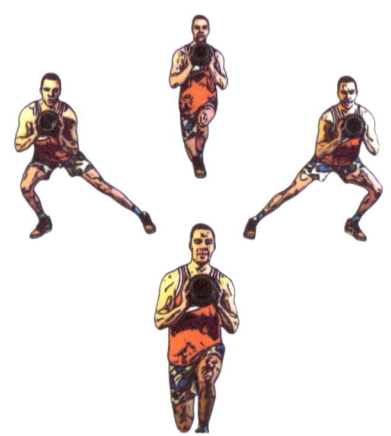

110. Clock Lunges

	Single Bell	Double Bell
SLOW	✓	✗

Technical Difficulty	Movement Pattern	Recommended Load
1	Lunge	Medium Weight

PRIMARY BENEFIT	MULTI-DIRECTIONAL LEG STRENGTH AND STABILITY
TARGET MUSCLES	QUADRICEPS, GLUTES, HAMSTRINGS, ADDUCTORS, ABDUCTORS

Hold the kettlebell securely in both hands. Begin with a forward lunge, then push off your forward foot and move it to the side, into a lateral lunge, followed by a reverse lunge—all on one side. You can then repeat in the opposite order on the other side, mimicking the motion of clock hands. Maintain proper lunge alignment throughout: chest up, hips back, and knees tracking the toes. ▶ PROKETTLEBELL.COM/110

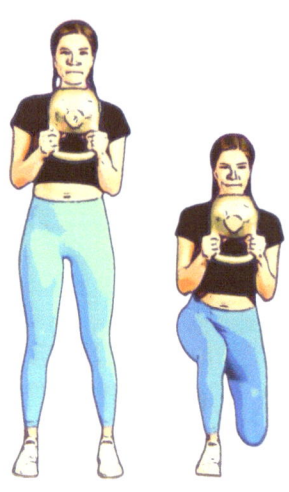

111. Horn Hold Reverse Lunge

	Single Bell	Double Bell
SLOW	✓	✗

Technical Difficulty	Movement Pattern	Recommended Load
1	Lunge	Medium Weight

PRIMARY BENEFIT	LEG STRENGTH AND CORE STABILITY
TARGET MUSCLES	GLUTES, QUADRICEPS, HAMSTRINGS, CORE, UPPER BACK, BICEPS

Hold the kettlebell by the horns, bottom up or down. Step back into a reverse lunge, ensuring your feet are shoulder-width apart and your feet, knee, and hip stay aligned. Keep your torso upright and the kettlebell close to your chest or slightly forward for added core engagement. You can alternate legs or focus on one side at a time. ▶ PROKETTLEBELL.COM/111

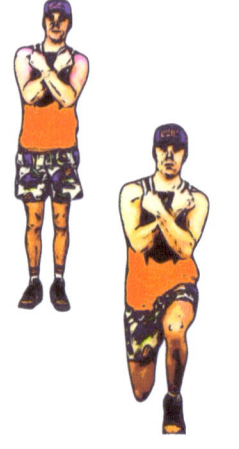

112. Hug Lunges

▶ PROKETTLEBELL.COM/112

	Single Bell	Double Bell
SLOW	✓	✗

Technical Difficulty	Movement Pattern	Recommended Load
1	Lunge	Medium Weight

PRIMARY BENEFIT	ANTERIOR LOAD LEG AND CORE STRENGTH
TARGET MUSCLES	QUADRICEPS, GLUTES, ERECTORS, CORE, UPPER BACK

Hold the kettlebell at chest height and wrap your arms around it, cradling it close. Step forward into a lunge. As with all lunges, keep your hip, knee and ankle joints aligned. Drive through the forward heel to push yourself back to standing. Alternate legs or focus on one side. Avoid rounding your back and ensure knees track toes.

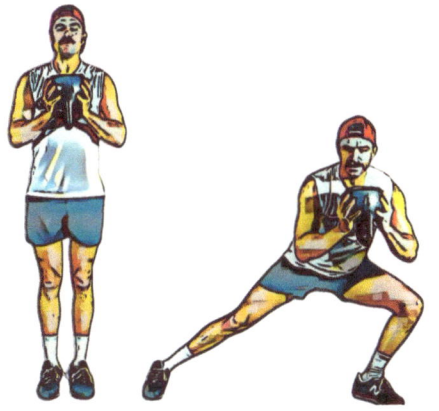

113. Lateral Lunges (Goblet Hold)

	Single Bell	Double Bell
	✓	✗

Technical Difficulty	Movement Pattern	Recommended Load
1	Lunge	Medium Weight

PRIMARY BENEFIT: LATERAL LEG STRENGTH AND HIP MOBILITY

TARGET MUSCLES: GLUTES, ADDUCTORS, QUADRICEPS, HAMSTRINGS, ABDUCTORS

Hold the kettlebell in front of your chest using a goblet grip. Step out laterally, slightly turning out the stepping foot so the knee can track over the toes. Sit back into the lunge while keeping the opposite leg straight and the chest tall by retracting your shoulder blades. Drive through the bent leg to return to standing, maintaining a neutral spine throughout the movement. ▶ PROKETTLEBELL.COM/113

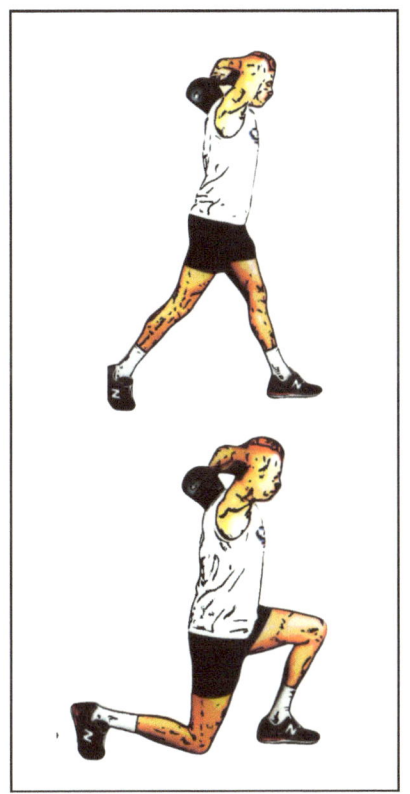

114. Loaded Stationary Lunge

	Single Bell	Double Bell
	✓	✓

Technical Difficulty	Movement Pattern	Recommended Load
1	Lunge	Medium Weight

PRIMARY BENEFIT: LEGS AND CORE STRENGTH

TARGET MUSCLES: GLUTES, QUADRICEPS, HAMSTRINGS, CORE

With the kettlebell resting behind your shoulders, take a long step forward into a split stance with feet about shoulder-width apart. Bend both legs, bringing the back knee as close to the ground as possible without touching, while keeping your weight evenly distributed. Drive through the front heel and back toe to return to standing.

▶ PROKETTLEBELL.COM/114

115. Lunge Pulse

▶ PROKETTLEBELL.COM/115

	Single Bell	Double Bell
	✓	✓

Technical Difficulty	Movement Pattern	Recommended Load
1	Lunge	Medium Weight

PRIMARY BENEFIT: ISOMETRIC AND END-RANGE LEG STRENGTH

TARGET MUSCLES: QUADRICEPS, GLUTES, HAMSTRINGS, ADDUCTORS, ERECTORS

Take a long step forward into a lunge stance and lower until your back knee hovers above the floor. Perform small pulses up and down, keeping your core tight and chest lifted. You can hold the kettlebell in the farmer carry, goblet, or behind-the-back position depending on preference. Ensure knees track toes and posture remains upright.

LUNGES

PROKETTLEBELL.COM/116

116. Overhead Lunge

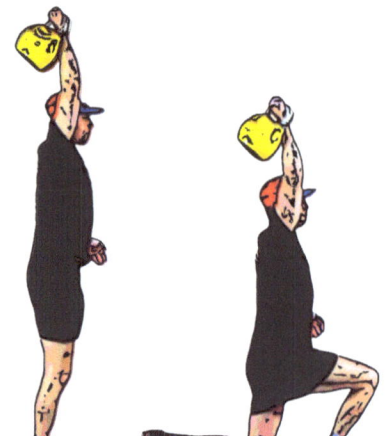

	Single Bell	Double Bell
SLOW	✓	✓

Technical Difficulty	Movement Pattern	Recommended Load
1	Lunge	Medium Weight

PRIMARY BENEFIT	SINGLE-LEG STRENGTH AND OVERHEAD STABILITY
TARGET MUSCLES	QUADRICEPS, GLUTES, HAMSTRINGS, SHOULDER STABILIZERS

Lock the kettlebell overhead with a straight arm, keeping the bicep aligned with your ear. Step forward into a lunge while maintaining the kettlebell stacked over your shoulder. Keep your torso upright, core braced, and knees tracking the toes. Drive through the front heel to return to standing. Alternate legs or complete all reps on one side.

117. Side Lunge Twist

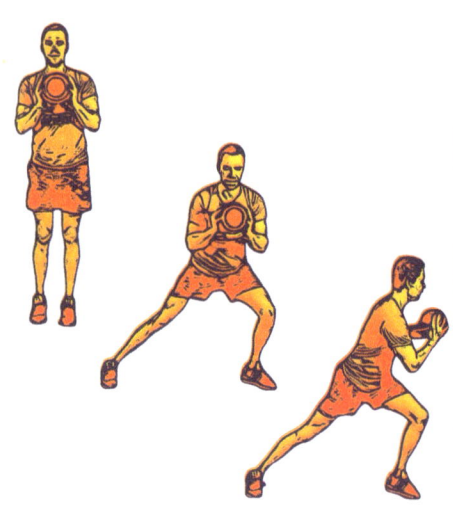

	Single Bell	Double Bell
SLOW	✓	✗

Technical Difficulty	Movement Pattern	Recommended Load
1	Lunge + Rotation	Medium Weight

PRIMARY BENEFIT	LEG, ROTATIONAL STRENGTH AND MOBILITY
TARGET MUSCLES	QUADRICEPS, GLUTES HAMSTRINGS, ABDUCTORS, ADDUCTORS, ERECTORS, OBLIQUES DELTOIDS, LATS

Hold the kettlebell at chest height. Step into a lateral lunge and rotate your torso toward the bent leg while keeping your chest tall and lumbar spine neutral. Push through the bent leg to return to standing, then repeat on the opposite side. Holding the bell closer increases control; extending it farther increases the challenge. PROKETTLEBELL.COM/117

118. Stationary Lunge Press, Two-Hand

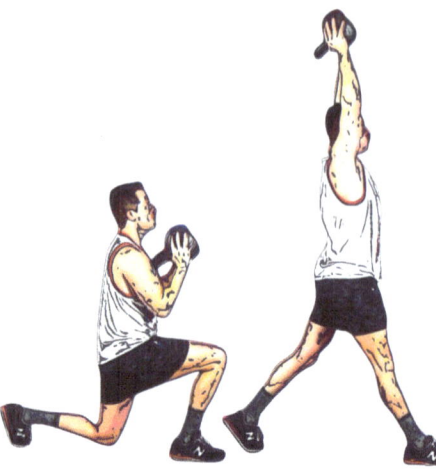

	Single Bell	Double Bell
SLOW	✓	✗

Technical Difficulty	Movement Pattern	Recommended Load
1	Push	Medium Weight

PRIMARY BENEFIT	LEGS, CORE AND ARM STRENGTH
TARGET MUSCLES	QUAD, GLUTES, HAMSTRINGS, ERECTORS, DELTOIDS, TRICEPS

Hold a kettlebell in both hands at chest level. Step into a lunge and, from the bottom position, press the kettlebell overhead. Lock out the arms, then return the kettlebell to your chest and stand up. Maintain alignment through the ankles, knees, and hips. Keep core engaged and chest upright. PROKETTLEBELL.COM/118

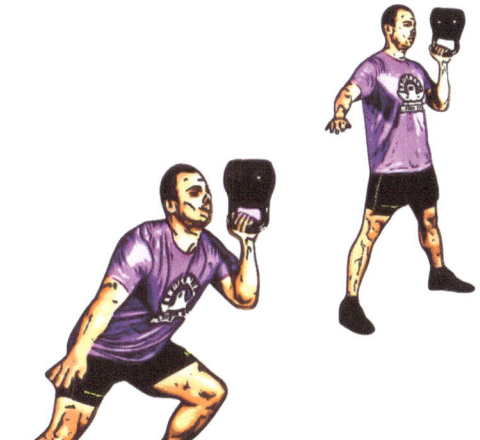

119. Bottoms-Up Side Lunge

	Single Bell	Double Bell
	✓	✓

Technical Difficulty	Movement Pattern	Recommended Load
2	Lunge	Medium Weight

PRIMARY BENEFIT	LATERAL LEG STRENGTH AND SHOULDER STABILITY
TARGET MUSCLES	QUADRICEPS, GLUTES, HAMSTRINGS, ERECTORS, BICEPS, FOREARMS

Hold a kettlebell in a bottoms-up grip, keeping the thumb and index finger close to the horn for control. Take a wide stance with both feet planted. Shift into a side lunge by bending one leg and pushing the hips back while keeping the opposite leg straight. Maintain an upright trunk and neutral lumbar spine. Drive through the bent leg to return to center and alternate sides.

▶ PROKETTLEBELL.COM/119

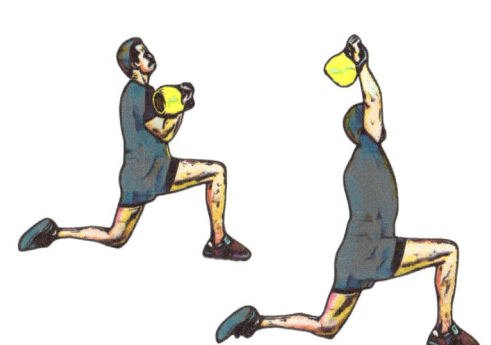

120. Deep Lunge Press

	Single Bell	Double Bell
	✓	✓

Technical Difficulty	Movement Pattern	Recommended Load
2	Push	Medium Weight

PRIMARY BENEFIT	INTEGRATED LUNGE AND OVERHEAD PRESS STRENGTH
TARGET MUSCLES	QUADRICEPS, GLUTES, HAMSTRINGS, ERECTORS, LATS, DELTOIDS, TRICEPS

Start in a half-kneeling runner's lunge with the kettlebell racked on the same side as the forward leg. Sink into the lunge to open the hip and groin, then press the kettlebell straight overhead, locking out the elbow with the bicep in line with the ear. Lower the kettlebell back to the rack and repeat for the desired number of presses before switching sides. The back knee may hover, rest on the floor, or the front foot can be elevated to deepen the stretch based on mobility.

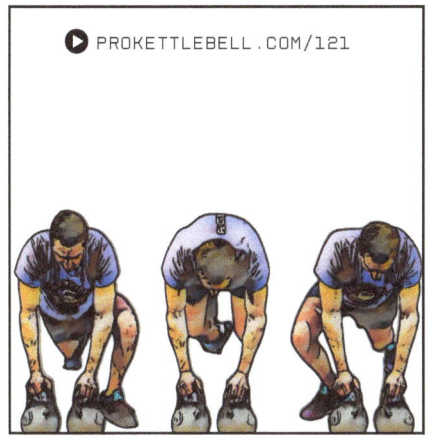

▶ PROKETTLEBELL.COM/121

121. Kettlebell Lunge Jumps

	Single Bell	Double Bell
	✗	✓

Technical Difficulty	Movement Pattern	Recommended Load
2	Lunge	Medium Weight

PRIMARY BENEFIT	EXPLOSIVE LUNGE POWER AND CORE STABILITY
TARGET MUSCLES	TRICEPS, LATS, ERECTORS, OBLIQUES, HIP FLEXORS

Start in a stable plank with your hands on a pair of kettlebells. Step one foot directly outside the kettlebell on the same side and establish balance. Explosively hop and switch legs in midair, driving through both feet. Land softly with a braced core, avoiding lumbar sag or sway. Using heavier kettlebells can increase stability during the movement.

LUNGES 59

122. Kettlebell Lunge Unders

	Single Bell	Double Bell
	✓	✗

Technical Difficulty	Movement Pattern	Recommended Load
2	Lunge	Medium Weight

PRIMARY BENEFIT	COORDINATED LUNGE STRENGTH AND CORE STABILITY
TARGET MUSCLES	QUADRICEPS, GLUTES, HAMSTRINGS, ADDUCTORS, OBLIQUES, ERECTORS

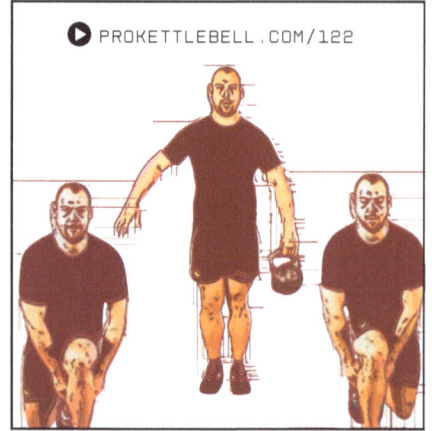

PROKETTLEBELL.COM/122

Hold a kettlebell in one hand and step forward with the opposite leg. As you lunge, pass the kettlebell under your front thigh to the other hand. Once you've completed the pass, return to both feet together. Repeat. Keep your torso upright and spine neutral throughout. This move works your legs, core, and coordination. Adjust speed or weight based on your fitness level.

123. Lateral Lunge Row

	Single Bell	Double Bell
	✓	✗

Technical Difficulty	Movement Pattern	Recommended Load
2	Compound	Medium Weight

PRIMARY BENEFIT	LATERAL LEG AND UPPER BODY STRENGTH
TARGET MUSCLES	GLUTES, ADDUCTORS, QUADRICEPS, HAMSTRINGS, LATS, RHOMBOIDS, BICEPS

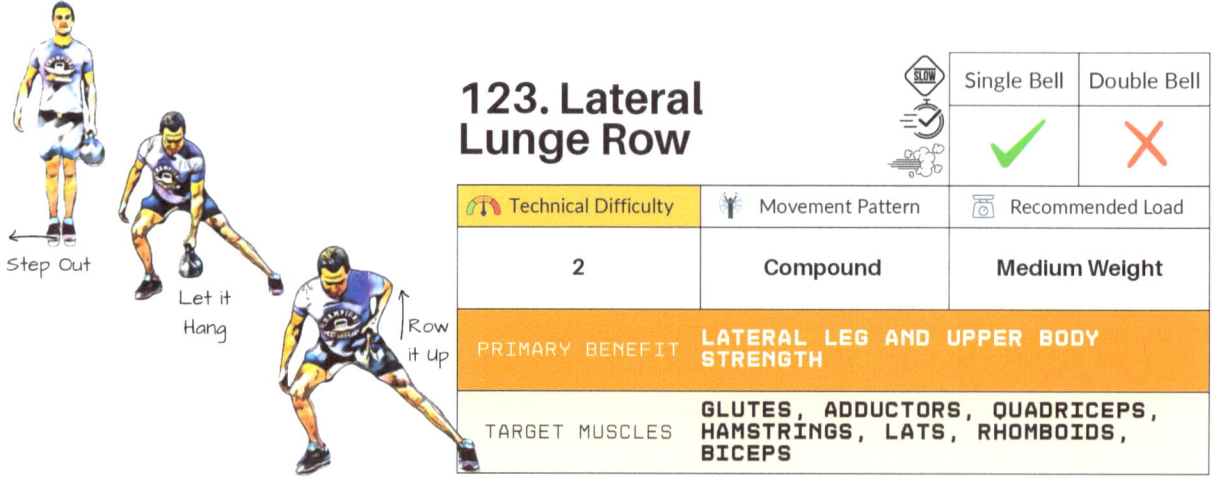

Hold a kettlebell in one hand on the side opposite the stepping leg. Step out laterally and load the bent leg while keeping the kettlebell-side leg straight. Allow the kettlebell to hang naturally beneath your shoulder, then perform a row by pulling it toward your ribcage. Squeeze briefly at the top. Lower the kettlebell with control, return to standing, and repeat. Maintain a neutral spine throughout the movement. ▶ PROKETTLEBELL.COM/123

124. Lateral Lunge Slingers

	Single Bell	Double Bell
	✓	✗

Technical Difficulty	Movement Pattern	Recommended Load
2	Lunge	Medium Weight

PRIMARY BENEFIT	LATERAL STRENGTH AND ROTATIONAL COORDINATION
TARGET MUSCLES	GLUTES, ADDUCTORS, QUADRICEPS, HAMSTRINGS, OBLIQUES, ERECTORS, BICEPS

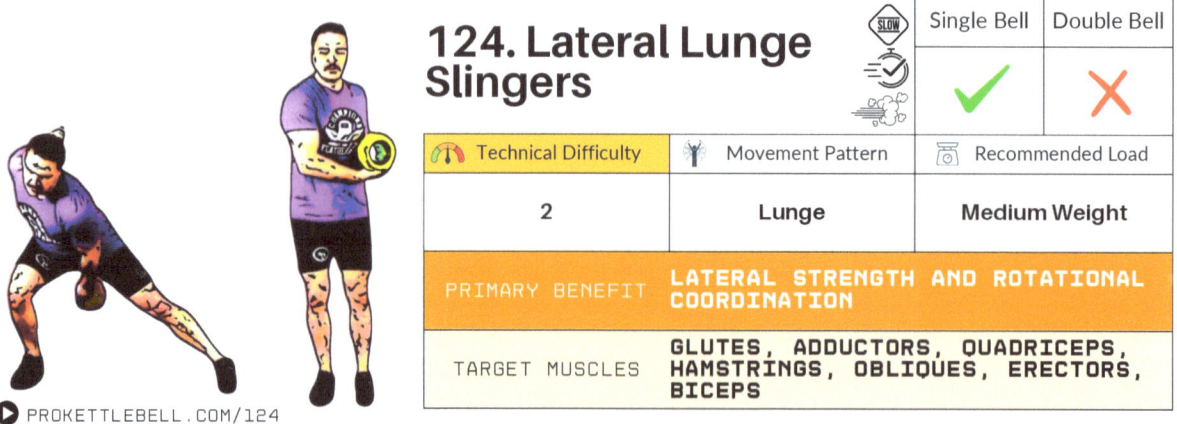

PROKETTLEBELL.COM/124

Start with the kettlebell holstered to one side, elbow by your ribs, holding the kettlebell with thumb pointed to the sky and supported by your free hand. Step out laterally with the opposite leg while swinging the kettlebell backward, high between your legs. Load the moving leg, swing forward and re-holster the kettlebell as you return to standing.

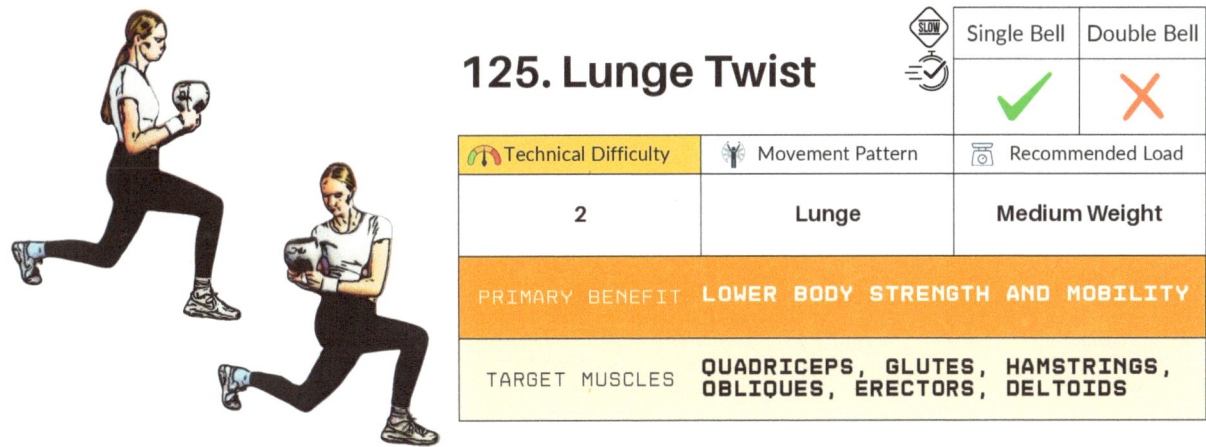

125. Lunge Twist

	Single Bell	Double Bell
SLOW	✓	✗

Technical Difficulty	Movement Pattern	Recommended Load
2	Lunge	Medium Weight

PRIMARY BENEFIT	LOWER BODY STRENGTH AND MOBILITY
TARGET MUSCLES	QUADRICEPS, GLUTES, HAMSTRINGS, OBLIQUES, ERECTORS, DELTOIDS

Hold the kettlebell at chest height securely. Step forward into a lunge, then twist your torso toward the front leg before returning to center and stepping back. You can alternate legs or perform all reps on one side. Maintain proper posture and joint alignment throughout the movement. ▶ PROKETTLEBELL.COM/125

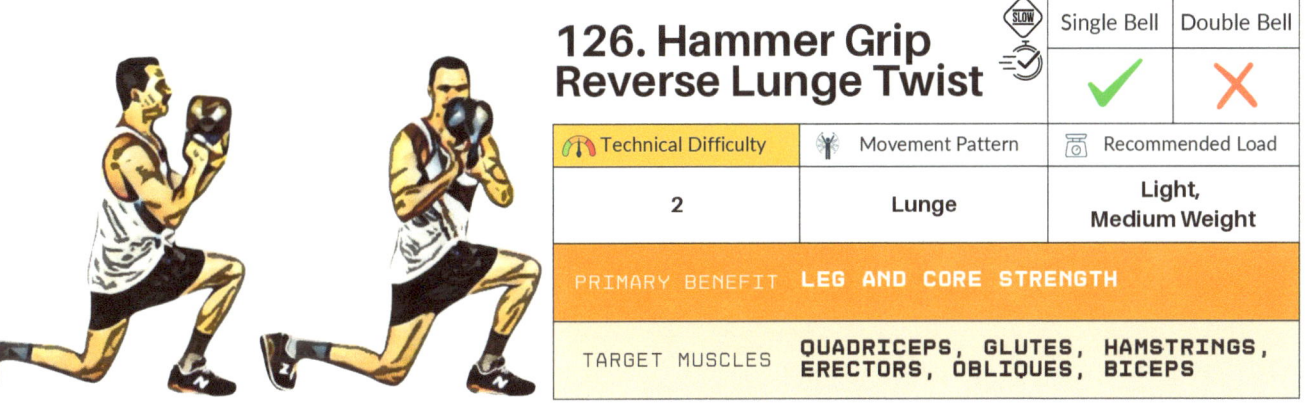

126. Hammer Grip Reverse Lunge Twist

	Single Bell	Double Bell
SLOW	✓	✗

Technical Difficulty	Movement Pattern	Recommended Load
2	Lunge	Light, Medium Weight

PRIMARY BENEFIT	LEG AND CORE STRENGTH
TARGET MUSCLES	QUADRICEPS, GLUTES, HAMSTRINGS, ERECTORS, OBLIQUES, BICEPS

Hold the kettlebell in a hammer grip with fists stacked vertically. Step into a reverse lunge and rotate your torso toward the front leg. Return to center and stand. Alternate legs or stay on one side. This move targets core, legs, and grip strength while maintaining upright posture. ▶ PROKETTLEBELL.COM/126

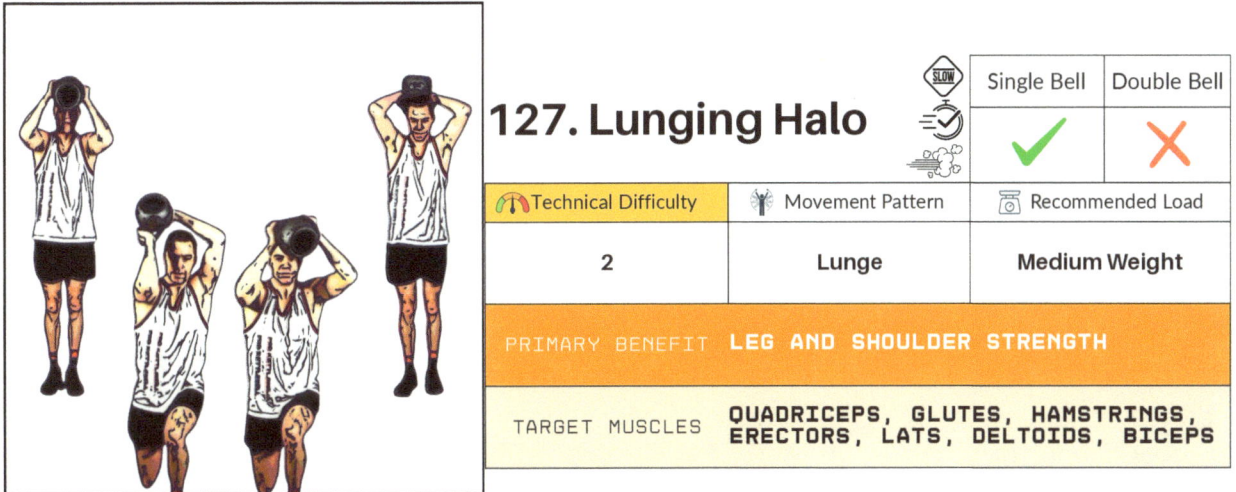

127. Lunging Halo

	Single Bell	Double Bell
SLOW	✓	✗

Technical Difficulty	Movement Pattern	Recommended Load
2	Lunge	Medium Weight

PRIMARY BENEFIT	LEG AND SHOULDER STRENGTH
TARGET MUSCLES	QUADRICEPS, GLUTES, HAMSTRINGS, ERECTORS, LATS, DELTOIDS, BICEPS

Grasp the kettlebell with both hands and hold it at forehead height. Step forward into a lunge while simultaneously haloing the kettlebell around your head in the direction of the stepping leg. Alternate the direction of the halo with each leg. Keep your torso upright and use a light weight for control. ▶ PROKETTLEBELL.COM/127

LUNGES

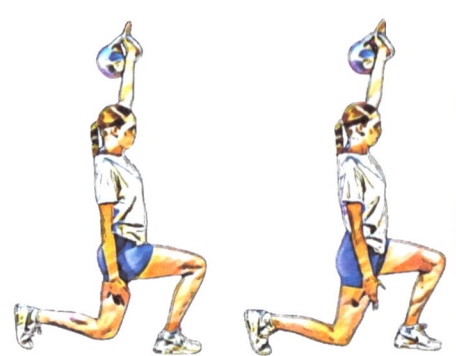

128. Overhead Walking Lunge

	Single Bell	Double Bell
SLOW	✓	✓

Technical Difficulty	Movement Pattern	Recommended Load
2	Lunge	Medium Weight

PRIMARY BENEFIT	FULL-BODY STRENGTH AND MOBILITY
TARGET MUSCLES	QUADRICEPS, GLUTES, HAMSTRINGS ERECTORS, LATS, DELTOIDS, TRICEPS

With one or two kettlebells locked out overhead, walk forward into lunges while keeping the weight stacked over your shoulder and hip. Maintain upright posture and don't rush. Use a single kettlebell for moderate difficulty or doubles for added challenge. Keep core braced throughout. ▶ PROKETTLEBELL.COM/128

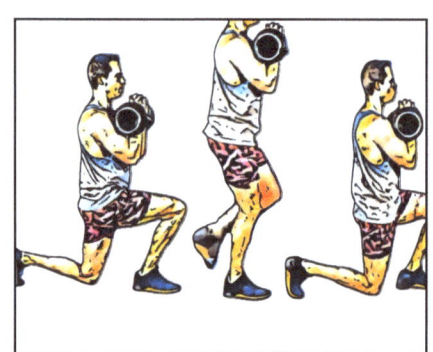

129. Rack Step-Thru Lunge

	Single Bell	Double Bell
SLOW	✓	✗

Technical Difficulty	Movement Pattern	Recommended Load
2	Lunge	Medium Weight

PRIMARY BENEFIT	LEG AND SHOULDER STRENGTH
TARGET MUSCLES	QUADRICEPS, GLUTES, HAMSTRINGS, ERECTORS, LATS, DELTOIDS, BICEPS

▶ PROKETTLEBELL.COM/129

With one or two kettlebells in the rack position, step forward into a lunge, then immediately step that same leg back into a reverse lunge. Repeat without returning to center. Keep your weight stacked over your hips, maintain proper alignment, and use a balanced stance to stay stable.

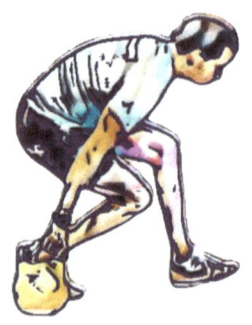

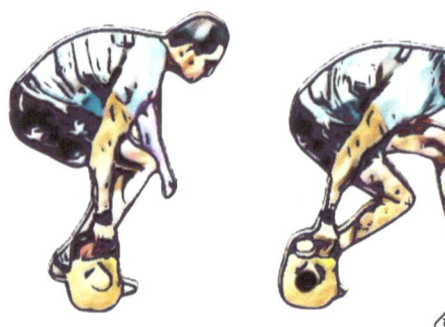

130. Shuffle Lunge

▶ PROKETTLEBELL.COM/130

	Single Bell	Double Bell
SLOW	✓	✓

Technical Difficulty	Movement Pattern	Recommended Load
2	Lunge	Medium Weight

PRIMARY BENEFIT	LOWER BODY STRENGTH
TARGET MUSCLES	QUADRICEPS, GLUTES, HAMSTRINGS, ERECTORS

Begin in a low crouched stance with the kettlebell on one side. Step forward with the opposite leg and shuffle the kettlebell and back leg up. Repeat in a forward crawling motion. Keep your back flat and weight over your hips. This mimics movement in tight spaces and builds endurance and leg strength.

131. Side Lunge Ribbons

	Single Bell	Double Bell
	✓	✗

Technical Difficulty	Movement Pattern	Recommended Load
2	Lunge	Medium Weight

PRIMARY BENEFIT	UPPER BODY AND LOWER BODY STRENGTH
TARGET MUSCLES	QUADRICEPS, GLUTES, HAMSTRINGS, ERECTORS, LATS, DELTOIDS, BICEPS

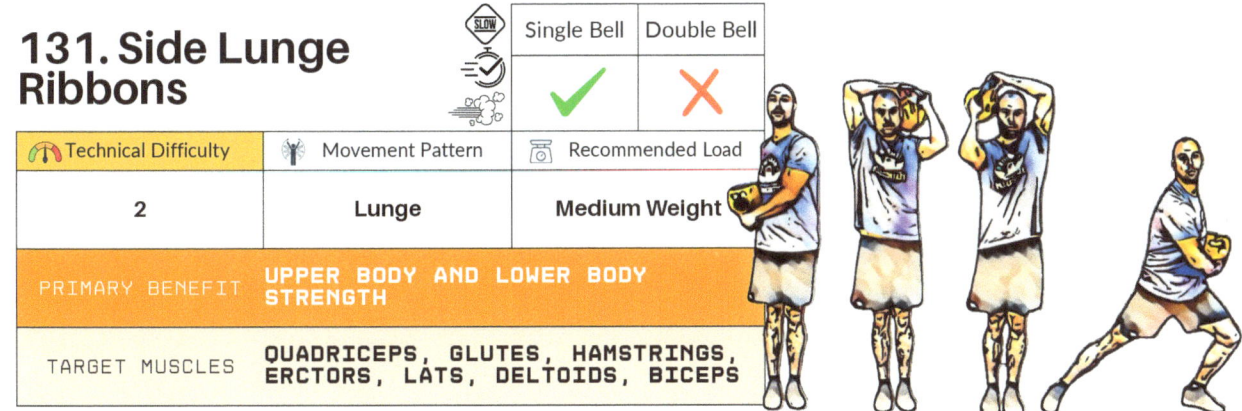

Start with the kettlebell on one hip. Step laterally to the opposite side and simultaneously move the kettlebell around your head and back down to the lunging side. Keep the kettlebell controlled, elbows tucked, and your posture upright. This move targets legs, obliques, shoulders, and coordination. ▶ PROKETTLEBELL.COM/131

132. Side Lunge Toss

	Single Bell	Double Bell
	✓	✗

Technical Difficulty	Movement Pattern	Recommended Load
2	Lunge	Medium Weight

PRIMARY BENEFIT	LEG, CORE STRENGTH AND COORDINATION
TARGET MUSCLES	GLUTES, QUADRICEPS, HAMSTRINGS, ADDUCTORS, ABDUCTORS, ERECTORS

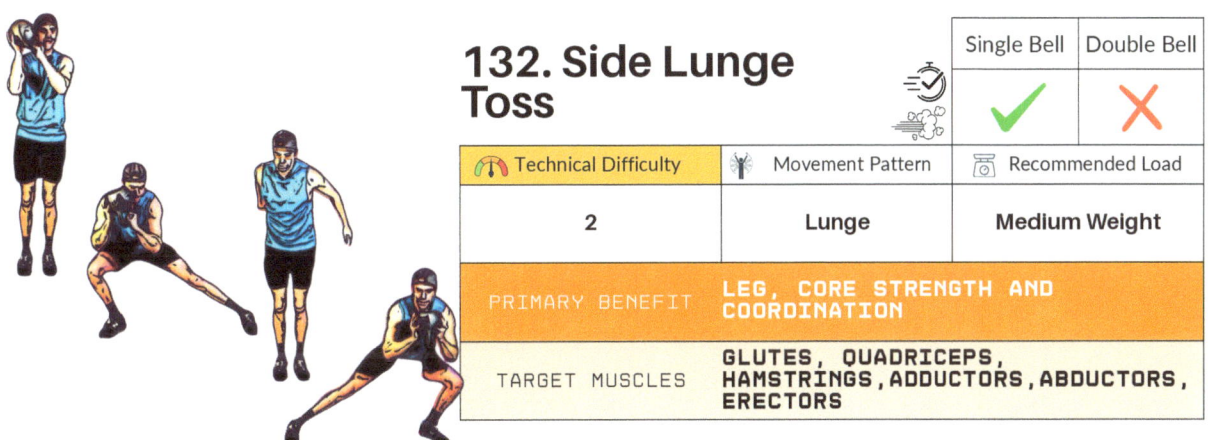

Hold the kettlebell between your palms, bottom side up. Swing the kettlebell across the body as you lunge to one side, catching it with the opposite hand. Load the bent leg while keeping your chest up and lumbar flat. Alternate sides while maintaining controlled form. ▶ PROKETTLEBELL.COM/132

133. Slingshot Reverse Lunge

	Single Bell	Double Bell
	✓	✗

Technical Difficulty	Movement Pattern	Recommended Load
2	Lunge	Medium Weight

PRIMARY BENEFIT	LEG AND CORE STRENGTH
TARGET MUSCLES	QUADRICEPS, GLUTES, HAMSTRINGS, ERECTORS, BICEPS, DELTOIDS

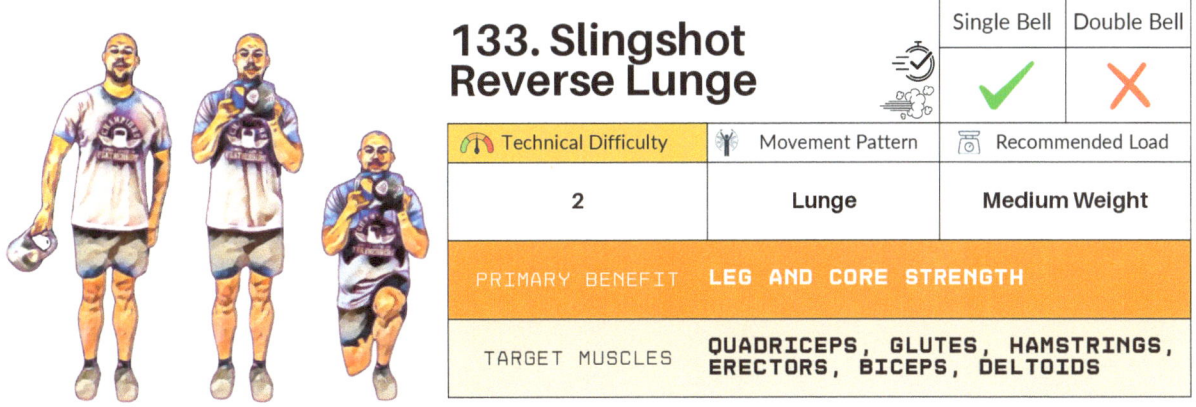

Wrap the kettlebell around your waist, catch it in front, and step back into a reverse lunge. Return to standing, sling the bell the other direction, and reverse lunge with the opposite leg. This dynamic move enhances coordination, shoulder mobility, and leg strength while keeping the core engaged. ▶ PROKETTLEBELL.COM/133

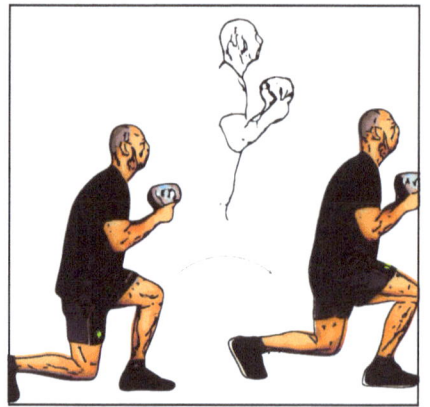

134. Split Lunge Jumps

	Single Bell	Double Bell
	✓	✗

Technical Difficulty	Movement Pattern	Recommended Load
2	Lunge	Medium Weight

PRIMARY BENEFIT — LEG STRENGTH AND STABILITY

TARGET MUSCLES — QUADRICEPS, GLUTES, HAMSTRINGS, CALVES

PROKETTLEBELL.COM/134

Hold a kettlebell by the horns, bottom side up, at your chest. Jump and land in a split lunge with a wide, stable base. Keep your chest lifted and spine neutral. For a low-impact version, perform alternating reverse lunges. Use a weight that allows control and balance throughout.

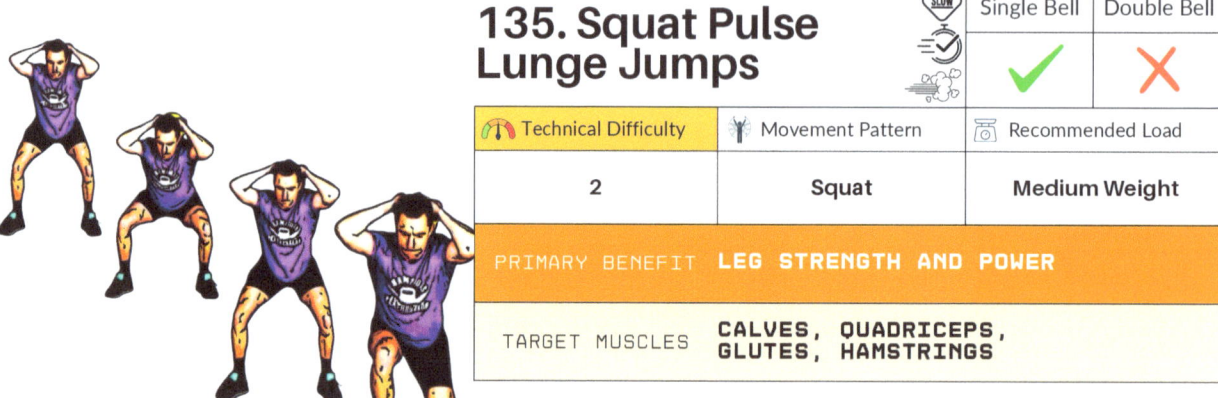

135. Squat Pulse Lunge Jumps

	Single Bell	Double Bell
	✓	✗

Technical Difficulty	Movement Pattern	Recommended Load
2	Squat	Medium Weight

PRIMARY BENEFIT — LEG STRENGTH AND POWER

TARGET MUSCLES — CALVES, QUADRICEPS, GLUTES, HAMSTRINGS

PROKETTLEBELL.COM/135

With the kettlebell behind your shoulders, perform a squat pulse and then explode into a split lunge jump. Jump back to feet parallel for another two squat pulses and repeat with a split lunge forward with the opposite leg. Keep the kettlebell pressed firmly against your upper back to prevent bouncing. Maintain a flat back and knee alignment throughout.

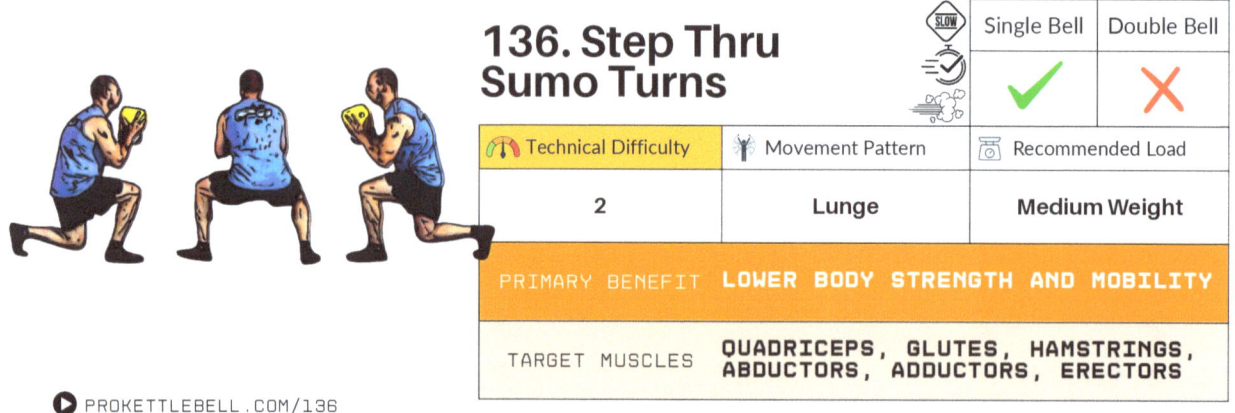

136. Step Thru Sumo Turns

	Single Bell	Double Bell
	✓	✗

Technical Difficulty	Movement Pattern	Recommended Load
2	Lunge	Medium Weight

PRIMARY BENEFIT — LOWER BODY STRENGTH AND MOBILITY

TARGET MUSCLES — QUADRICEPS, GLUTES, HAMSTRINGS, ABDUCTORS, ADDUCTORS, ERECTORS

PROKETTLEBELL.COM/136

Hold a kettlebell in the goblet position and stand in a wide sumo stance. Perform a quarter turn and lunge in that direction, stepping fully through. Complete a full circle (4-quarter turns) to make one rep. Maintain upright posture and stacked joints. You can vary grip and speed for added challenge.

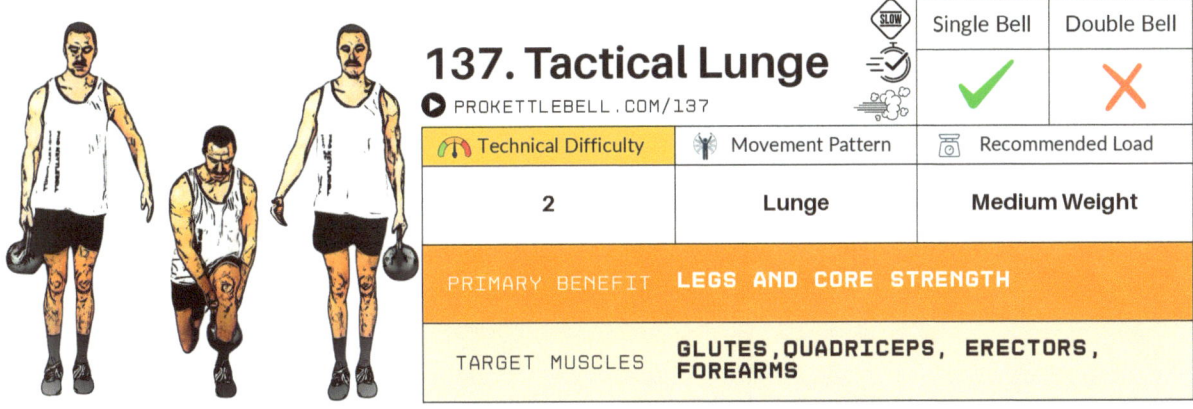

137. Tactical Lunge
PROKETTLEBELL.COM/137

	Single Bell	Double Bell
	✓	✗

Technical Difficulty	Movement Pattern	Recommended Load
2	Lunge	Medium Weight

PRIMARY BENEFIT	LEGS AND CORE STRENGTH
TARGET MUSCLES	GLUTES, QUADRICEPS, ERECTORS, FOREARMS

Start with the kettlebell beside one foot. Pick it up and step into a reverse lunge on the same side. Pass the kettlebell under the forward leg to the opposite hand, then stand. Repeat with the opposite side. Stay upright and control the pass to work core stability and leg coordination.

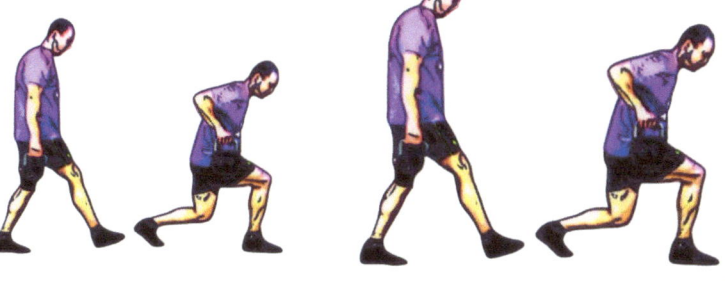

138. Walking Lunge Row
PROKETTLEBELL.COM/138

	Single Bell	Double Bell
	✓	✓

Technical Difficulty	Movement Pattern	Recommended Load
2	Pull	Medium Weight

PRIMARY BENEFIT	FULL-BODY STRENGTH
TARGET MUSCLES	QUADRICEPS, GLUTES, HAMSTRINGS, ERECTORS, LATS, BICEPS

Start with a kettlebell hanging from each hand and step forward into a lunge. From the low position row up, then lower the bells to hover near the floor. Pick up your back foot and take a full step forward, ending in another lunge and subsequent row. Continue the pattern. Keep your spine neutral and avoid using momentum to lift the kettlebells. If space is restricted, you can lunge forward and back in place, still alternating legs each rep.

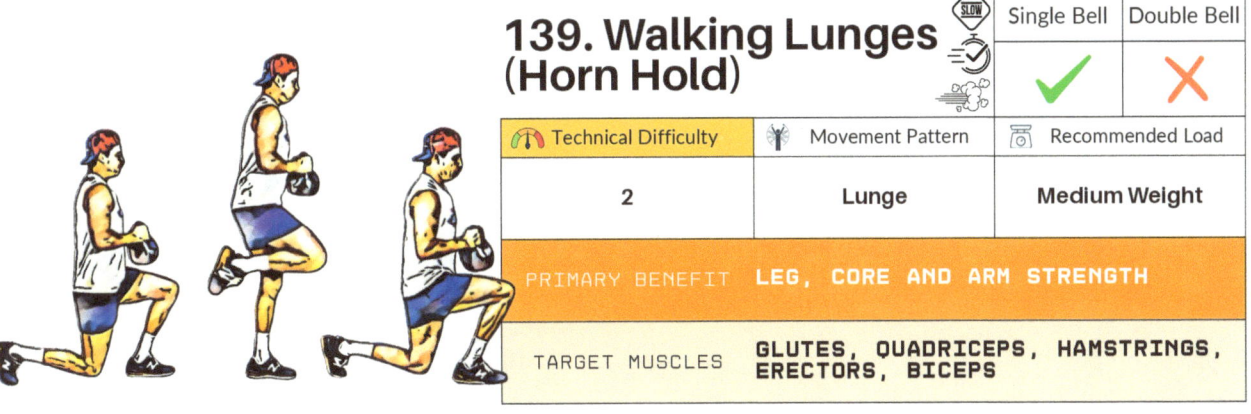

139. Walking Lunges (Horn Hold)

	Single Bell	Double Bell
	✓	✗

Technical Difficulty	Movement Pattern	Recommended Load
2	Lunge	Medium Weight

PRIMARY BENEFIT	LEG, CORE AND ARM STRENGTH
TARGET MUSCLES	GLUTES, QUADRICEPS, HAMSTRINGS, ERECTORS, BICEPS

Hold the kettlebell by the horns at chest height. Step forward into a lunge, keeping your torso upright and weight stacked over your hips. Ensure your front knee stays in line with your toes. Walk forward continuously, alternating legs, and keeping your chest lifted throughout. PROKETTLEBELL.COM/139

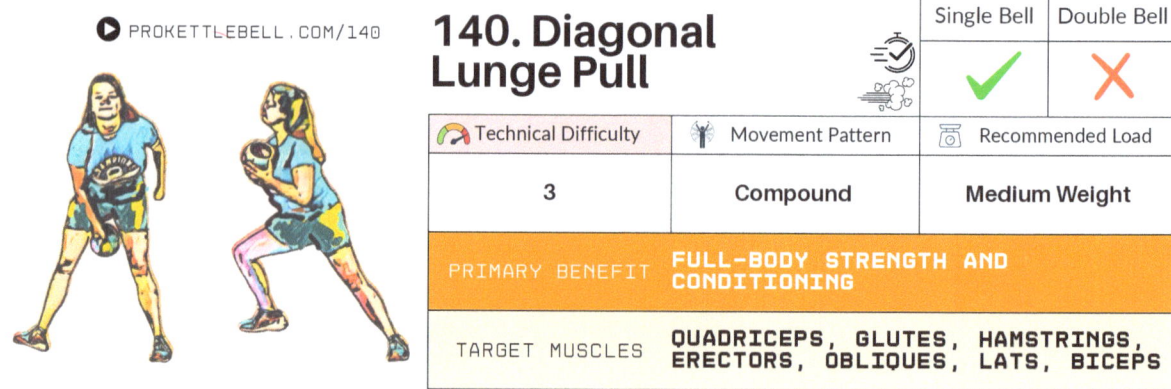

▶ PROKETTLEBELL.COM/140

140. Diagonal Lunge Pull

	Single Bell	Double Bell
	✓	✗

Technical Difficulty	Movement Pattern	Recommended Load
3	Compound	Medium Weight

PRIMARY BENEFIT	FULL-BODY STRENGTH AND CONDITIONING
TARGET MUSCLES	QUADRICEPS, GLUTES, HAMSTRINGS, ERECTORS, OBLIQUES, LATS, BICEPS

Visualize a square around you with the kettlebell at the front center. Swing it between your legs with your right hand. After the backswing, as it rises, step diagonally to the back-right corner with your right leg, rotating to face the right side of the square while rowing the kettlebell toward your body and catching it with your free hand. Launch the next swing as you bring your right foot back to the front and repeat multiple reps before switching sides.

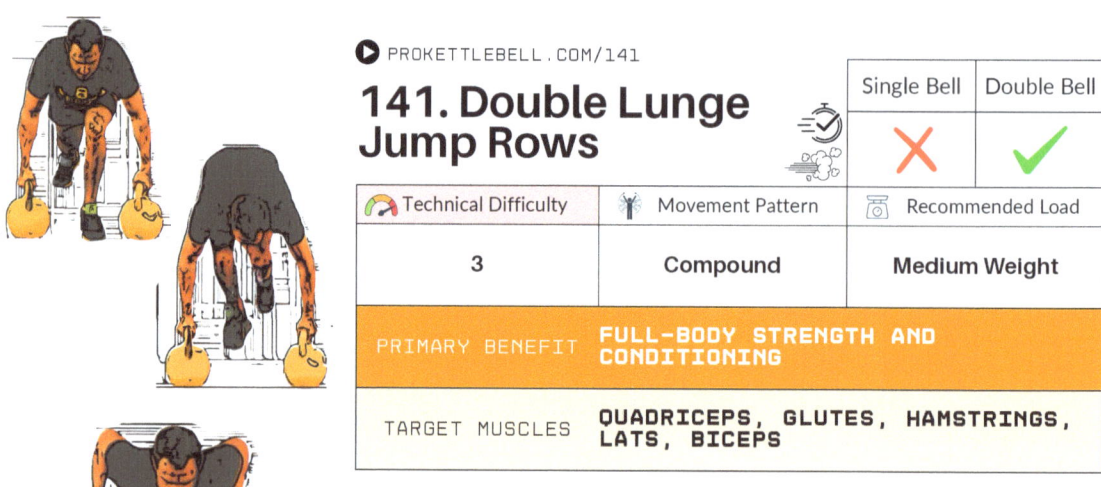

▶ PROKETTLEBELL.COM/141

141. Double Lunge Jump Rows

	Single Bell	Double Bell
	✗	✓

Technical Difficulty	Movement Pattern	Recommended Load
3	Compound	Medium Weight

PRIMARY BENEFIT	FULL-BODY STRENGTH AND CONDITIONING
TARGET MUSCLES	QUADRICEPS, GLUTES, HAMSTRINGS, LATS, BICEPS

Place two kettlebells shoulder-width apart and start in a lunge with one leg forward, foot planted between them. Lean into the lunge and row both kettlebells, keeping elbows tight. With the bells back on the ground, quickly switch legs, either by jumping or stepping, and repeat. Keep your chest up and core engaged to avoid momentum-based lifting. This move strengthens both the upper and lower body simultaneously.

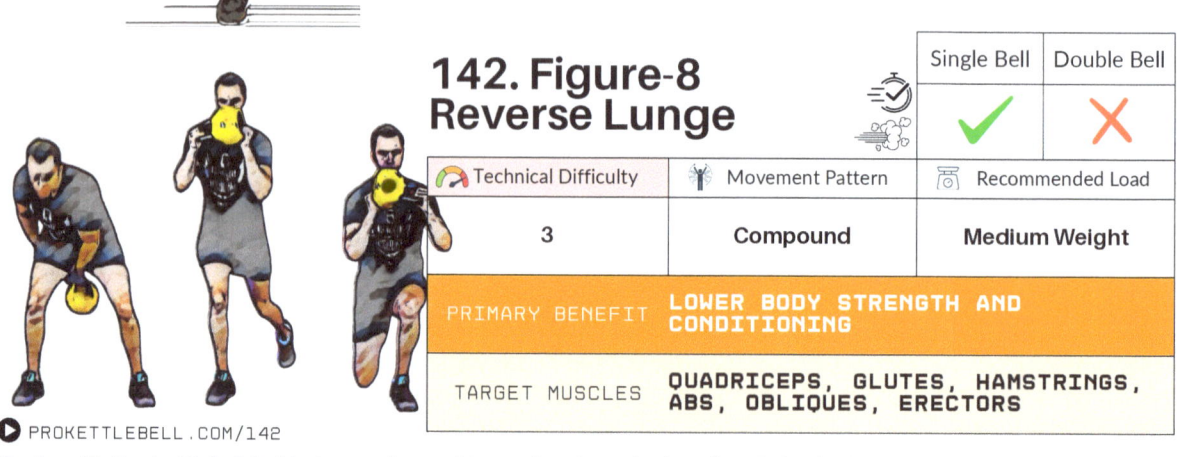

142. Figure-8 Reverse Lunge

	Single Bell	Double Bell
	✓	✗

Technical Difficulty	Movement Pattern	Recommended Load
3	Compound	Medium Weight

PRIMARY BENEFIT	LOWER BODY STRENGTH AND CONDITIONING
TARGET MUSCLES	QUADRICEPS, GLUTES, HAMSTRINGS, ABS, OBLIQUES, ERECTORS

▶ PROKETTLEBELL.COM/142

Begin with the kettlebell held at your chest with one hand on the handle. Circle the kettlebell behind the planted leg and pass it to the other hand as the opposite leg steps into a reverse lunge. After the hand switch behind the knee, catch the bell in front of you, return the back leg to start, and mirror the movement on the other side.

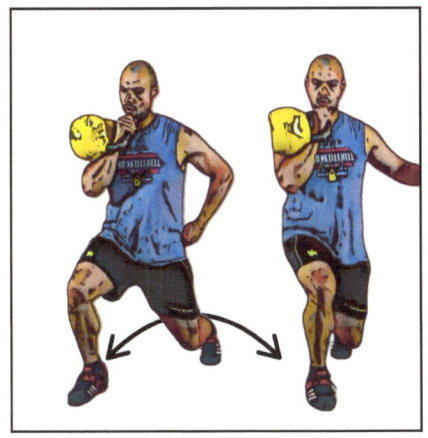

143. Racked Lunge Hops

	Single Bell	Double Bell
	✓	✗

Technical Difficulty	Movement Pattern	Recommended Load
3	Lunge	Medium Weight

PRIMARY BENEFIT	EXPLOSIVE LEG STRENGTH AND BALANCE
TARGET MUSCLES	QUADRICEPS, CALVES, DELTOIDS, ERECTORS

Hold the kettlebell in the rack position. Lunge forward with the same side leg, then perform small hops side-to-side from that lunge stance. Keep your back upright and core engaged. Be sure your stride is long enough to maintain knee alignment. ▶ PROKETTLEBELL.COM/143

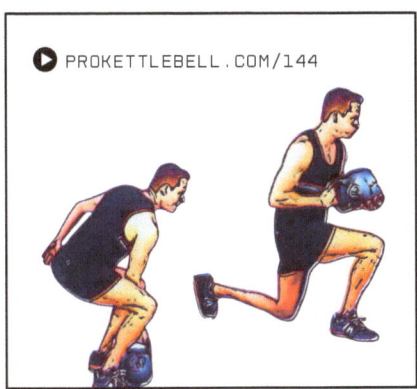

144. Shotgun Reverse Lunge

	Single Bell	Double Bell
	✓	✗

Technical Difficulty	Movement Pattern	Recommended Load
3	Lunge	Medium Weight

PRIMARY BENEFIT	FULL-BODY STRENGTH AND CONDITIONING
TARGET MUSCLES	QUADRICEPS, GLUTES, HAMSTRINGS, ERECTORS, LATS, BICEPS

▶ PROKETTLEBELL.COM/144

Hold the kettlebell in one hand between your feet. Step back into a reverse lunge as you quickly row the kettlebell up toward your body, catching it with the free hand while sliding your elbow along the same-side rib cage. Keep your knee just off the floor and your spine upright. Return the bell and back leg to start and repeat. You may alternate arms each rep, or alternate legs while keeping the same rowing arm before switching sides.

145. Slingshot Side Lunge

	Single Bell	Double Bell
	✓	✗

Technical Difficulty	Movement Pattern	Recommended Load
3	Lunge	Medium Weight

PRIMARY BENEFIT	LOWER BODY STRENGTH AND CONDITIONING
TARGET MUSCLES	QUADRICEPS, GLUTES, HAMSTRINGS, ERECTORS, OBLIQUES, BICEPS

Slingshot the kettlebell around your waist and lunge in the direction it's swinging AFTER you've switched hands behind you. Lunge deeply with your torso upright and hips back, ensuring the knee tracks the toe. The momentum of the bell helps guide the movement. Alternate sides while maintaining alignment and control.

▶ PROKETTLEBELL.COM/145

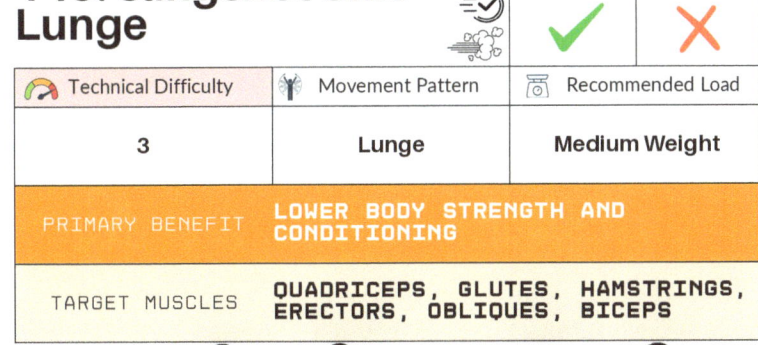
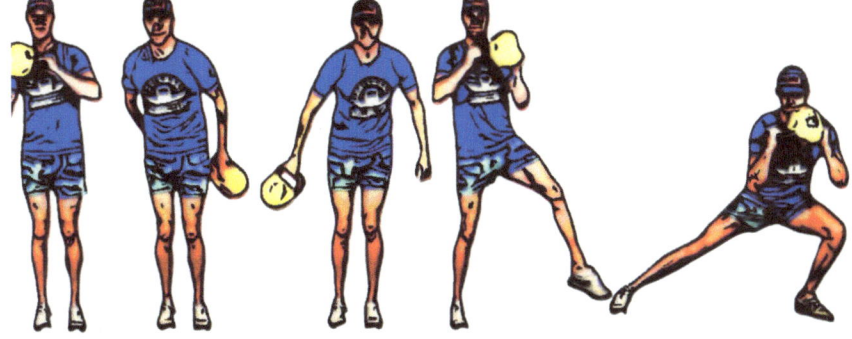

146. Figure-4 Glute Bridge

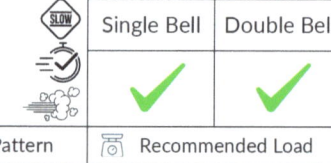

	Single Bell	Double Bell
	✓	✓

Technical Difficulty	Movement Pattern	Recommended Load
1	Compound	Medium Weight

PRIMARY BENEFIT	GLUTE STRENGTH AND HIP MOBILITY
TARGET MUSCLES	GLUTES, HAMSTRINGS, ERECTORS, QUADRICEPS, ABDUCTORS

Lie on your back with a kettlebell held above or on your shoulder. Cross one ankle over the opposite knee to create a figure-4. Drive through the grounded heel and lift your hips as high as possible. Hold or perform repetitions, then switch sides. Maintain alignment and control.

▶ PROKETTLEBELL.COM/146

147. Marching Glute Bridge

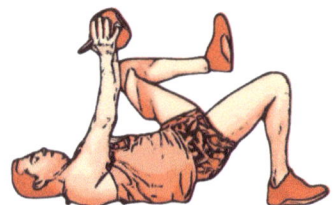

	Single Bell	Double Bell
	✓	✓

Technical Difficulty	Movement Pattern	Recommended Load
1	Compound	Medium Weight

PRIMARY BENEFIT	HIP MOBILITY AND STRENGTH
TARGET MUSCLES	GLUTES, HAMSTRINGS, HIP FLEXORS

Lie on your back with a kettlebell held overhead or on your hips. Bridge up by driving through your heels, then alternate lifting each foot in a marching motion. Keep hips high and stable, ensuring your shoulders and heels bear your weight. Adjust kettlebell placement for difficulty.

▶ PROKETTLEBELL.COM/147

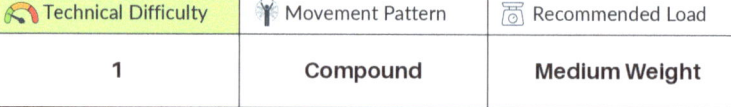

148. Kettlebell Leg Extensions

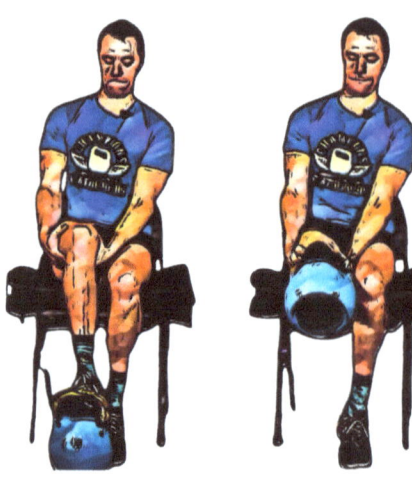

	Single Bell	Double Bell
	✓	✗

Technical Difficulty	Movement Pattern	Recommended Load
1	Push	Light Weight

PRIMARY BENEFIT	LEG STRENGTH
TARGET MUSCLES	QUADRICEPS, HIP FLEXORS

Sit upright and loop your foot through the kettlebell handle. Support your leg under the knee with your hands, then slowly extend and lower the leg. Use a light weight and perform with control to protect the knee joint. This isolates the quadriceps and is great for rehab or strength building. ▶ PROKETTLEBELL.COM/148

PROKETTLEBELL.COM/149

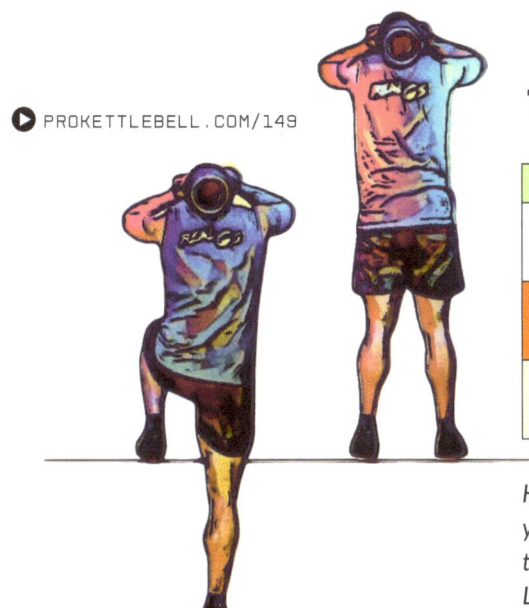

149. Step Ups

	Single Bell	Double Bell
SLOW	✓	✓

Technical Difficulty	Movement Pattern	Recommended Load
1	Lunge	Medium Weight

PRIMARY BENEFIT	LEG STRENGTH
TARGET MUSCLES	QUADRICEPS, GLUTES, HAMSTRINGS

Hold the kettlebell between your shoulder blades (not on your neck). Place your full foot on a sturdy elevated surface and step up, driving through the heel. Maintain a flat back, chest up, and align the knee with the toe. Lower back down under control and repeat. Start bodyweight-only if needed. Alternate the leading leg or repeat for reps prior to switching.

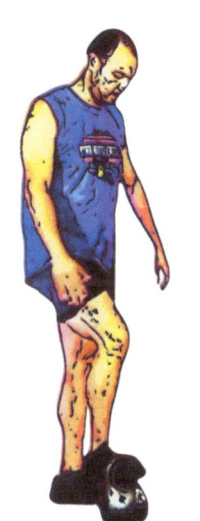

150. Toe Lifts

	Single Bell	Double Bell
SLOW	✓	✗

Technical Difficulty	Movement Pattern	Recommended Load
1	Pull	Light Weight

PRIMARY BENEFIT	LOWER BODY STRENGTH
TARGET MUSCLES	HIP FLEXORS

Hook your toes under the kettlebell handle and lift your knee up toward hip height or higher. Use a light kettlebell for control and full range of motion. Lower slowly and repeat. Add a rainbow arc to increase difficulty and hip mobility. This is a great movement for hip flexor strength and rehab. PROKETTLEBELL.COM/150

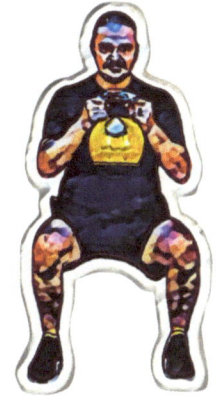

151. Weighted Wall Sit

	Single Bell	Double Bell
SLOW	✓	✗

Technical Difficulty	Movement Pattern	Recommended Load
1	Squat	Medium Weight

PRIMARY BENEFIT	LEG STRENGTH
TARGET MUSCLES	QUADRICEPS, GLUTES, HAMSTRINGS

Sit against a wall with knees at a 90-degree angle. Hold a kettlebell in a comfortable position—by the horns, on your thighs, or in the rack. Keep your back flat against the wall and hold the position for time. Adjust weight and hand position based on your strength level. PROKETTLEBELL.COM/151

COMPOUND & MISC. LOWER BODY

Core Exercises

---— Section Three ---—

Sit-Ups, Twists, & Crunches
Core-Focused Planks
Windmills

Core & More

1. Sit-Ups, Twists & Crunches	
Ab Circles	73
Anchored Racked Sit-Ups	73
Anchored Wiper Crunch	73
Anchored Leg Raise	74
Armbar Bicycles	74
Armbar Reverse Crunch	74
Boat Pose Kicks	75
Butt Kicker Sit-Up	75
CPR Crunch	75
Escape Punch	76
Frogger Sit-Up	76
Golden Arches	76
Halo Sit-Up	77
Hollow Hold Crunch	77
Kettlebell Kayaks	77
L-Sit-Up	78
Pull-Over Tucks	78
Racked Trunk Twists	78
Russian Twist	79
Sit-Up Getup	79
Sit-Up Twist	79
Star Pullover	80
Twisted Pull-Over	80
Twisted Punch	80
Wood Chopper Sit-Up	81
Anchored Side Cycles	81
Armbar Sit-Up	81
Armbar Sit-Up + Press	82
Sideways V-Up	82
Turkish Sit-Up	82
Turkish Kick n' Sit	83
Anchored Plow	83
L-Sit	83
Sideways V-Ups (Dbl Alternating)	84

2. Core-Focused Planks	
KB Mountain Climbers	85
KB Mountain Climb Twist	85
KB Shoulder Touches	85
Pull-Under	86
Cross-Overs	86
Crouching Pull Across	86
Crab Kick Dips	87
KB Side Plank	87
Turkish Planks	87

3. Windmills	
Kneeling Windmill	88
Kneeling Windmill > Side Plank	88
Windmill	88
Low Windmill	89
Double Windmill	89
Windmill Cleans	89

152. Ab Circles

PROKETTLEBELL.COM/152

	Single Bell	Double Bell
SLOW	✓	✗

Technical Difficulty	Movement Pattern	Recommended Load
1	Compound	Medium Weight

PRIMARY BENEFIT — CORE STRENGTH

TARGET MUSCLES — ABS, OBLIQUES

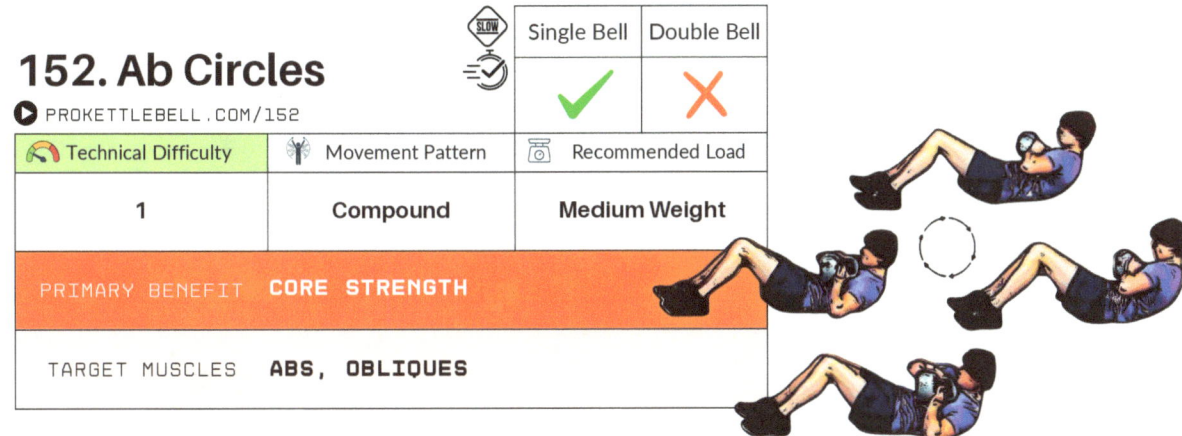

Lie on your back holding a kettlebell at your chest. Create small circles with your upper body by lifting one shoulder blade at a time. Circle in one direction for reps or time, then reverse. Keep the movement controlled and your abs engaged. Moving the kettlebell farther from your core increases difficulty. Start without weight if needed to master the range of motion.

153. Anchored Racked Sit-Ups

	Single Bell	Double Bell
SLOW	✗	✓

Technical Difficulty	Movement Pattern	Recommended Load
1	Compound	Light, Medium Weight

PRIMARY BENEFIT — CORE STRENGTH

TARGET MUSCLES — ABS

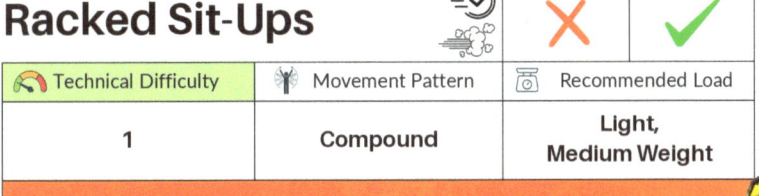

PROKETTLEBELL.COM/153

Anchor your feet under heavy kettlebells, a bench, or a partner's assistance. Sit holding two kettlebells in the rack position at shoulder level. Perform a controlled sit-up without pushing the kettlebells forward. Initiate the sit-up by squeezing your abs to protect your back. Start with light weights and maintain tension through the core, especially the lumbar region.

154. Anchored Wiper Crunch

	Single Bell	Double Bell
SLOW	✗	✓

Technical Difficulty	Movement Pattern	Recommended Load
1	Compound	Light, Medium Weight

PRIMARY BENEFIT — CORE STRENGTH

TARGET MUSCLES — ABS, OBLIQUES

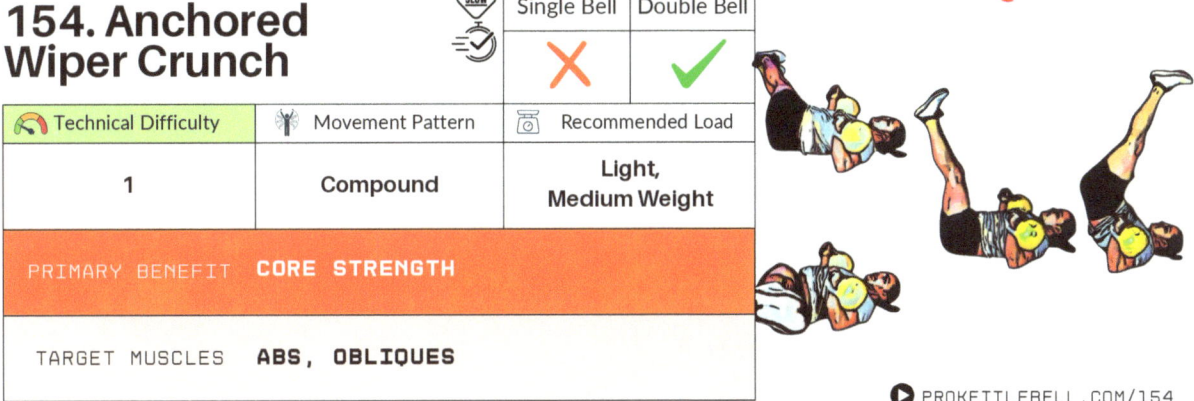

PROKETTLEBELL.COM/154

Lie on your back holding two kettlebells with bent arms—forearms upright and the backs of your arms on the floor. Raise your legs straight up and perform a windshield wiper to one side. Return to center, lift your hips off the floor by pushing your heels toward the sky (reverse crunch), then lower and wiper to the opposite side. Repeat. Move slowly and with control; keep your legs straight if possible, or bend them to reduce difficulty.

SIT-UPS, TWISTS & CRUNCHES

155. Anchored Leg Raise

	SLOW	Single Bell	Double Bell
		✗	✓

Technical Difficulty	Movement Pattern	Recommended Load
1	Compound	Medium, Heavy Weight

PRIMARY BENEFIT	CORE STRENGTH
TARGET MUSCLES	ABS

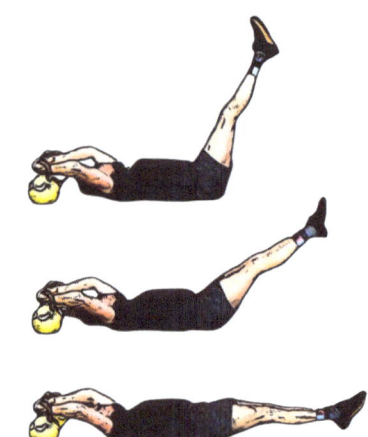

● PROKETTLEBELL.COM/155

Lie on your back with your hands anchored behind you by holding kettlebells overhead. Keep your upper body grounded and raise your legs while keeping them straight (if needed, bend your knees slightly to reduce lumbar tension). Lower the legs slowly and repeat. Focus on isolating the abs during each lift.

156. Armbar Bicycles

	SLOW	Single Bell	Double Bell
		✓	✓

Technical Difficulty	Movement Pattern	Recommended Load
1	Compound	Medium, Heavy Weight

PRIMARY BENEFIT	SHOULDER, HIP FLEXOR AND CORE STRENGTH
TARGET MUSCLES	ABS, OBLIQUES, DELTOIDS, TRICEPS

● PROKETTLEBELL.COM/156

Lie flat holding a kettlebell overhead in one arm. Keep the arm locked and perform a controlled bicycle motion with your legs. Resist hip movement and avoid rocking side to side as you cycle. Repeat and reverse direction as desired. Maintain alignment and stability in the armbar position to maximize core, shoulder, and hip flexor engagement.

157. Armbar Reverse Crunch

	SLOW	Single Bell	Double Bell
		✓	✓

Technical Difficulty	Movement Pattern	Recommended Load
1	Compound	Medium, Heavy Weight

PRIMARY BENEFIT	CORE AND ARM STRENGTH
TARGET MUSCLES	ABS, DELTOIDS, TRICEPS

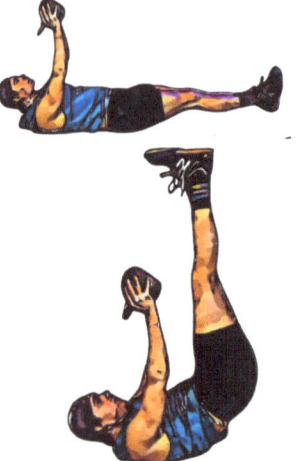

● PROKETTLEBELL.COM/157

Lie on your back holding a kettlebell overhead with both hands, arms locked out. Keep the kettlebell steady as you raise your legs, then drive your heels upward to lift your hips using core control—not momentum. Lower with control and repeat. Bend your knees or omit the hip lift to reduce strain if needed and maintain full control of the kettlebell throughout.

158. Boat Pose Kicks

Technical Difficulty	Movement Pattern	Recommended Load
1	Compound	Medium Weight

Single Bell	Double Bell
✓	✗

PRIMARY BENEFIT — CORE AND HIP FLEXOR STRENGTH

TARGET MUSCLES — ABS, ERECTORS, HIP FLEXORS, QUADRICEPS, HAMSTRINGS

▶ PROKETTLEBELL.COM/158

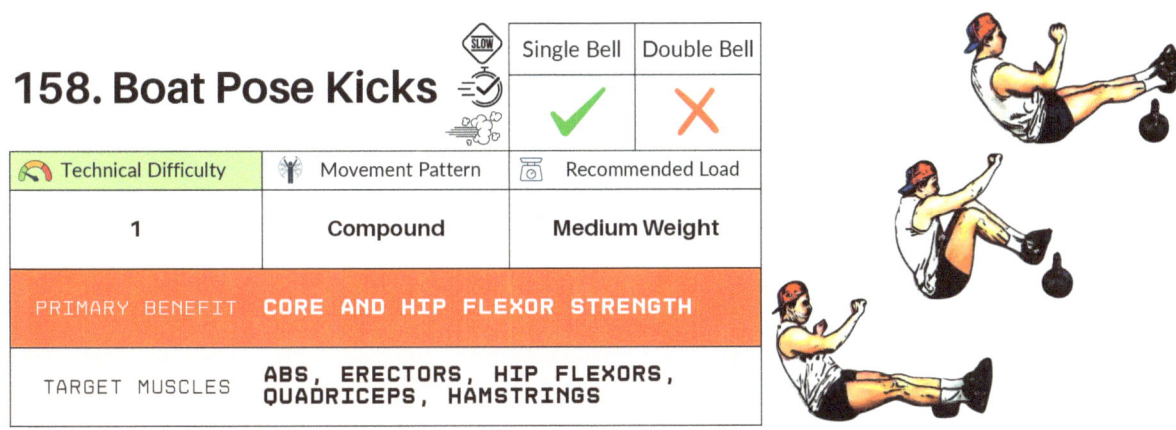

Sit with a kettlebell in front of you, hands placed behind your body. Pull your knees toward your chest and kick your feet to one side of the kettlebell, then to the other, keeping your feet elevated and pulling your knees to your chest between each kick. Adjust the kettlebell's position to change difficulty. Keep your chest upright and lumbar spine flat; support this by planting your hands on the floor, or lift them to increase the challenge.

159. Butt Kicker Sit-Up

Technical Difficulty	Movement Pattern	Recommended Load
1	Compound	Medium, Heavy Weight

Single Bell	Double Bell
✓	✗

PRIMARY BENEFIT — CORE STRENGTH AND MOBILITY

TARGET MUSCLES — ABS, OBLIQUES, DELTOIDS

▶ PROKETTLEBELL.COM/159

Start lying back with a kettlebell held at your chest and both legs extended. As you sit up, kick one heel toward your butt, then return and repeat with the other leg. Alternate sides and keep the movement controlled. Use a light kettlebell to ensure proper form without excessive momentum.

160. CPR Crunch

Technical Difficulty	Movement Pattern	Recommended Load
1	Compound	Medium, Heavy Weight

Single Bell	Double Bell
✓	✗

PRIMARY BENEFIT — CORE AND ARM STRENGTH

TARGET MUSCLES — ABS, LATS, DELTOIDS, TRICEPS

▶ PROKETTLEBELL.COM/160

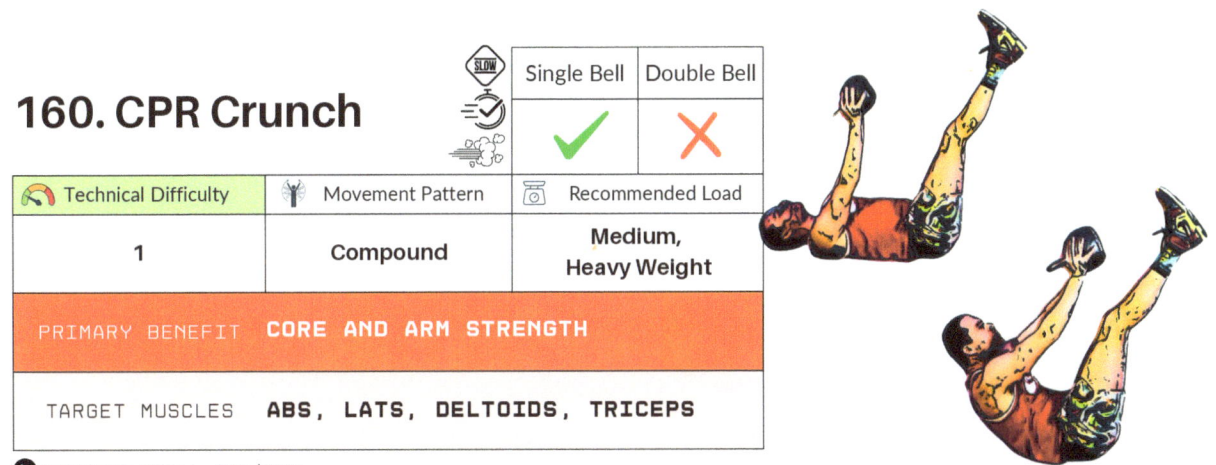

Lie on your back holding a kettlebell overhead with both arms locked, similar to CPR arm positioning. Raise your legs off the ground and crunch forward, bringing the kettlebell toward your feet. Resist collapsing to the floor as you return to your back between each crunch. Focus on keeping arms and legs straight and feet high throughout.

161. Escape Punch

PROKETTLEBELL.COM/161

	Single Bell	Double Bell
	✓	✗

Technical Difficulty	Movement Pattern	Recommended Load
1	Compound	Medium Weight

PRIMARY BENEFIT: FULL-BODY STRENGTH AND CONDITIONING

TARGET MUSCLES: QUADRICEPS, GLUTES, HAMSTRINGS, OBLIQUES, LATS, PECS, DELTOIDS, TRICEPS

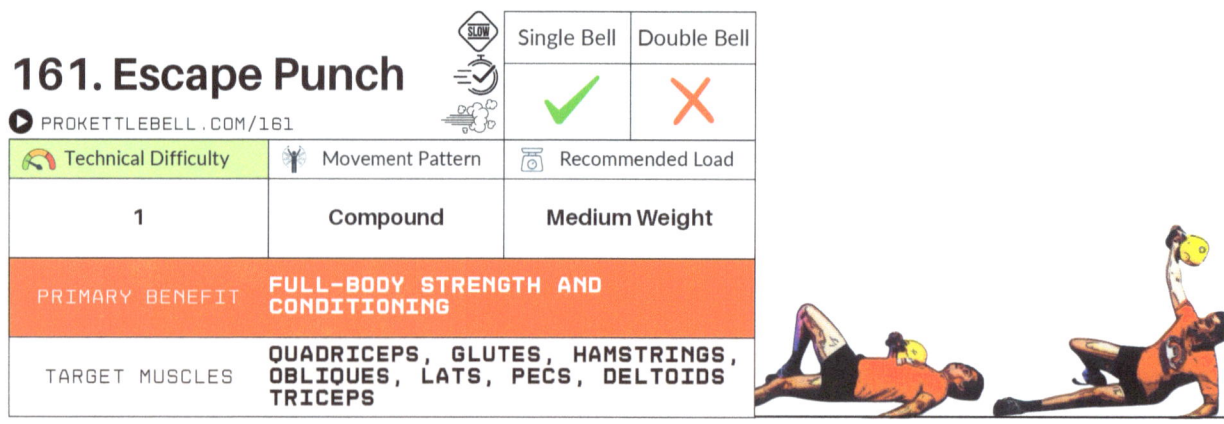

Lie flat with a kettlebell racked on the same side which your knee is bent. Place the other leg straight and your free hand out at a 45-degree angle. Explosively punch the kettlebell straight upward while rolling onto your free elbow. Return under control and repeat, keeping the weight aligned directly over your shoulder.

162. Frogger Sit-Up

	Single Bell	Double Bell
	✓	✗

Technical Difficulty	Movement Pattern	Recommended Load
1	Compound	Medium, Heavy Weight

PRIMARY BENEFIT: CORE STRENGTH AND GROIN MOBILITY

TARGET MUSCLES: ABS

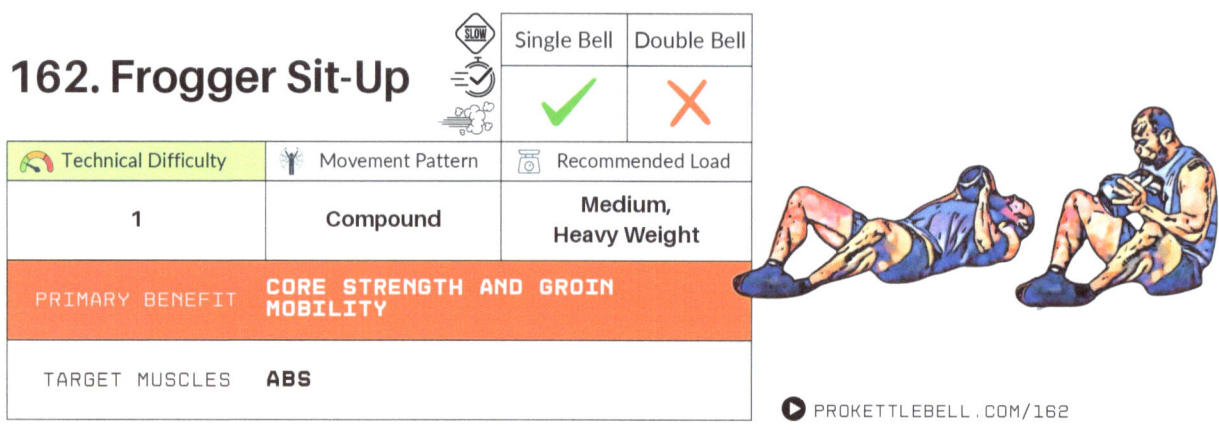

PROKETTLEBELL.COM/162

Lie back with the soles of your feet together, letting your knees fall open. Hold a kettlebell at your chest and perform a controlled sit-up while actively pressing your feet together. This foot position increases groin engagement and core activation. Perform with or without a kettlebell based on strength and experience.

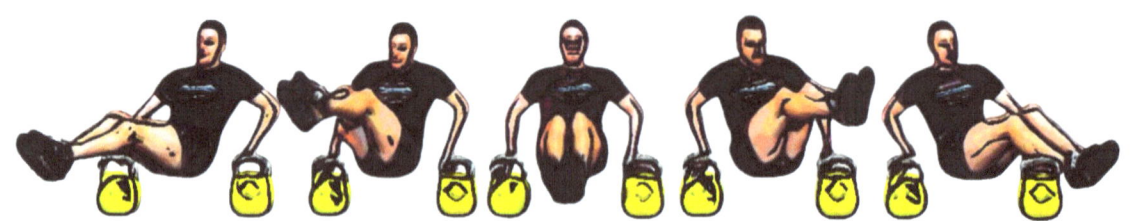

163. Golden Arches

PROKETTLEBELL.COM/163

	Single Bell	Double Bell
	✗	✓

Technical Difficulty	Movement Pattern	Recommended Load
1	Compound	Heavy Weight

PRIMARY BENEFIT: CORE STRENGTH

TARGET MUSCLES: HIP FLEXORS, ABS, OBLIQUES, ERECTORS

Sit between two kettlebells placed just outside your feet. With your hands planted behind you and your torso upright, lift your legs and sweep them over one kettlebell, then over the other, without letting your feet touch the ground. The leg path should trace the shape of the McDonald's "M" logo—hence the name Golden Arches. Keep your lumbar spine flat, chest lifted, and legs elevated throughout to maintain constant core tension.

164. Halo Situp

PROKETTLEBELL.COM/164

Single Bell	Double Bell
✓	✗

Technical Difficulty	Movement Pattern	Recommended Load
1	Compound	Light, Medium Weight

PRIMARY BENEFIT	CORE AND ARM STRENGTH

TARGET MUSCLES	ABS, DELTOIDS, LATS, ERECTORS, FOREARMS

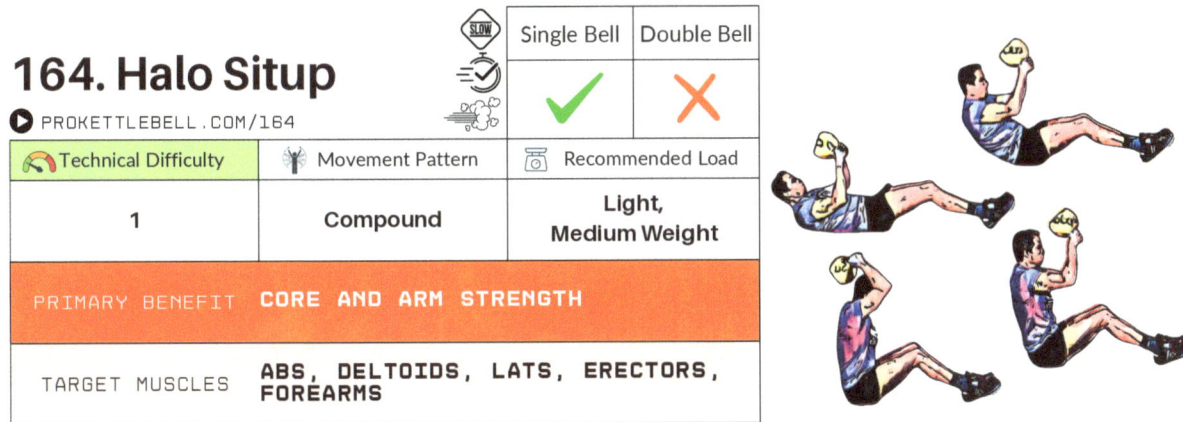

Sit holding a kettlebell upside down by the horns at forehead height. Circle the kettlebell around your head in one direction, then the other, performing a halo. After each full halo, complete a sit-up. Keep the kettlebell close to your head, elbows tight, and move with control throughout.

165. Hollow Hold Crunch

Single Bell	Double Bell
✓	✗

Technical Difficulty	Movement Pattern	Recommended Load
1	Compound	Light, Medium Weight

PRIMARY BENEFIT	CORE AND ARM STRENGTH

TARGET MUSCLES	HIP FLEXORS, ABS, LATS, TRICEPS

PROKETTLEBELL.COM/165

Lie on your back holding a kettlebell overhead. Raise your arms, legs, and shoulders to enter a hollow hold, tucking your chin slightly. Hold for time while keeping your abs engaged and your lumbar spine pressed into the floor. Bend your knees or elbows to shorten the lever and reduce difficulty if needed.

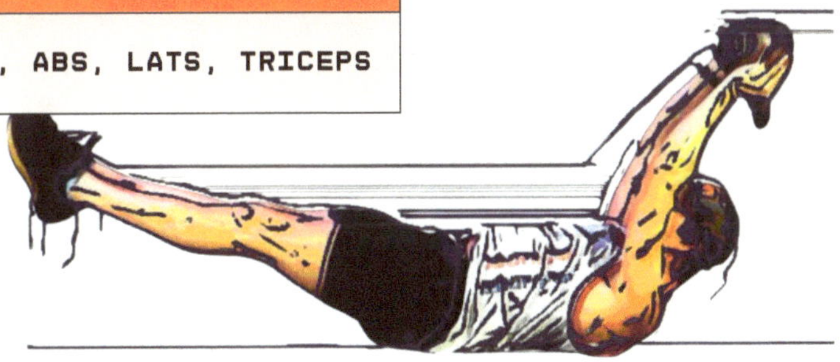

166. Kettlebell Kayaks

Single Bell	Double Bell
✓	✗

Technical Difficulty	Movement Pattern	Recommended Load
1	Compound	Light Weight

PRIMARY BENEFIT	UPPER BODY AND CORE STRENGTH

TARGET MUSCLES	ABS, OBLIQUES, BICEPS, DELTOIDS

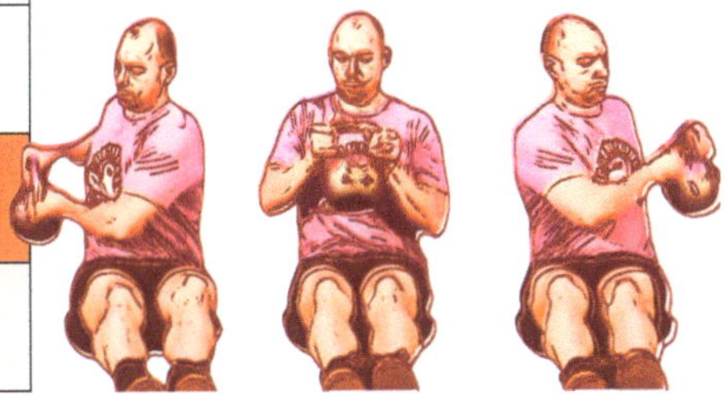

Sit upright holding a kettlebell with both hands. Rotate your torso while mimicking a kayaking motion, paddling the kettlebell from one side to the other. Keep your elbows close, chest proud, and avoid leaning back. Maintain tension in your biceps and core as you alternate strokes. PROKETTLEBELL.COM/166

SIT-UPS, TWISTS & CRUNCHES

167. L-Sit-Up

PROKETTLEBELL.COM/167

	Single Bell	Double Bell
	✗	✓

Technical Difficulty	Movement Pattern	Recommended Load
1	Compound	Light, Medium Weight

PRIMARY BENEFIT	SHOULDER, CORE STRENGTH AND STABILITY
TARGET MUSCLES	ABS, HIP FLEXORS, DELTOIDS, TRICEPS

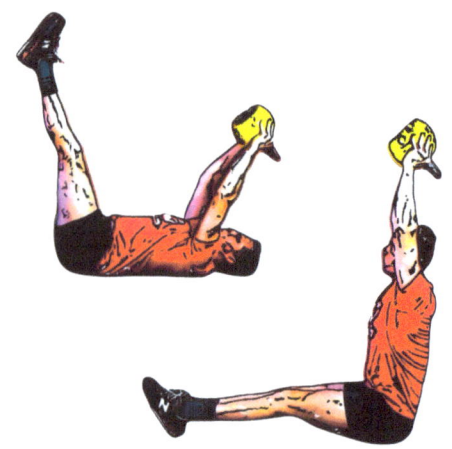

Begin in an L-sit with legs extended and a kettlebell locked overhead. Rock backward until your back is on the floor while maintaining the "L" shape, then sit up with minimal momentum, initiating the movement by squeezing your abdominals. Keep your arms elevated throughout. Maintain straight knees and pointed toes, and keep the kettlebell stacked directly over your head for balance and safety.

168. Pull-Over Tucks

PROKETTLEBELL.COM/168

	Single Bell	Double Bell
	✓	✗

Technical Difficulty	Movement Pattern	Recommended Load
1	Compound	Medium Weight

PRIMARY BENEFIT	CORE AND HIP FLEXOR STRENGTH
TARGET MUSCLES	ABS, HIP FLEXORS, OBLIQUES, LATS

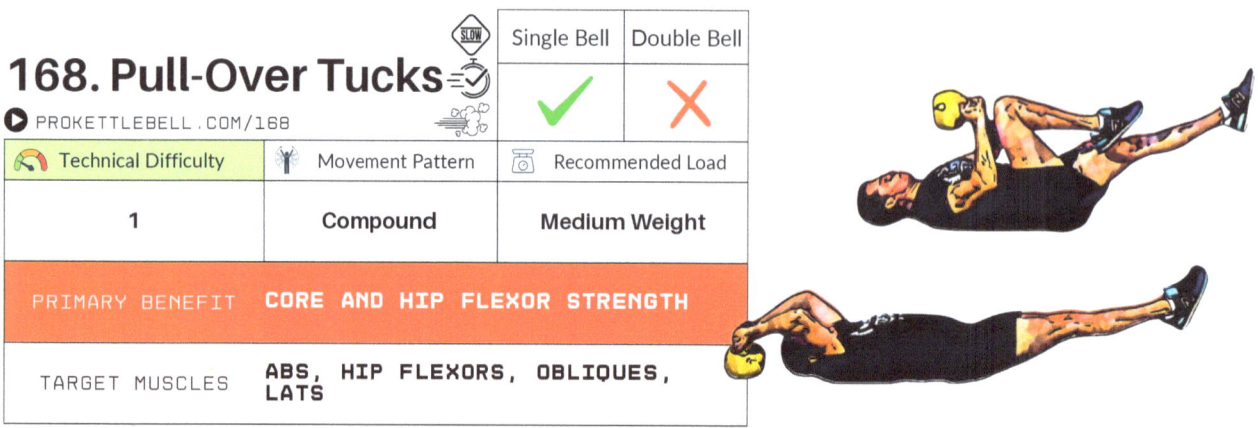

Lie flat holding a kettlebell by the horns on the floor behind your head. Lift your legs slightly off the floor and keep them straight. Pull the kettlebell from overhead to your chest as you draw both knees—or one knee—toward the kettlebell. Return the kettlebell overhead as your legs extend back to the elevated start position. Repeat.

169. Racked Trunk Twists

	Single Bell	Double Bell
	✗	✓

Technical Difficulty	Movement Pattern	Recommended Load
1	Rotate	Medium Weight

PRIMARY BENEFIT	CORE STRENGTH AND MOBILITY
TARGET MUSCLES	ABS, OBLIQUES

Hold two kettlebells in the rack position. With your feet grounded, twist your upper body to one side, pivoting your back foot slightly, then twist to the other side. Perform the motion slowly to target your obliques and warm up or cool down your spine.

PROKETTLEBELL.COM/169

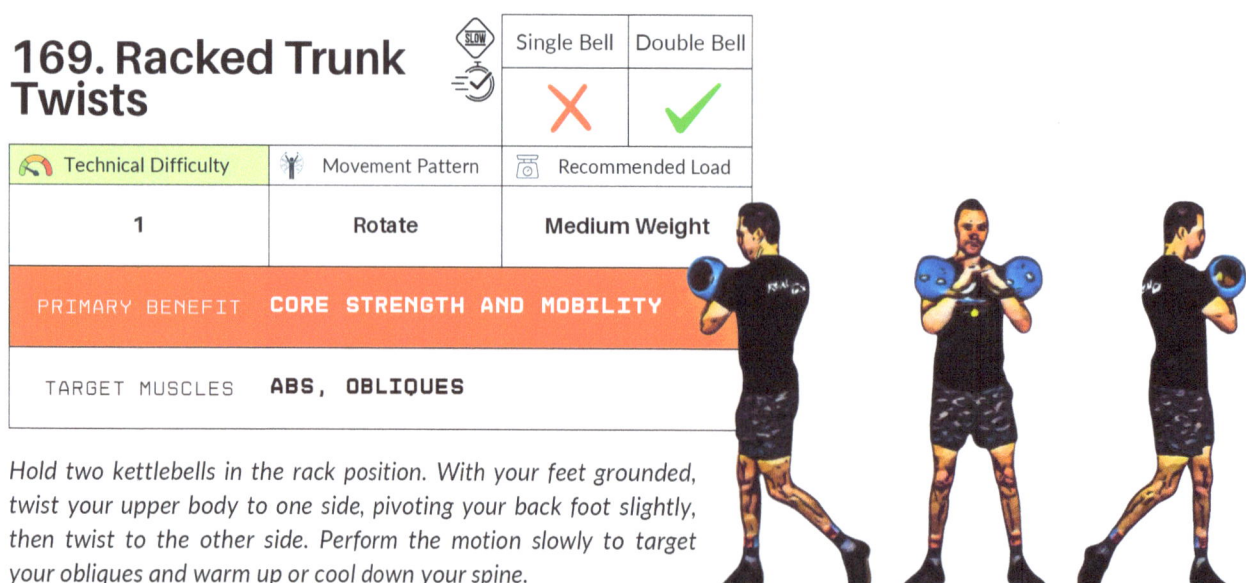

170. Russian Twist

▶ PROKETTLEBELL.COM/170

	Single Bell	Double Bell
	✓	✗

Technical Difficulty	Movement Pattern	Recommended Load
1	Rotate	Medium Weight

PRIMARY BENEFIT	CORE STRENGTH
TARGET MUSCLES	ERECTORS, OBLIQUES, ABS, SHOULDERS, BICEPS

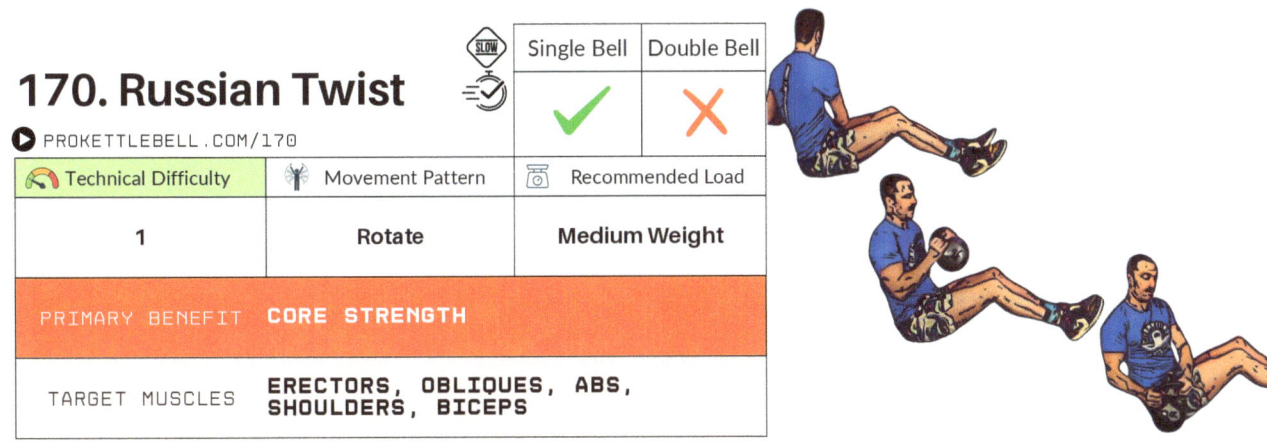

Sit with a kettlebell in both hands, knees bent and feet either on the floor or elevated. Twist your torso to tap the kettlebell beside one hip, then twist the other way. Keep your spine upright and avoid rounding the back. Perform under control for maximum oblique engagement.

171. Sit-Up Getup

▶ PROKETTLEBELL.COM/171

	Single Bell	Double Bell
	✓	✗

Technical Difficulty	Movement Pattern	Recommended Load
1	Compound	Light, Medium Weight

PRIMARY BENEFIT	CORE STRENGTH
TARGET MUSCLES	ABS, SHOULDERS, TRICEPS

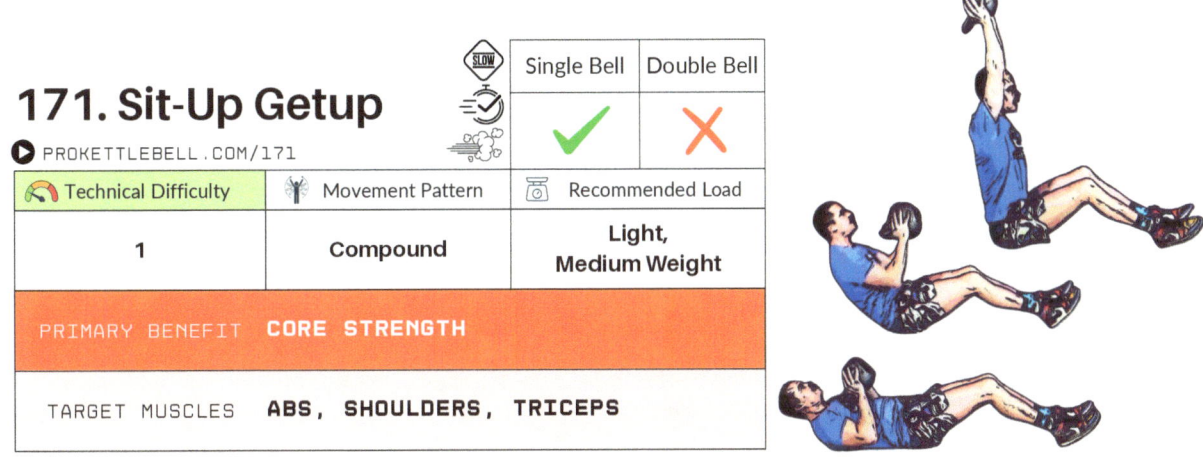

Lie back holding a kettlebell at your chest with both hands. Perform a full sit-up and press the kettlebell overhead at the top of the motion. Return to the start and repeat. Ensure the overhead press ends with arms locked and the kettlebell directly over the head.

172. Sit-Up Twist

▶ PROKETTLEBELL.COM/172

	Single Bell	Double Bell
	✓	✗

Technical Difficulty	Movement Pattern	Recommended Load
1	Compound	Light, Medium Weight

PRIMARY BENEFIT	CORE, ARM STRENGTH AND MOBILITY
TARGET MUSCLES	ABS, ERECTORS, OBLIQUES, BICEPS

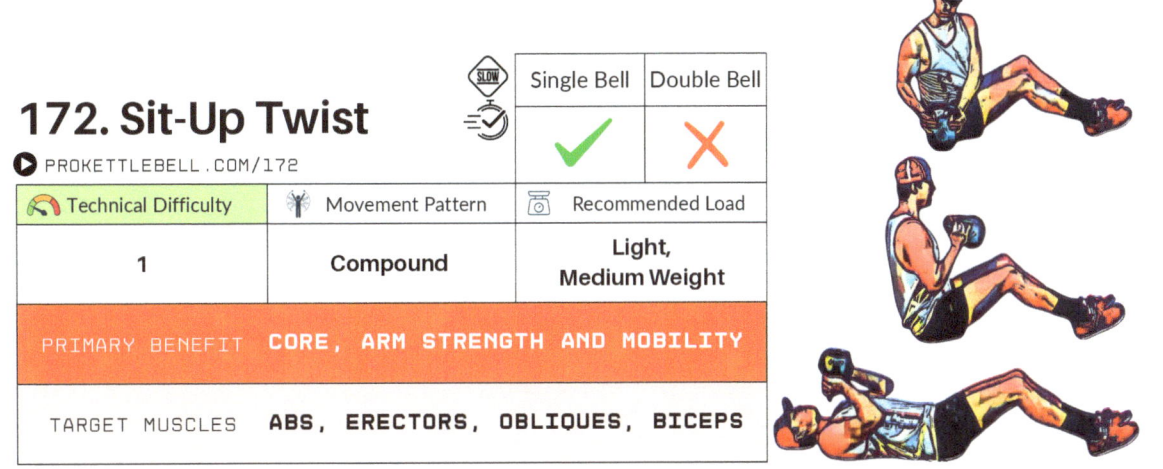

Start in a sit-up position holding a kettlebell close to your chest. Perform a sit-up, rotate to one side, and touch the kettlebell to the floor—or hover it just above. Return to center, lower with control, and repeat. Avoid momentum and keep the movement controlled. You may twist to each side between sit-ups or perform a sit-up between each twist.

SIT-UPS, TWISTS & CRUNCHES

173. Star Pullover

PROKETTLEBELL.COM/173

	Single Bell	Double Bell
	✓	✗

Technical Difficulty	Movement Pattern	Recommended Load
1	Compound	Light Weight

PRIMARY BENEFIT	CORE STRENGTH
TARGET MUSCLES	ABS, ERECTORS, OBLIQUES, DELTOIDS, TRAPS

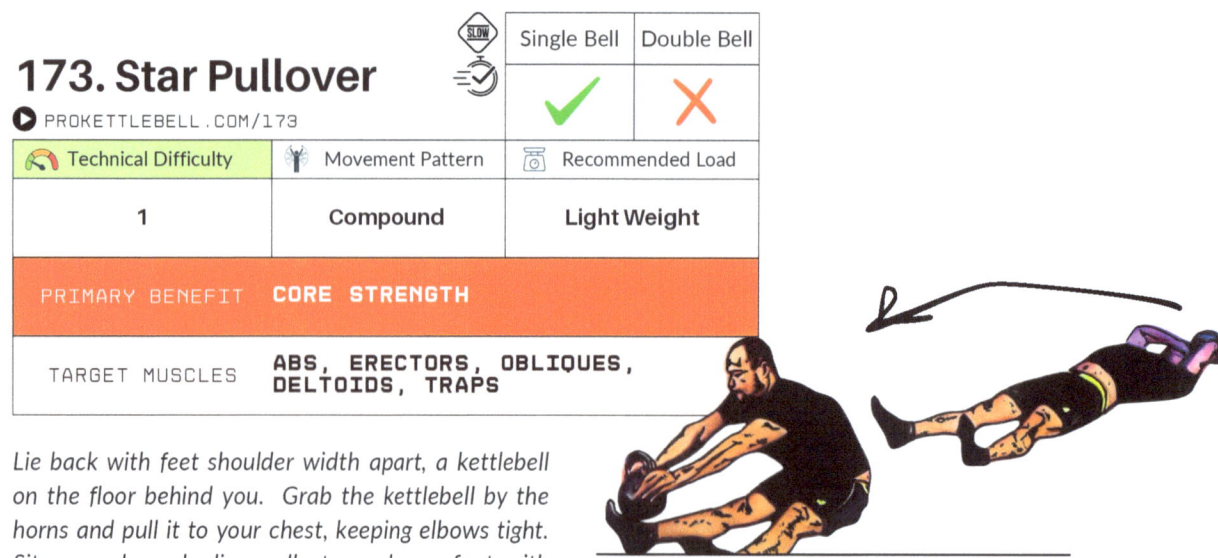

Lie back with feet shoulder width apart, a kettlebell on the floor behind you. Grab the kettlebell by the horns and pull it to your chest, keeping elbows tight. Sit up and reach diagonally toward one foot with your kettlebell. Lie back, repeat the pullover, and reach to the opposite foot. Focus on controlled movement and full-body engagement.

174. Twisted Pull-Over

	Single Bell	Double Bell
	✓	✗

Technical Difficulty	Movement Pattern	Recommended Load
1	Compound	Medium Weight

PRIMARY BENEFIT	CORE AND LAT STRENGTH
TARGET MUSCLES	OBLIQUES, LATS, LOWER CHEST

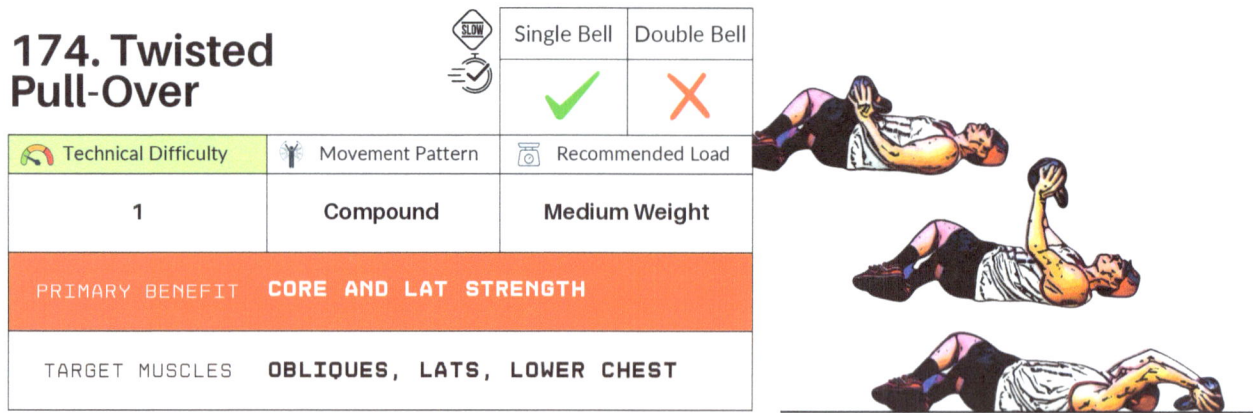

Lie on your back with a kettlebell at one hip and knees twisted to one side. Perform a pullover from your hip to overhead in a C-shaped arc. Keep forearms parallel and tension in your lats. Perform slowly for maximum muscle engagement, adjusting grip and weight based on mobility. PROKETTLEBELL.COM/174

175. Twisted Punch

	Single Bell	Double Bell
	✓	✗

Technical Difficulty	Movement Pattern	Recommended Load
1	Compound	Medium Weight

PRIMARY BENEFIT	CORE AND ARM STRENGTH
TARGET MUSCLES	ABS, OBLIQUES, DELTOIDS, TRICEPS

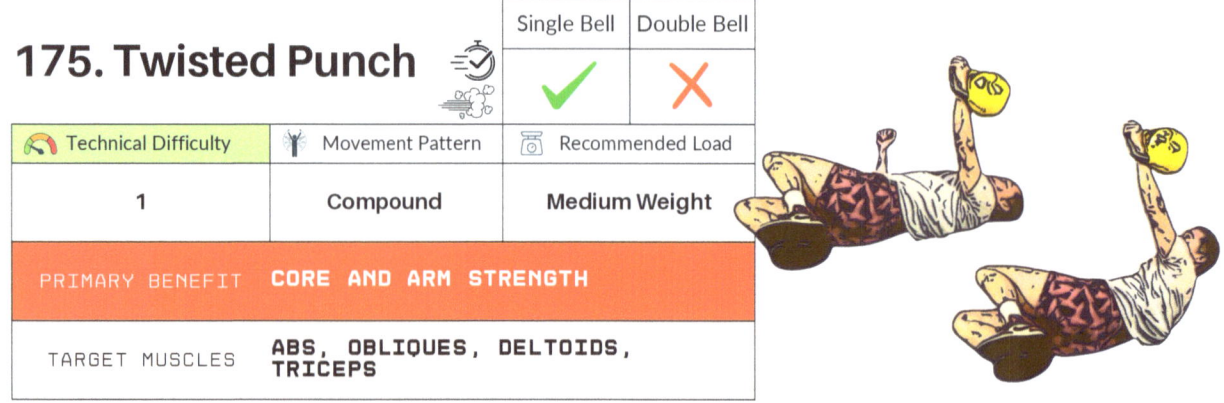

Lie back in a sit-up position with a kettlebell at your chest. Rotate your knees to the opposite side and press the kettlebell vertically, lifting only the shoulder blade on the kettlebell side off the floor. Return and repeat. The motion should be small and focused on oblique engagement. PROKETTLEBELL.COM/175

176. Wood Chopper Sit-Up

	Single Bell	Double Bell
	✓	✗

Technical Difficulty	Movement Pattern	Recommended Load
1	Compound	Light, Medium Weight

PRIMARY BENEFIT CORE STRENGTH

TARGET MUSCLES ABS, OBLIQUES, LATS

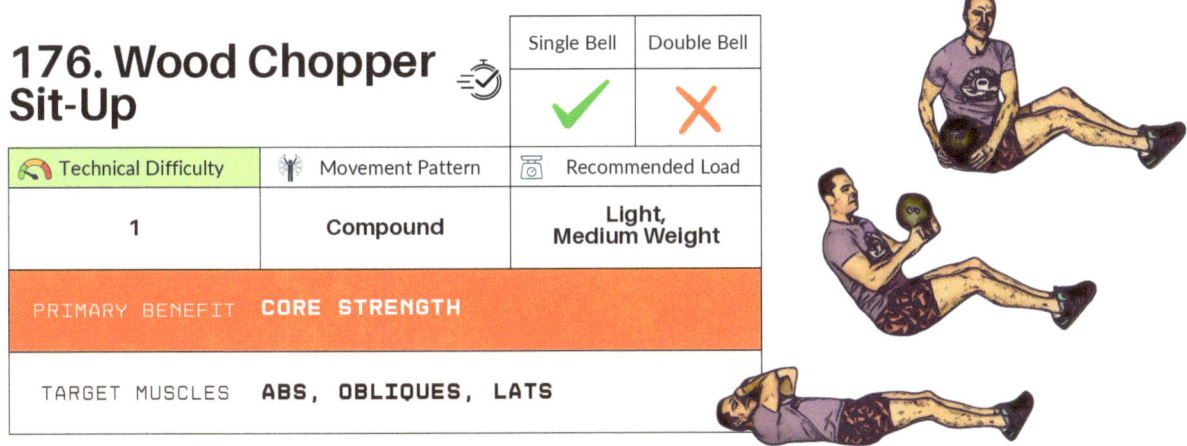

Lie on your back with a kettlebell beside one shoulder. Grab it by the horns with both hands and swing it diagonally across your body as you perform a sit-up, bringing it to the outside of the opposite hip in a chopping motion. Reverse the movement and return the kettlebell to the starting position without using momentum. Complete all reps on one side before switching and matching the same number of reps on the other side. ▶ PROKETTLEBELL.COM/176

177. Anchored Side Cycles

	Single Bell	Double Bell
	✗	✓

Technical Difficulty	Movement Pattern	Recommended Load
2	Rotation	Medium, Heavy Weight

PRIMARY BENEFIT CORE STRENGTH

TARGET MUSCLES ABS, OBLIQUES

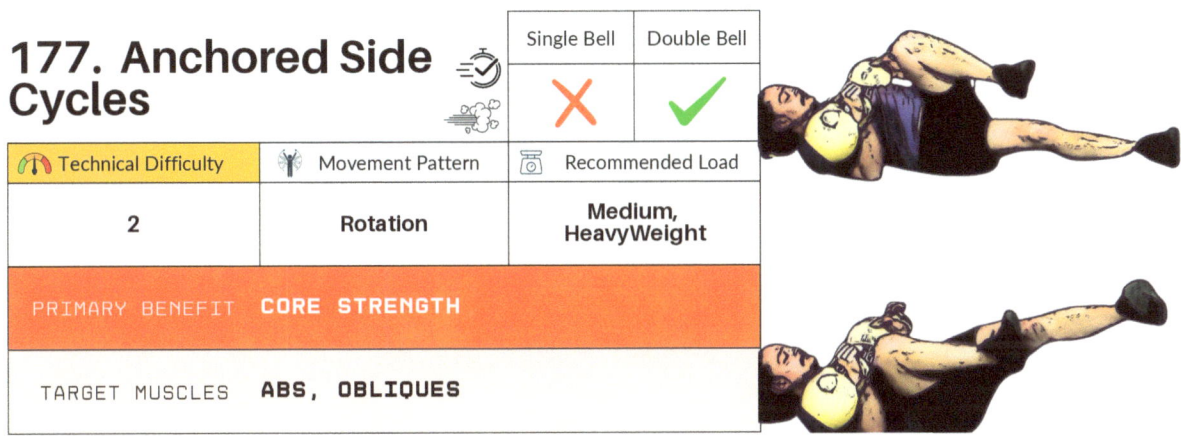

Lie on your back between two kettlebells and hold them with elbows out at a 45-degree angle, forearms perpendicular to the floor, bells balanced. Lift your legs and rotate them to one side, then begin a cycling motion in this position. After completing reps or time, switch sides and repeat. Keep your upper back still and abs engaged throughout. ▶ PROKETTLEBELL.COM/177

178. Armbar Sit-Up

▶ PROKETTLEBELL.COM/178

	Single Bell	Double Bell
	✓	✓

Technical Difficulty	Movement Pattern	Recommended Load
2	Compound	Light, Medium Weight

PRIMARY BENEFIT CORE AND ARM STRENGTH

TARGET MUSCLES ABS, ERECTORS, SHOULDERS, TRICEPS

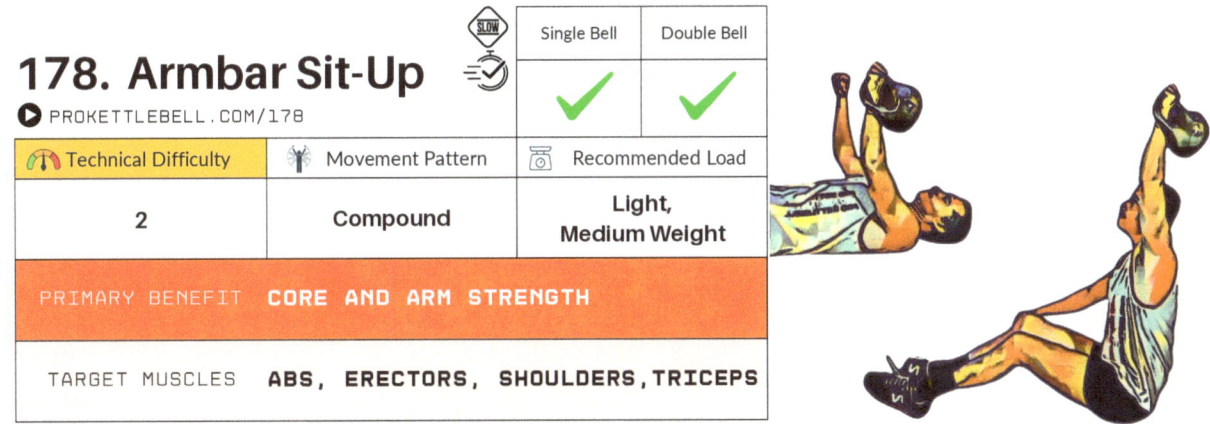

Lie down and press a kettlebell into the armbar position, arm locked out directly over your shoulder. Squeeze your abs to protect your lower back and perform a full sit-up while keeping the kettlebell steady and stacked over your shoulder throughout. Pause briefly at the top before lowering back down. Use your free hand to assist if needed.

SIT-UPS, TWISTS & CRUNCHES

179. Armbar Sit-Up + Press

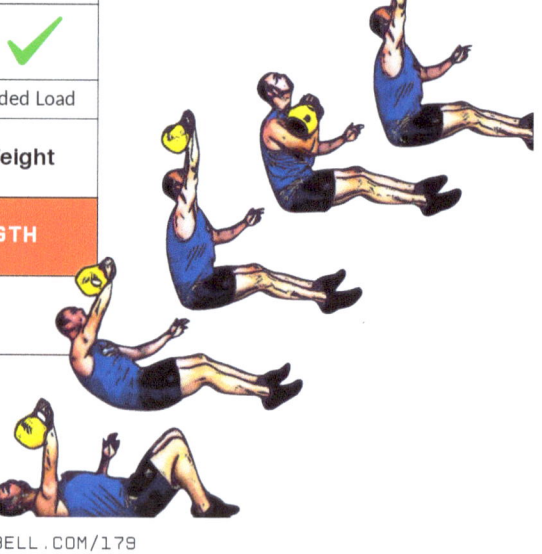

	Single Bell	Double Bell
SLOW	✓	✓

Technical Difficulty	Movement Pattern	Recommended Load
2	Compound	Medium Weight

PRIMARY BENEFIT	CORE AND UPPER BODY STRENGTH
TARGET MUSCLES	ABS, DELTOIDS, TRICEPS

A variation of the standard Armbar Sit-Up (Exercise #178), this combo increases core and shoulder strength and stability by returning the kettlebell to your chest and pressing it from the seated position before descending back to the floor. Legs may be straight or bent, depending on comfort. ▶ PROKETTLEBELL.COM/179

180. Sideways V-Up

▶ PROKETTLEBELL.COM/180

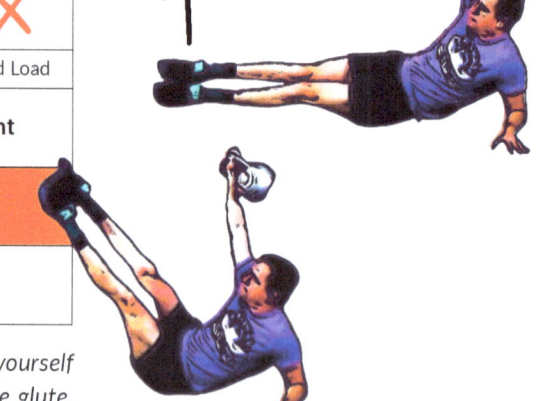

	Single Bell	Double Bell
SLOW	✓	✗

Technical Difficulty	Movement Pattern	Recommended Load
2	Compound	Light Weight

PRIMARY BENEFIT	CORE STRENGTH
TARGET MUSCLES	ABS, ERECTORS, OBLIQUES, DELTOIDS, TRICEPS

Lie on your side with a kettlebell pressed out on the top side. Prop yourself slightly on your lower arm and extend both legs, balancing on one glute. Keeping feet together, lift both legs toward the kettlebell. Keep the weight still and stacked over your shoulder and focus on engaging your obliques.

181. Turkish Sit-Up

▶ PROKETTLEBELL.COM/181

	Single Bell	Double Bell
SLOW	✓	✗

Technical Difficulty	Movement Pattern	Recommended Load
2	Compound	Light, Medium Weight

PRIMARY BENEFIT	CORE, SHOULDER, ELBOW STRENGTH AND STABILITY
TARGET MUSCLES	ABS, OBLIQUES, ERECTORS, LATS, DELTOIDS, TRICEPS

Lie in a fetal position next to a kettlebell. Insert your hand through the window of the handle and roll the bell onto your chest. With the same-side leg bent, press the kettlebell overhead and sit up onto your elbow, then straighten your arm to finish in a seated position. Reverse the movement and repeat before switching sides.

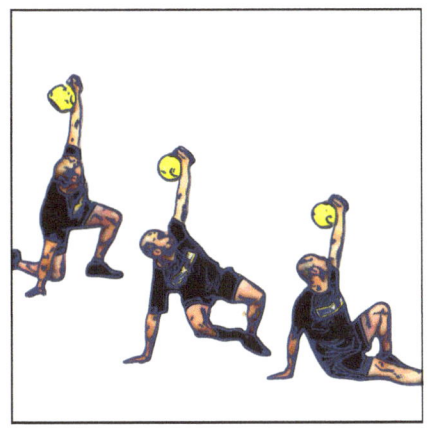

182. Turkish Kick n' Sit

	Single Bell	Double Bell
SLOW	✓	✗

Technical Difficulty	Movement Pattern	Recommended Load
2	Compound	Medium Weight

PRIMARY BENEFIT	CORE STRENGTH
TARGET MUSCLES	OBLIQUES, ERECTORS, LATS, DELTS, TRICEPS, QUADS, HAMSTRINGS

▶ PROKETTLEBELL.COM/182

Begin in a kneeling position with the front leg on the same side as the kettlebell. Press the kettlebell overhead and plant the opposite hand firmly outside your hip to form a tripod position. Once stable, pick up the back leg and kick it straight through to the seated position. Lift the hips and slide the leg back behind you to return to the original kneeling position. Move slowly and with control, keeping the kettlebell stacked overhead and your hand placed far enough from the hip to allow leg clearance.

183. Anchored Plow

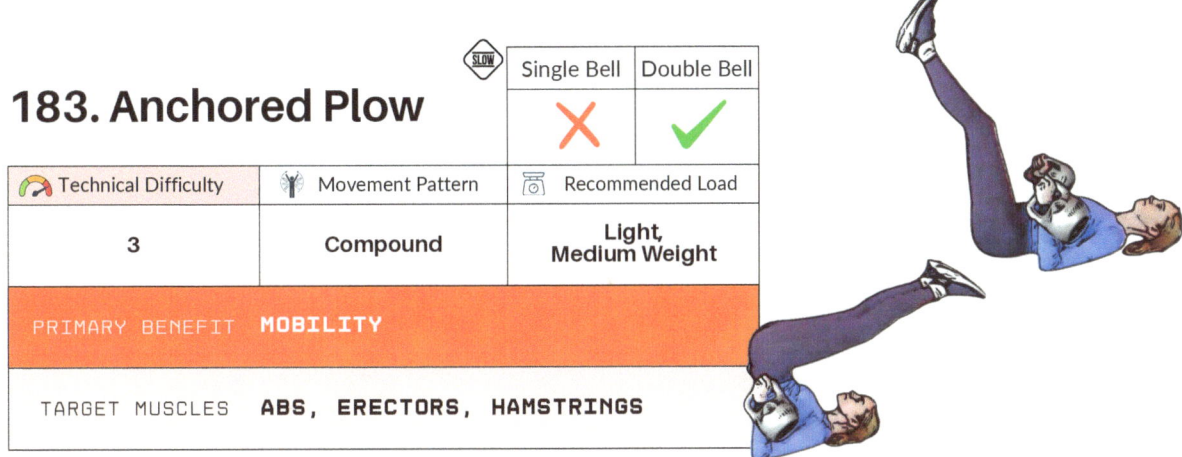

	Single Bell	Double Bell
SLOW	✗	✓

Technical Difficulty	Movement Pattern	Recommended Load
3	Compound	Light, Medium Weight

PRIMARY BENEFIT	MOBILITY
TARGET MUSCLES	ABS, ERECTORS, HAMSTRINGS

Lie on your back between two kettlebells and hold them with forearms vertical, anchoring your upper arms to the ground. Straighten your legs and bring them up and over your head, as far as possible without shifting weight onto your neck. Keep legs as straight as possible and hold. Lower with control. ▶ PROKETTLEBELL.COM/183

184. L-Sit

▶ PROKETTLEBELL.COM/184

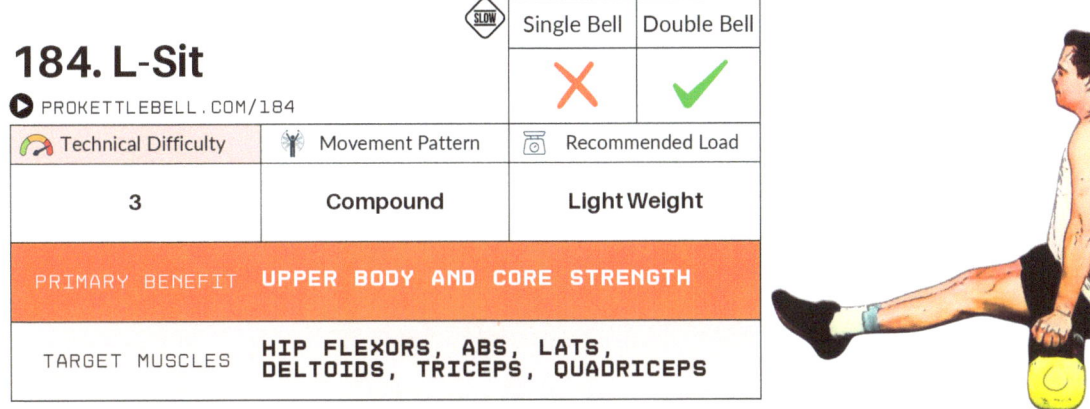

	Single Bell	Double Bell
SLOW	✗	✓

Technical Difficulty	Movement Pattern	Recommended Load
3	Compound	Light Weight

PRIMARY BENEFIT	UPPER BODY AND CORE STRENGTH
TARGET MUSCLES	HIP FLEXORS, ABS, LATS, DELTOIDS, TRICEPS, QUADRICEPS

Place two stable kettlebells beside and slightly forward of your hips. Extend your legs forward into an L position. Press down on the handles and lift your body off the ground with toes pointed. Hold the position, keeping shoulders, elbows, and wrists aligned. Begin with bent knees if needed, progressing to full extension.

SIT-UPS, TWISTS & CRUNCHES

185. Sideways V-Ups (Double Alternating)

Single Bell	Double Bell
✗	✓

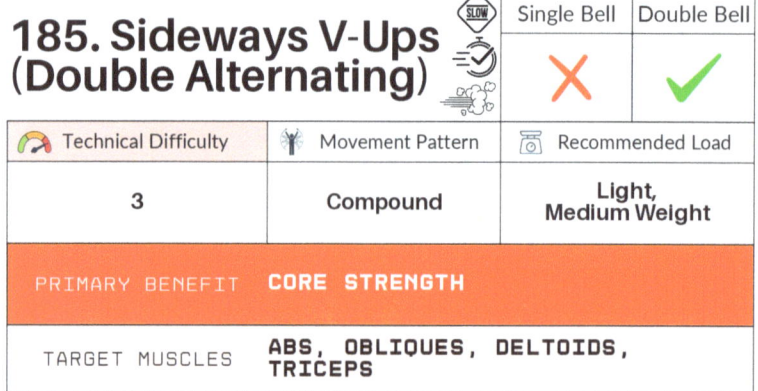

Technical Difficulty	Movement Pattern	Recommended Load
3	Compound	Light, Medium Weight

PRIMARY BENEFIT	**CORE STRENGTH**
TARGET MUSCLES	**ABS, OBLIQUES, DELTOIDS, TRICEPS**

PROKETTLEBELL.COM/185

Begin on your back, holding kettlebells in both hands – upper arms resting on the floor, elbows bent and forearms vertical. Keeping your feet together, rotate your legs to one side and lift them while sitting up and pressing the opposite side kettlebell toward your feet. Return to the center as you lower the bell. Alternate sides with fluidity. Sit up as tall as you can at the top of each repetition. Protect your back and neck by keeping your core muscles engaged throughout the movement.

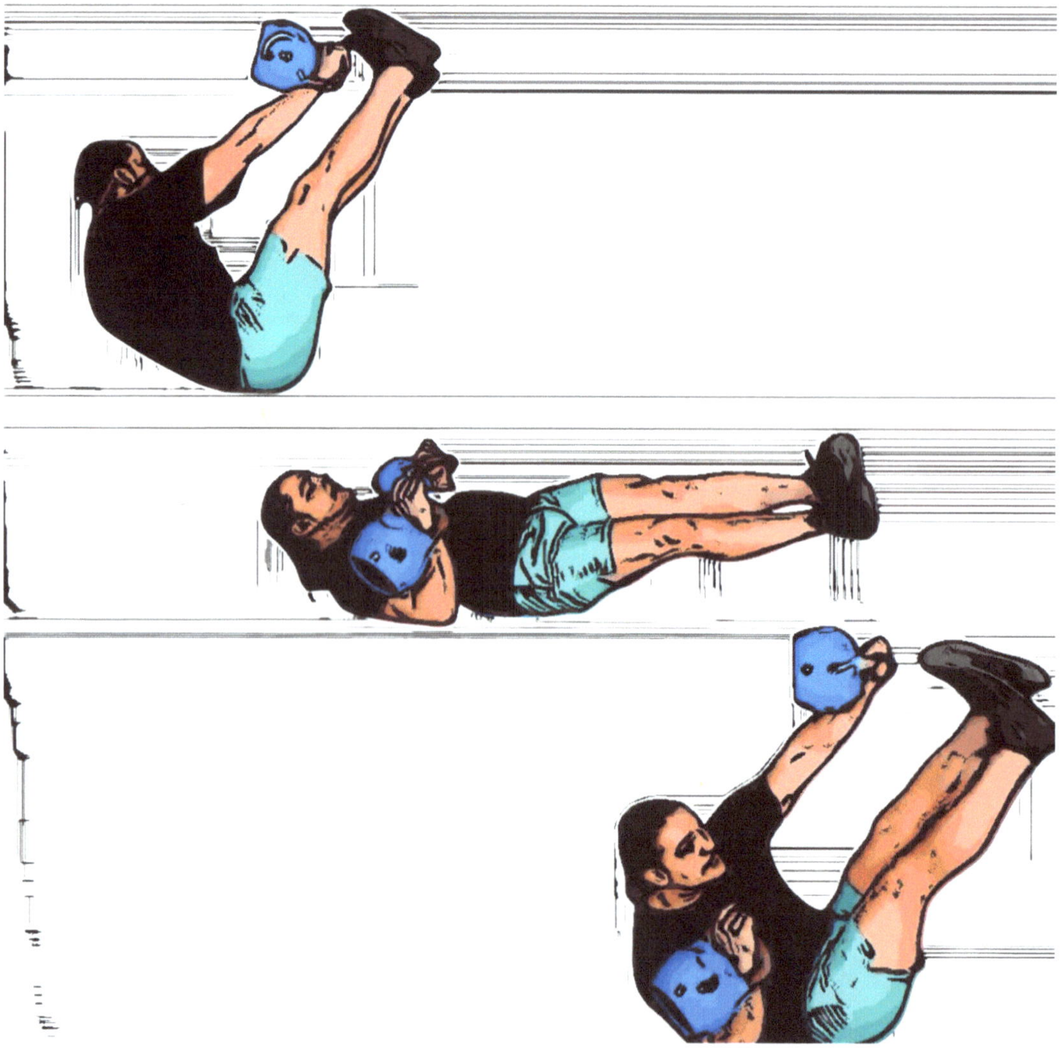

186. KB Mountain Climbers

	SLOW	Single Bell	Double Bell
		✗	✓

Technical Difficulty	Movement Pattern	Recommended Load
1	Compound	Heavy Weight

PRIMARY BENEFIT	UPPER BODY, CORE STRENGTH AND CARDIO
TARGET MUSCLES	DELTOIDS, TRICEPS, ABS, OBLIQUES, HIP FLEXORS

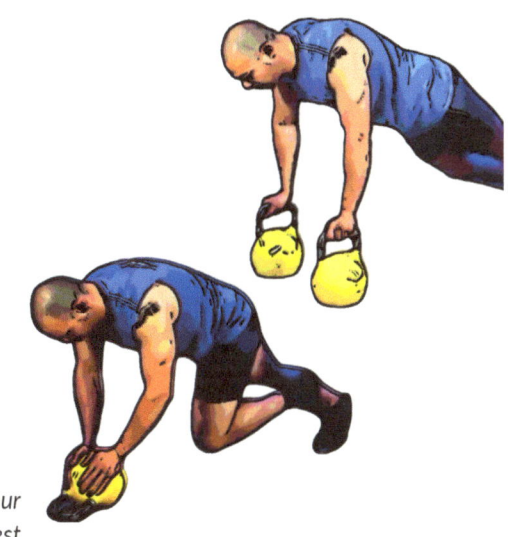

With both hands placed on stable kettlebell handles directly under your shoulders, assume a plank position. Begin running your knees toward your chest one at a time while keeping your back flat and hips low. Maintain a fast but controlled pace, focusing on core stability and minimizing movement in the upper body. Modify by placing hands directly on the floor if kettlebells are unstable.

▶ PROKETTLEBELL.COM/186

187. KB Mountain Climber Twist

	SLOW	Single Bell	Double Bell
		✗	✓

Technical Difficulty	Movement Pattern	Recommended Load
1	Compound	Heavy Weight

PRIMARY BENEFIT	CORE STRENGTH AND CONDITIONING
TARGET MUSCLES	ABS, OBLIQUES, ERECTORS, DELTOIDS, TRICEPS

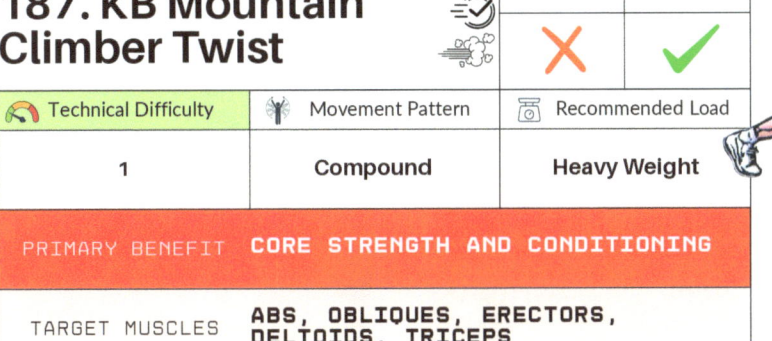

Start in a plank position with both hands on stable kettlebells. From here, drive one knee diagonally across your body toward the opposite elbow. Alternate knees in a twisting motion, engaging the obliques with each rep. Keep your core tight and shoulders still throughout. ▶ PROKETTLEBELL.COM/187

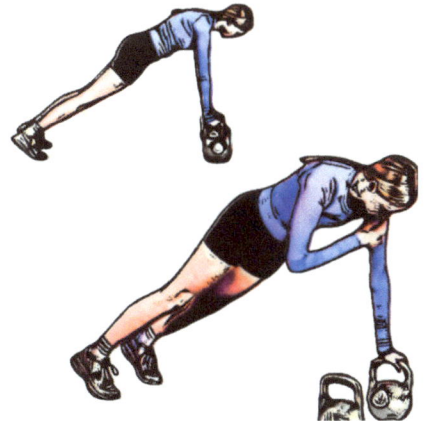

188. KB Shoulder Touches

	SLOW	Single Bell	Double Bell
		✗	✓

Technical Difficulty	Movement Pattern	Recommended Load
1	Compound	Heavy Weight

PRIMARY BENEFIT	FULL-BODY STRENGTH AND CONDITIONING
TARGET MUSCLES	QUADRICEPS, GLUTES, HAMSTRINGS, ERECTORS, LATS, DELTOIDS, TRICEPS

Assume a strong plank position with hands on kettlebells placed shoulder-width apart. Keep your hips stable and core braced as you alternate tapping your shoulders with the opposite hand. Move slowly and avoid twisting or sagging through the torso. A wider stance offers more balance, while a narrow one increases the challenge. Modify by performing the movement on your knees. ▶ PROKETTLEBELL.COM/188

*Recommended load is heavy because heavier bells are more stable to plank on

189. Pull-Under

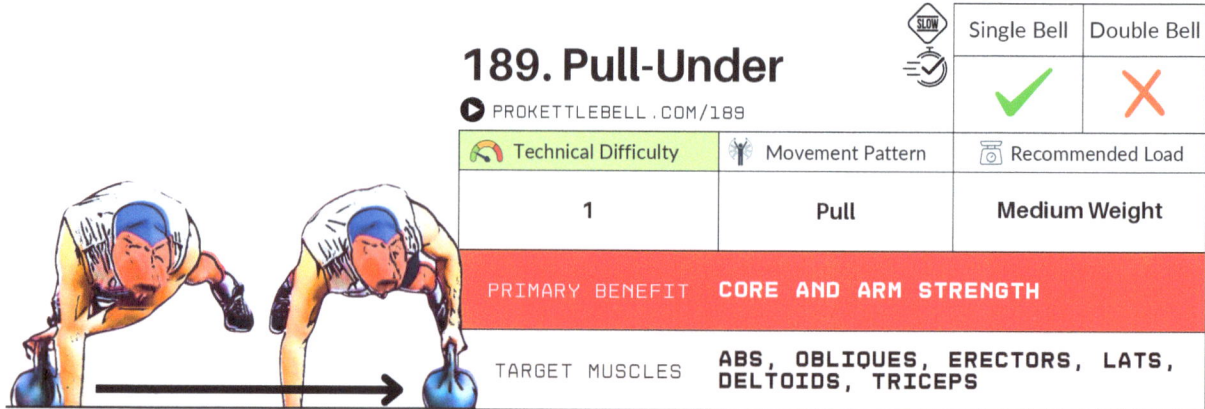

PROKETTLEBELL.COM/189

		Single Bell	Double Bell
		✓	✗

Technical Difficulty	Movement Pattern	Recommended Load
1	Pull	Medium Weight

PRIMARY BENEFIT — CORE AND ARM STRENGTH

TARGET MUSCLES — ABS, OBLIQUES, ERECTORS, LATS, DELTOIDS, TRICEPS

Start in a plank with the kettlebell placed to one side of your body. Reach under with the far hand and drag the kettlebell across to the opposite side. Keep your hips and shoulders square to the ground, focusing on control. Repeat by pulling it back across using the other hand. Maintain a strong plank throughout and avoid rushing the movement.

190. Cross-Overs

PROKETTLEBELL.COM/190

	Single Bell	Double Bell
	✓	✗

Technical Difficulty	Movement Pattern	Recommended Load
1	Compound	Light, Medium Weight

PRIMARY BENEFIT — CORE STRENGTH

TARGET MUSCLES — ABS, QUADRICEPS, GLUTES, DELTOIDS, BICEPS

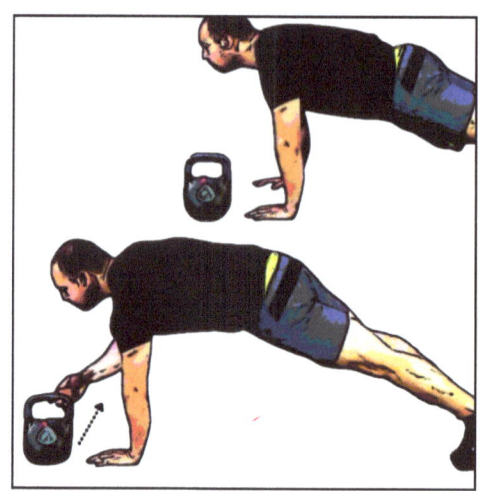

Start in a plank with the kettlebell in front of your body. Reach one hand across to drag the kettlebell to the opposite side. Alternate sides with each rep, keeping your chest up and core engaged. Avoid shifting your weight excessively. This movement emphasizes trunk rotation and stability through the shoulders, obliques, and lower body.

From a wide crouched stance, place the kettlebell just in front of your toes. Keeping your chest lifted and back flat, reach across to pull the kettlebell to one side, tap the ground, and pull it back across. Keep the movement close to your body and controlled. Counterbalance by keeping your hips back and weight in your heels. Keep strong core engagement throughout the exercise.

PROKETTLEBELL.COM/191

191. Crouching Pull Across

	Single Bell	Double Bell
	✓	✗

Technical Difficulty	Movement Pattern	Recommended Load
1	Compound	Light, Medium Weight

PRIMARY BENEFIT — LEGS AND CORE STRENGTH

TARGET MUSCLES — QUADRICEPS, GLUTES, HAMSTRINGS, ABS, OBLIQUES, ERECTORS, DELTOIDS

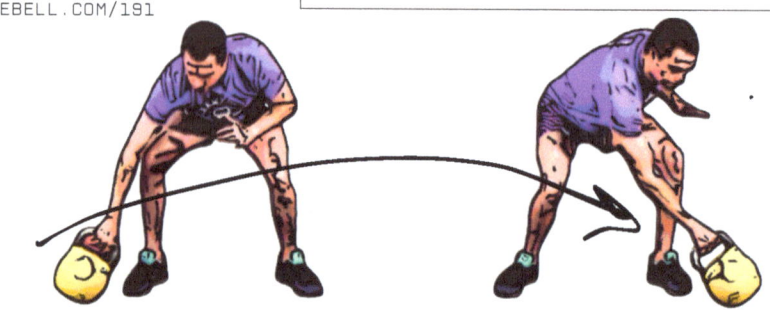

192. Crab Kick Dips

▶ PROKETTLEBELL.COM/192

	Single Bell	Double Bell
	✓	✓

Technical Difficulty	Movement Pattern	Recommended Load
2	Push	Heavy Weight

PRIMARY BENEFIT	ARMS AND CORE
TARGET MUSCLES	ABS, ERECTORS, DELTOIDS, TRICEPS

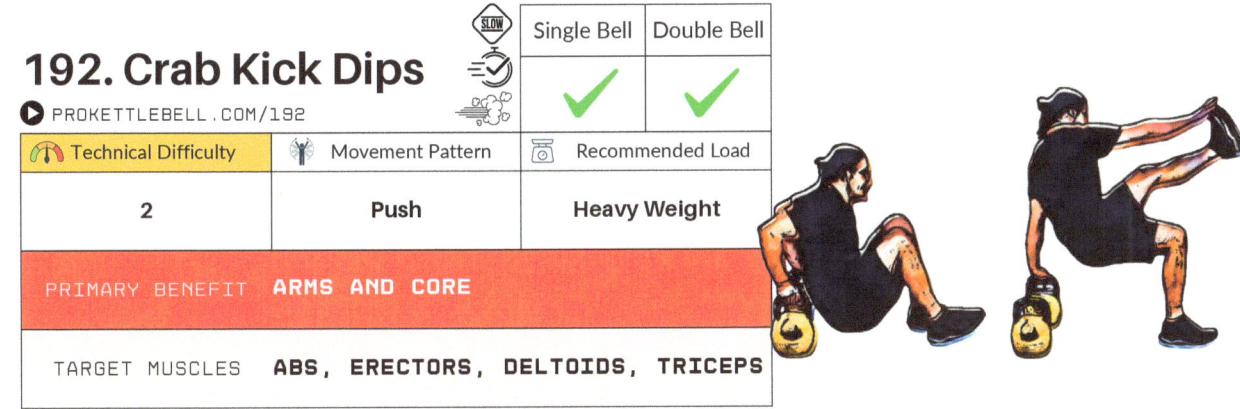

Sit in a crab position between two kettlebells with your hands on the handles. Straighten your elbows, lift your hips and kick one leg up while reaching across with the opposite hand to touch the toe. Bend your arms to return to start (the "dip") and alternate sides. Keep your hips elevated and your movement controlled throughout to activate your triceps, core, and hip flexors while maintaining balance.

193. Side Plank

	Single Bell	Double Bell
	✓	✗

Technical Difficulty	Movement Pattern	Recommended Load
2	Compound	Medium Weight

PRIMARY BENEFIT	CORE, LEG AND ARM STRENGTH
TARGET MUSCLES	OBLIQUES, TRANSVERSE ABS, GLUTES, QUADRICEPS, ADDUCTORS, ERECTORS, DELTOIDS, LATS, TRICEPS

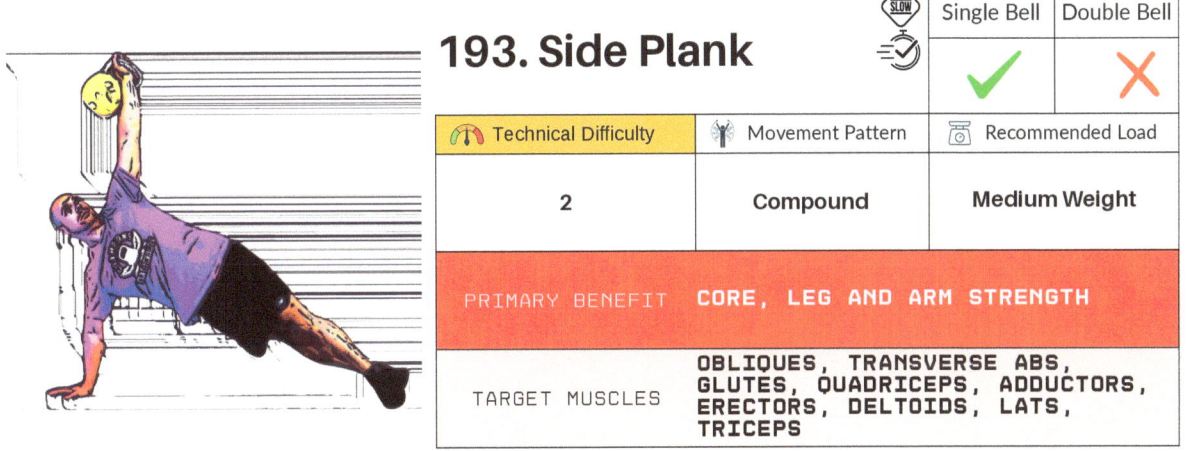

Enter the kettlebell side plank from a half-kneeling position. Press a kettlebell overhead (same side as the "up" knee), then bring your free hand to the floor. Extend the bottom leg. For more challenge, extend and stack the top leg. Maintain a straight trunk, keeping the kettlebell directly above your shoulder. Return to kneeling by reversing the movement carefully. ▶ PROKETTLEBELL.COM/193

194. Turkish Planks

▶ PROKETTLEBELL.COM/194

	Single Bell	Double Bell
	✓	✗

Technical Difficulty	Movement Pattern	Recommended Load
2	Compound	Medium Weight

PRIMARY BENEFIT	CORE AND ARM STRENGTH
TARGET MUSCLES	GLUTES, HAMSTRINGS, QUADRICEPS, OBLIQUES, ABS, ERECTORS, DELTOIDS, TRICEPS

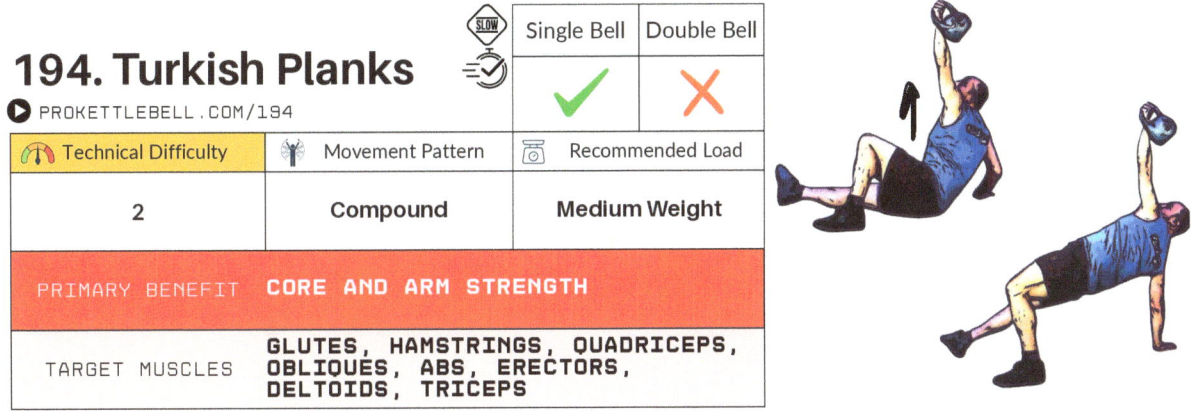

Begin on your back with the kettlebell pressed overhead on one side and the same-side leg bent. Use that leg to drive your body up onto your opposite elbow, then hand. Raise your hips into a reverse plank while keeping the kettlebell stacked over the shoulder. Lower back down step-by-step. Focus on slow, controlled movement throughout.

CORE-FOCUSED PLANKS

195. Kneeling Windmill

	Single Bell	Double Bell
SLOW	✓	✗

Technical Difficulty	Movement Pattern	Recommended Load
2	Rotate	Light, Medium Weight

PRIMARY BENEFIT	CORE, SHOULDER STRENGTH AND MOBILITY
TARGET MUSCLES	ABS, ERECTORS, OBLIQUES, LATS, DELTOIDS, TRICEPS

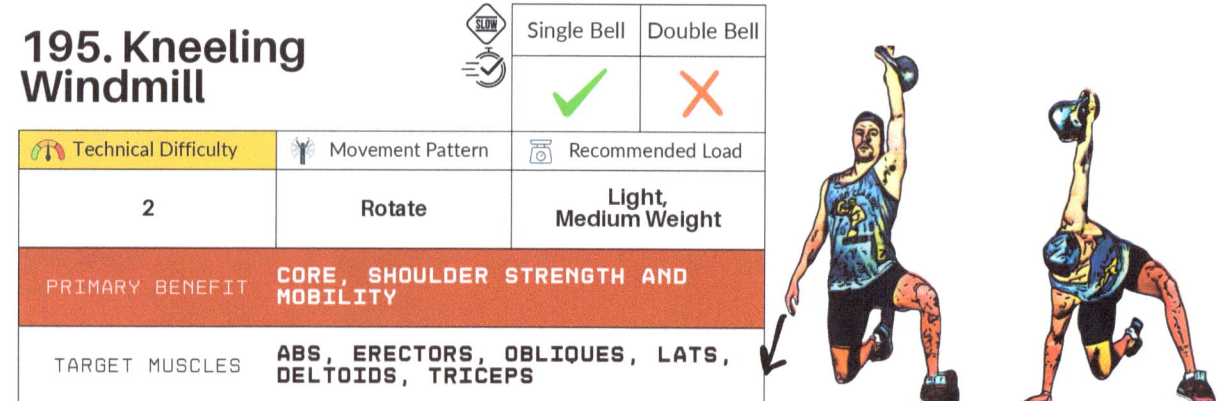

Begin in a half-kneeling position with the kettlebell in the rack on the up-leg side. Press it overhead and keep it stacked over your shoulder. Reach your free hand toward the ground, forming a tripod with your foot and knee. Move slowly and control your descent, hinging at the hips. Return to upright while keeping the kettlebell steady and your body aligned. ▶ PROKETTLEBELL.COM/195

196. Kneeling Windmill > Side Plank

	Single Bell	Double Bell
SLOW	✗	✓

Technical Difficulty	Movement Pattern	Recommended Load
2	Rotate	Light, Medium Weight

PRIMARY BENEFIT	FULL-BODY STRENGTH AND MOBILITY
TARGET MUSCLES	ABS, OBLIQUES, ERECTORS, LATS, DELTOIDS, TRICEPS

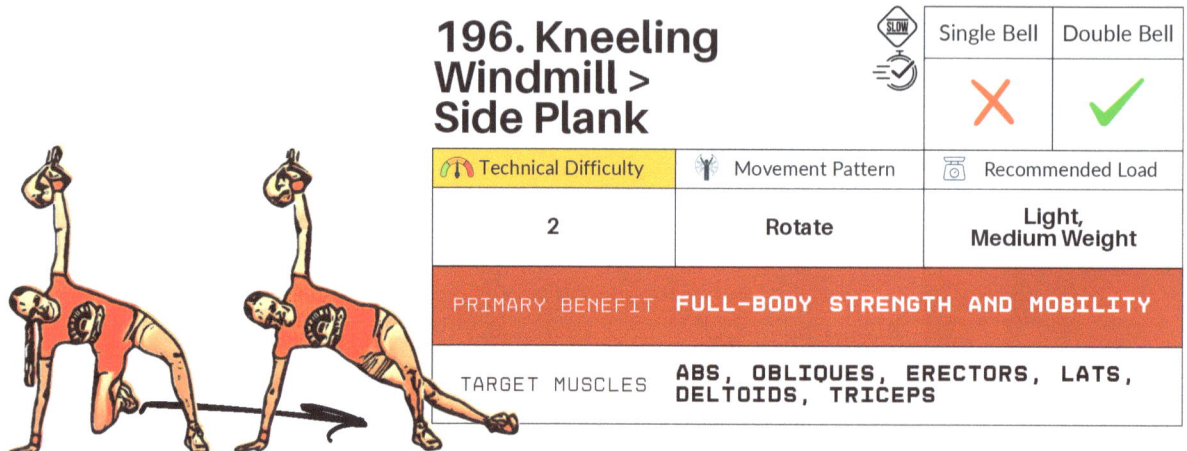

From the kneeling windmill setup, establish a wide, stable base. Press the kettlebell overhead and lower your free hand to the floor. Kick out your down leg to extend into a side plank, keeping the kettlebell stacked over the shoulder. Reverse the movement to return to kneeling. Repeat, making sure to complete the same amount of repetitions on each side.
▶ PROKETTLEBELL.COM/196

197. Windmill

	Single Bell	Double Bell
SLOW	✓	✓

▶ PROKETTLEBELL.COM/197

Technical Difficulty	Movement Pattern	Recommended Load
2	Rotate	Light, Medium Weight

PRIMARY BENEFIT	CORE STRENGTH AND MOBILITY
TARGET MUSCLES	ABS, OBLIQUES, ERECTORS, LATS, DELTOIDS, TRICEPS

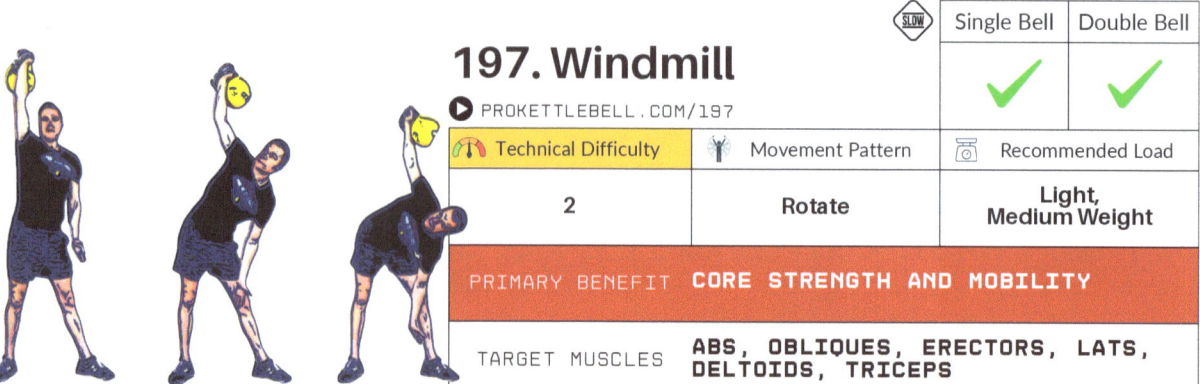

Stand with a kettlebell in the rack, then press it overhead. Turn your feet slightly away from the kettlebell side and hinge your hips in that direction. Keep your arm locked out and your gaze on the kettlebell as you lower your free hand along the opposite leg toward the floor. Return upright slowly, ensuring the kettlebell stays vertical over your shoulder. Repeat for multiple repetitions prior to mirroring the exercise on the opposite side.

198. Low Windmill

PROKETTLEBELL.COM/198

	SLOW	Single Bell	Double Bell
		✓	✓

Technical Difficulty	Movement Pattern	Recommended Load
2	Rotate	Light Weight

PRIMARY BENEFIT	CORE STRENGTH, HIP, HAMSTRING AND SHOULDER MOBILITY
TARGET MUSCLES	HAMSTRINGS, GLUTES, OBLIQUES, ERECTORS

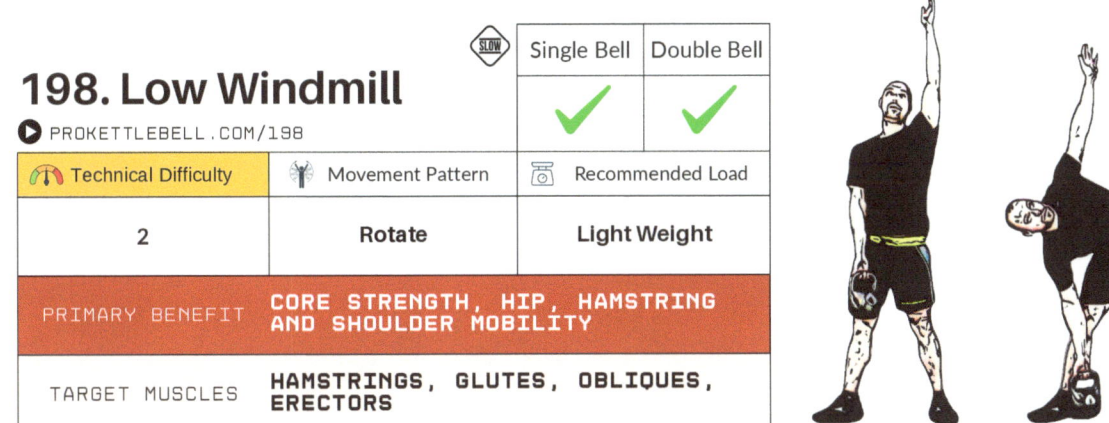

Hold the kettlebell in your lower hand and take a wide stance with the toes of the kettlebell side turned out. Hinge at your hips, keeping your top arm extended and eyes looking up. Lower the kettlebell close to the inside of your leg. Without bending your arms, raise and lower the kettlebell repeatedly, focusing on keeping a flat back and legs straight throughout. This variation emphasizes inner thigh and hamstring mobility.

199. Double Windmill

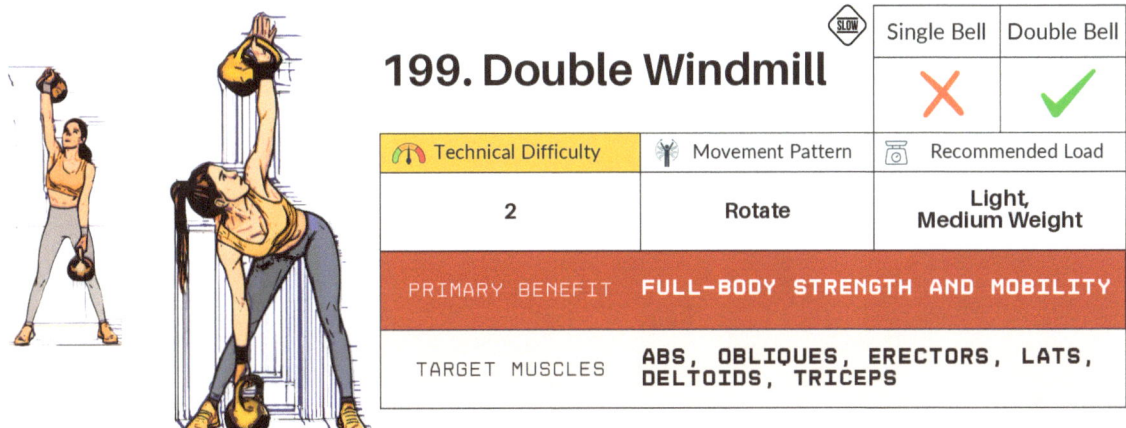

	SLOW	Single Bell	Double Bell
		✗	✓

Technical Difficulty	Movement Pattern	Recommended Load
2	Rotate	Light, Medium Weight

PRIMARY BENEFIT	FULL-BODY STRENGTH AND MOBILITY
TARGET MUSCLES	ABS, OBLIQUES, ERECTORS, LATS, DELTOIDS, TRICEPS

Hold one kettlebell overhead and one in the opposite hand at your side. With your feet set wide and the foot on the lower-bell side turned out, hinge at the hips and lower toward the floor. Aim to stack the kettlebells vertically when the low bell is on the ground. Allow your torso to rotate naturally. Move slowly— especially during the rising, emphasizing core stability and hip mobility.

PROKETTLEBELL.COM/199

200. Windmill Cleans

PROKETTLEBELL.COM/200

	SLOW	Single Bell	Double Bell
		✓	✗

Technical Difficulty	Movement Pattern	Recommended Load
3	Rotate	Heavy Weight

PRIMARY BENEFIT	FULL-BODY STRENGTH AND MOBILITY
TARGET MUSCLES	QUADRICEPS, GLUTES, HAMSTRINGS, ERECTORS, BICEPS, DELTOIDS, TRICEPS

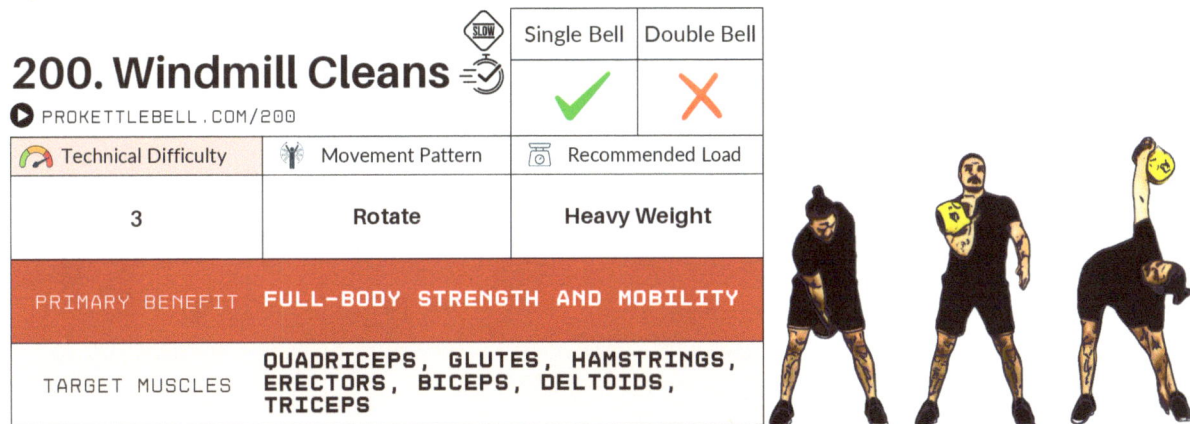

Start with a kettlebell in the rack position. Press the kettlebell overhead while immediately hinging at the hips into a windmill, allowing your free hand to slide down the inside of your leg. At the bottom position, aim to stack the kettlebell vertically over the shoulder with both shoulders aligned. Reverse the hinge to return to standing with the kettlebell still overhead, then lower it back to the rack to reset. Clean and repeat. Move slowly and deliberately, prioritizing shoulder stacking, control, and stable overhead positioning.

WINDMILLS

Full-Body & Compound Movements
Power & Conditioning

---------- Section Four ----------

Swings
Cleans
Snatches
Jerks

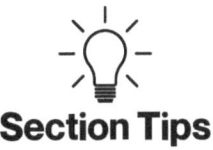

Section Tips

Learn the ballistic exercises in this chapter in sequence as follows:
Level-1 swings, level-1 cleans, level-1 snatches, level-1 jerks.
Develop comfort & muscle-memory prior to layering in levels 2 and 3.

**Recommended Sequence for Learning the
Two-Hand Kettlebell Swing:**

#202. Single-Hand Outside Swing
#214. Single Inside Swing
#206. Alternating Swing
#204. Two-Hand Swing

Power & Conditioning

1: Swings

Gunslinger	93
Single Hand Outside Swing	93
Figure-8s	93
Two Hand Swing	94
Alternating Lateral Swing	94
Alternating Swing	94
Battering Ram Swings (Crossbody)	95
Dropslingers	95
Float Swing	95
High Pull	96
Lat-Pull Swings	96
Rotational Swings (Golf Swing)	96
Scoop Swings	97
Single Kettlebell Inside Swing	97
Double Swings, Outside & Inside	97
Single-Arm Staggered Swing	98
Stop Swing	98
Step-Out Stop Swings	98
Swing + High Knee	99
Swinging Bottoms-Up Lunges	99
Backward Gunslingers	99
Side-Hop Swing	100
One-Arm Squat Swing	100
Walking Swings, Two-Hand	100

2: Cleans

Fireman Clean	101
Horn Clean	101
Horn Clean > Walkout Push-Up	101
Horn Clean + Press	102
Horn Clean + Squat Pulse	102
Sledgehammer Cleans	102
Bottoms Up-Cleans	103
Cleans, One-Arm	103
Cleans, Two-Arm	103
Curtsy Cleans	104
Dead Clean + High Knee	104
Dead Clean, One-Arm	104
Gorilla Cleans	105
Horn Clean + Tip Toe Squat	105
Horn Clean Squat Jack	105
Kneeling Clean	106
Kneeling Outside Cleans	106
Outside Clean + French Press	106
Outside Swing + Clean	107
Reverse Lunge Cleans	107
Split Lunge Dead Clean	107
Split Stance Dead Clean	108
Stop Clean	108
Walking Hang Cleans	108
Figure-8 Clean	109
Speed-Switch Swing n' Clean	109

3. Snatches

Assisted Hang Snatch	110
Bottoms-Up Snatch	110
Double Hand-Insertion Drill	110
Half-Snatch	111
Lo/Hi Swing-to-Snatch	111
Reverse Lunge Snatch	111
Snatch	112
Stop Snatch	112
Stop Snatch + Overhead Squat	112
Alternating Snatch	113
Speed-Switch Snatch	113
Curtsy Snatch	113
Double Half-Snatch	114
Double Snatch	114
Figure-8 Half-Snatch	114
Figure-8 Snatch	115
Stop Swing Switch-Snatch	115
Survival Snatch (Hang Snatch)	115

4. Jerks

3-Position Drill (2-Hand)	116
Jerk, Two-Hand	116
Bumps	116
Double 3-Position Drill	117
Jerk, One-Arm	117
Jerk, Two-Arm	117
Long Cycle (Clean + Jerk)	118
Speed-Switch Long Cycle	118
Split Jerk	118

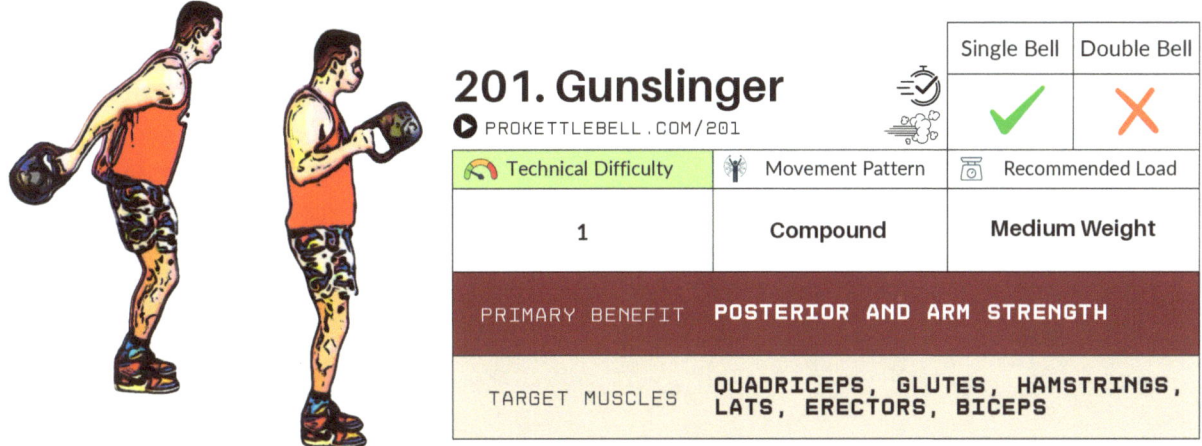

201. Gunslinger
● PROKETTLEBELL.COM/201

	Single Bell	Double Bell
	✓	✗

Technical Difficulty	Movement Pattern	Recommended Load
1	Compound	Medium Weight

PRIMARY BENEFIT	POSTERIOR AND ARM STRENGTH
TARGET MUSCLES	QUADRICEPS, GLUTES, HAMSTRINGS, LATS, ERECTORS, BICEPS

Feet together, thumb pointed upward throughout, begin with a single hand outside swing. As the bell rises in front of you, row it back toward your hip like holstering a pistol. Keep your elbow tight to your body. Once your hand reaches your body, push it forward to reinitiate the swing. Maintain tight control through the lats and biceps.

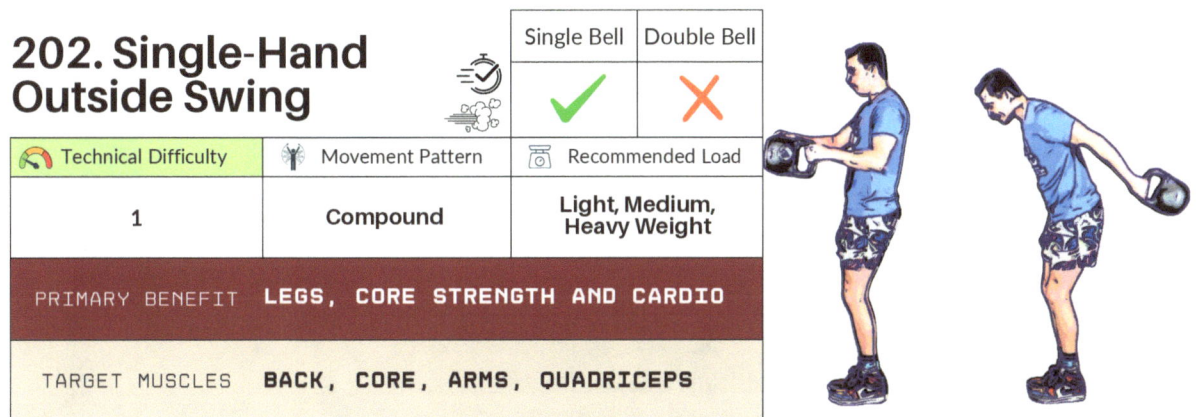

202. Single-Hand Outside Swing

	Single Bell	Double Bell
	✓	✗

Technical Difficulty	Movement Pattern	Recommended Load
1	Compound	Light, Medium, Heavy Weight

PRIMARY BENEFIT	LEGS, CORE STRENGTH AND CARDIO
TARGET MUSCLES	BACK, CORE, ARMS, QUADRICEPS

Stand with feet closer together and the kettlebell positioned outside your foot. Pick it up and swing it on the outside of your body, allowing full arc in both the front and back swing. Let the arm fully extend at the bottom, with a slight elbow bend at the top. Keep the bell close to the hip and hinge forward as the bell passes behind you. The free hand should mirror the kettlebell's path on the opposite side. ● PROKETTLEBELL.COM/202

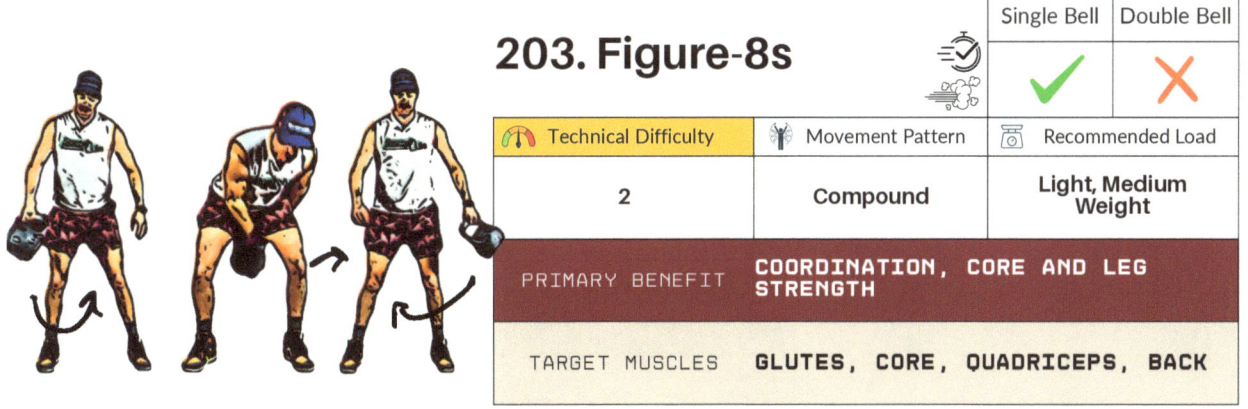

203. Figure-8s

	Single Bell	Double Bell
	✓	✗

Technical Difficulty	Movement Pattern	Recommended Load
2	Compound	Light, Medium Weight

PRIMARY BENEFIT	COORDINATION, CORE AND LEG STRENGTH
TARGET MUSCLES	GLUTES, CORE, QUADRICEPS, BACK

The figure eight swing involves passing the kettlebell in a figure-eight motion between your legs. Begin in a slightly wider than usual stance to allow the kettlebell to pass through the highest point between your thighs. Maintain a flat lumbar spine and upright chest. Keep your hips back and ensure the kettlebell handle stays above the knees. Avoid rounding your back. Variations including staying low or standing up between passes or contrasting passing the bell front-to-back with the reverse (behind-to-front). ● PROKETTLEBELL.COM/203

204. Two-Hand Swing

	Single Bell	Double Bell
	✓	✗

Technical Difficulty	Movement Pattern	Recommended Load
2	Compound	Light, Medium, Heavy Weight

PRIMARY BENEFIT	LEGS AND CORE STRENGTH
TARGET MUSCLES	HAMSTRINGS, GLUTES, QUADRICEPS, ERECTORS, FOREARMS

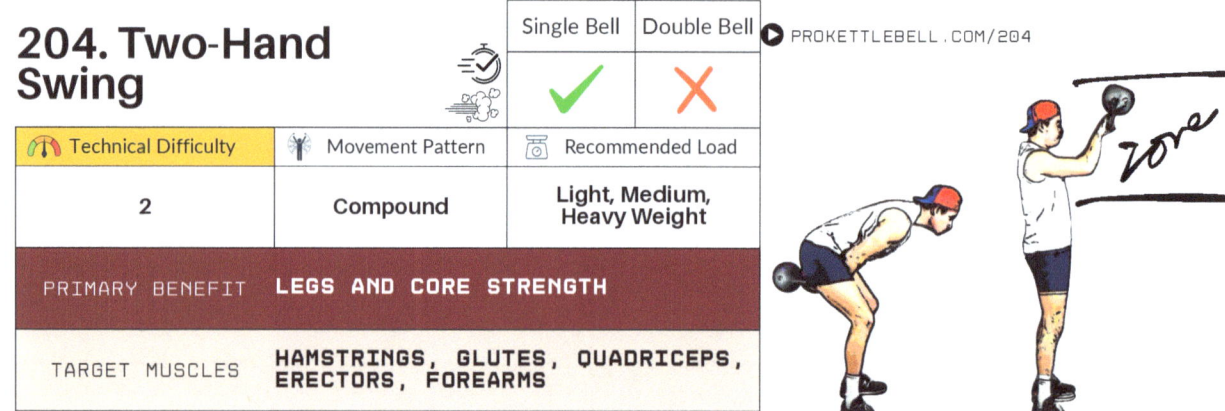

PROKETTLEBELL.COM/204

Start in an athletic stance with the kettlebell 12–18 inches in front of you. With a flat spine and heels grounded, sit low and hook your fingers around the handle. Hike the kettlebell high between your legs (using your lats). When the bell is as far back as it can go, drive through your legs to stand and accelerate the bell upward. Guide the kettlebell close to your body, and as it drops, wait until your arms reconnect with your torso before hinging forward. Always keep your wrists as high as possible when passing either direction between your legs, and don't hinge forward too soon! Let the legs and bodyweight do the work—they're the engine, your arms are just the steering wheel.

205. Alternating Lateral Swing

	Single Bell	Double Bell
	✓	✓

Technical Difficulty	Movement Pattern	Recommended Load
2	Compound	Light, Medium Weight

PRIMARY BENEFIT	FULL-BODY STRENGTH AND COORDINATION
TARGET MUSCLES	QUADRICEPS, GLUTES, HAMSTRINGS, ERECTORS, LATS

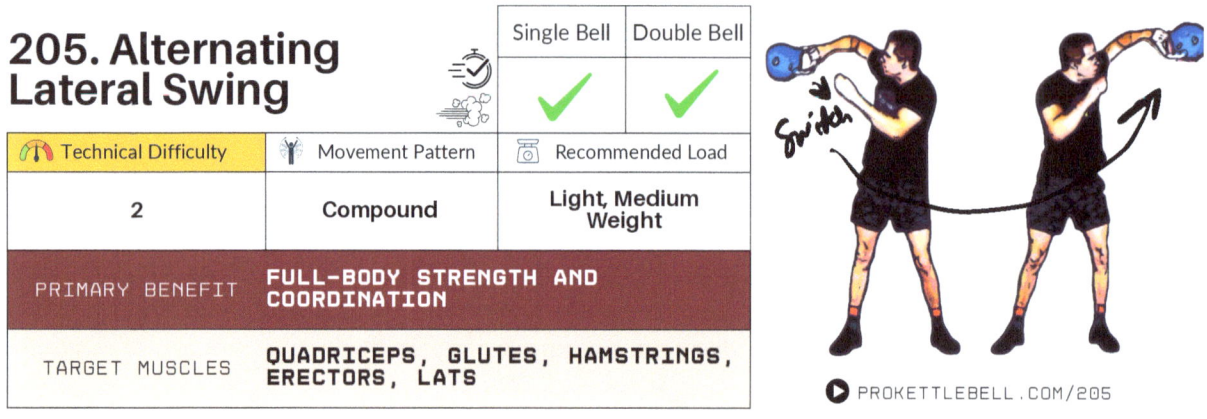

PROKETTLEBELL.COM/205

Set up with a wide, athletic stance (knees slightly bent, hips back). Swing the bell back and forth in front of you in a "U" shaped path, switching hands at the top of each swing. Stay slightly more upright than you would for golf swings (#212) and keep your eyes on the kettlebell throughout the movement. Avoid grazing your knees. Focus on core engagement. Perform in an environment where it's safe to let go of the kettlebell if you feel you might lose control. Swing higher and wider for increased challenge.

206. Alternating Swing

	Single Bell	Double Bell
	✓	✗

Technical Difficulty	Movement Pattern	Recommended Load
2	Compound	Light, Medium Weight

PRIMARY BENEFIT	LEGS AND CORE STRENGTH
TARGET MUSCLES	HAMSTRINGS, GLUTES, QUADRICEPS, ERECTORS, FOREARMS

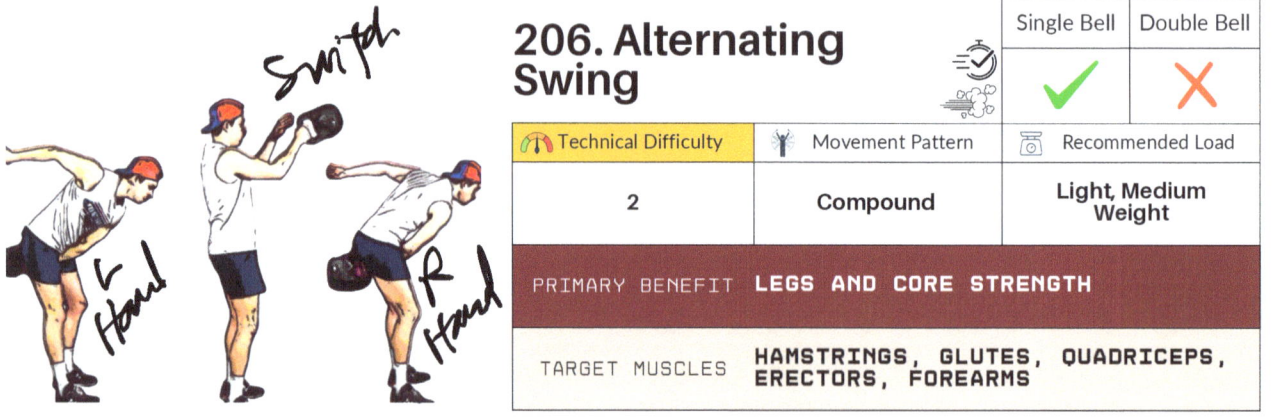

Begin with a standard single hand swing and switch hands at the top of each rep. Keep the kettlebell close to your body to control momentum and make the hand switch smoother. Follow all swing fundamentals including arm-body contact when the weight is under your hips and counterbalancing when it isn't. If the hand-switch doesn't feel safe, it's better to let go of the kettlebell than risk injury. PROKETTLEBELL.COM/206

207. Battering Ram Swings (Crossbody)

	Single Bell	Double Bell
	✓	✗

Technical Difficulty	Movement Pattern	Recommended Load
2	Compound	Light, Medium Weight

PRIMARY BENEFIT	FULL-BODY STRENGTH
TARGET MUSCLES	QUADRICEPS, GLUTES, HAMSTRINGS, ERECTORS, LATS, OBLIQUES, DELTOIDS, BICEPS, TRICEPS

▶ PROKETTLEBELL.COM/207

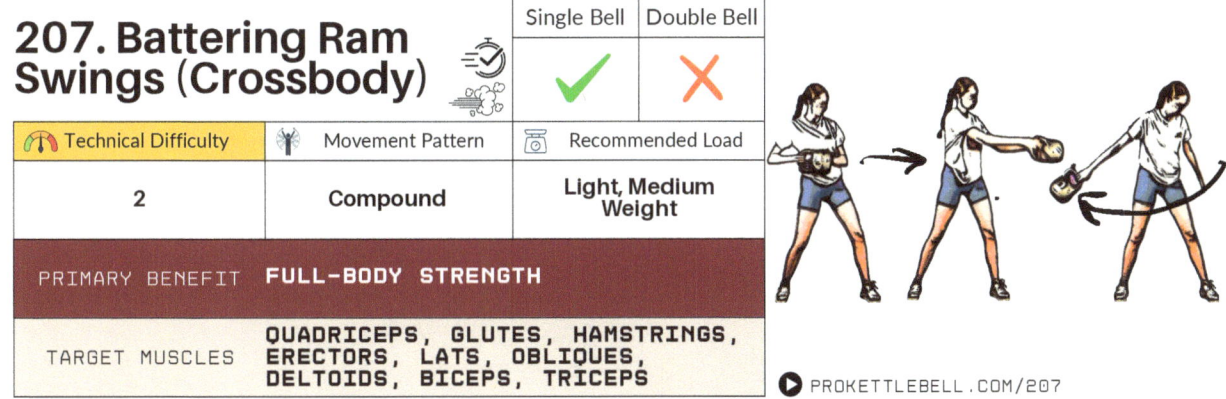

Assume a wide, grounded stance and swing the kettlebell laterally across your body. At the apex of the swing, catch it underneath with your free hand and pull it back using your lats, keeping the elbow close to the body. Then, push straight forward with both hands as if ramming a door. Release the bottom hand and let the bell fall into the swing again and repeat before switching sides. Maintain a flat lumbar spine flat, chest up, and avoid hitting your knees. This swing is ideal for building rotational strength and mimics tactical movement patterns.

208. Drop Slingers

▶ PROKETTLEBELL.COM/208

	Single Bell	Double Bell
	✓	✓

Technical Difficulty	Movement Pattern	Recommended Load
2	Compound	Light, Medium Weight

PRIMARY BENEFIT	LOWER BODY STRENGTH AND CONDITIONING
TARGET MUSCLES	QUADRICEPS, GLUTES, HAMSTRINGS, ERECTORS, LATS, BICEPS

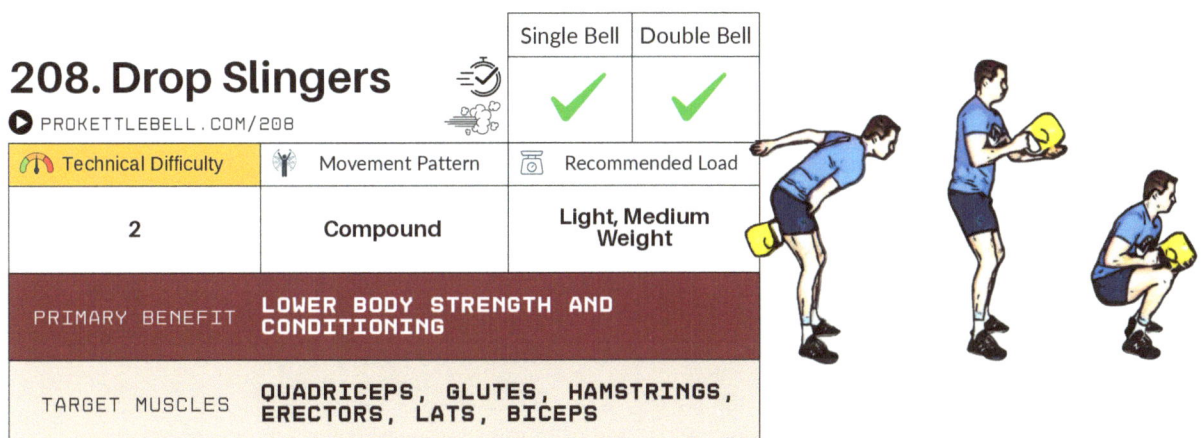

Start in your standard swing stance. As you hike the kettlebell back, swing it up and row the arm back tightly to your lats. Catch the bell's base with your free hand (on the outside of your body) while simultaneously dropping into a squat. Keep heels down, knees tracking toes, chest up, and lumbar flat. This compound movement targets both lower and upper body, emphasizing coordination and timing between the pull and squat.

209. Float Swing

▶ PROKETTLEBELL.COM/209

	Single Bell	Double Bell
	✓	✗

Technical Difficulty	Movement Pattern	Recommended Load
2	Compound	Light, Medium Weight

PRIMARY BENEFIT	POSTERIOR STRENGTH, CONDITIONING AND TECHNIQUE
TARGET MUSCLES	GLUTES, HAMSTRINGS, QUADRICEPS, ERECTORS, LATS, BICEPS

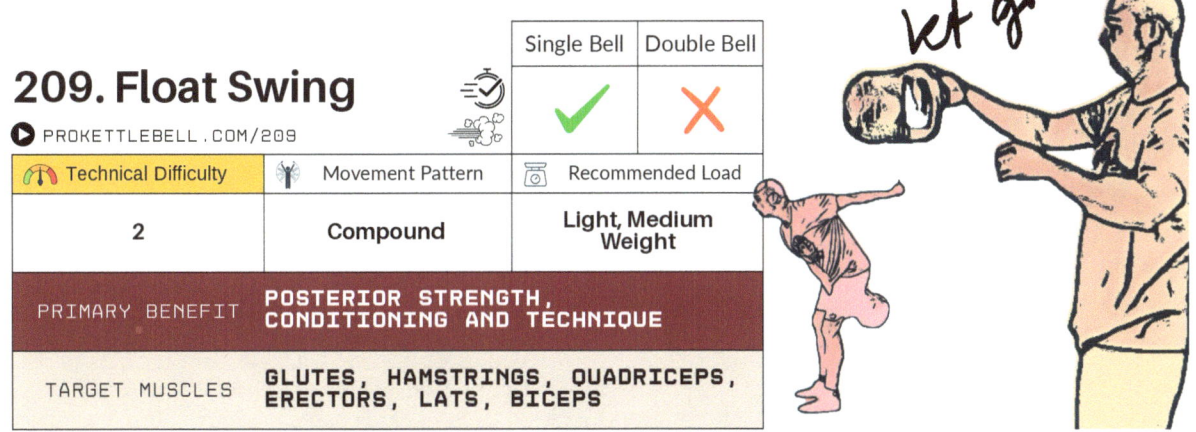

Start with a traditional one-arm swing. Keep the bell traveling on a vertical path as it rises from the hips. At chest height, briefly release the handle, then quickly regrip and guide the bell back into the downswing. The free arm tracks alongside the bell on the outside of the body. This drill builds timing, coordination, and confidence in the float phase, making it an excellent progression toward the snatch.

SWINGS

210. High Pull

PROKETTLEBELL.COM/210

	Single Bell	Double Bell
	✓	✗

Technical Difficulty	Movement Pattern	Recommended Load
2	Compound	Light, Medium Weight

PRIMARY BENEFIT	LEG, BACK, CORE AND ARM STRENGTH
TARGET MUSCLES	GLUTES, HAMSTRINGS, QUADRICEPS, ERECTORS, OBLIQUES, LATS, REAR DELTOIDS

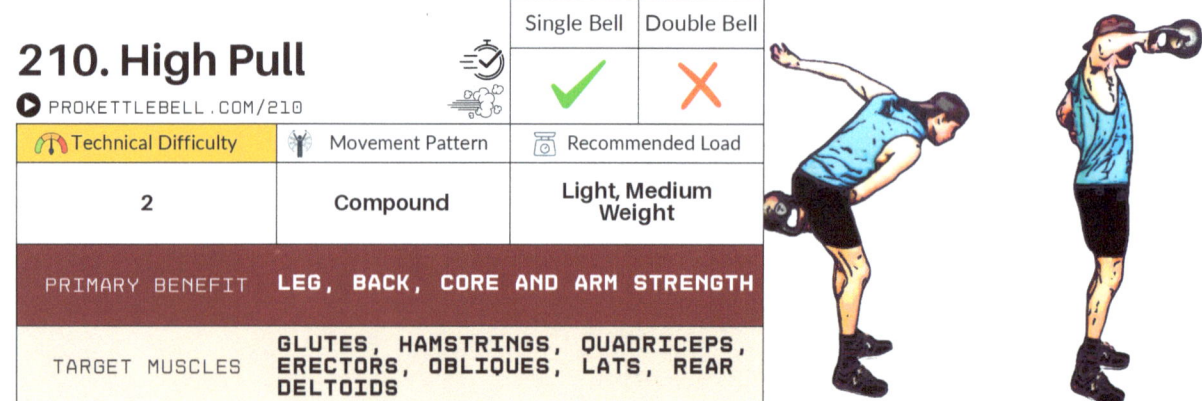

Start with a single hand swing. As the kettlebell nears shoulder height, row the elbow back until the shoulder, elbow, and hand align horizontally. To return to the swing, guide the kettlebell forward in a smooth arc. Avoid allowing the bell to flop. Keep the elbow high at the top of the pull. Maintain all standard swing fundamentals, especially arm-body contact and counterbalancing. The high pull enhances shoulder and upper back engagement.

211. Lat Pull Swings

	Single Bell	Double Bell
	✓	✗

Technical Difficulty	Movement Pattern	Recommended Load
2	Compound	Light, Medium Weight

PRIMARY BENEFIT	FULL-BODY STRENGTH
TARGET MUSCLES	QUADRICEPS, GLUTES, HAMSTRINGS, ERECTORS, LATS

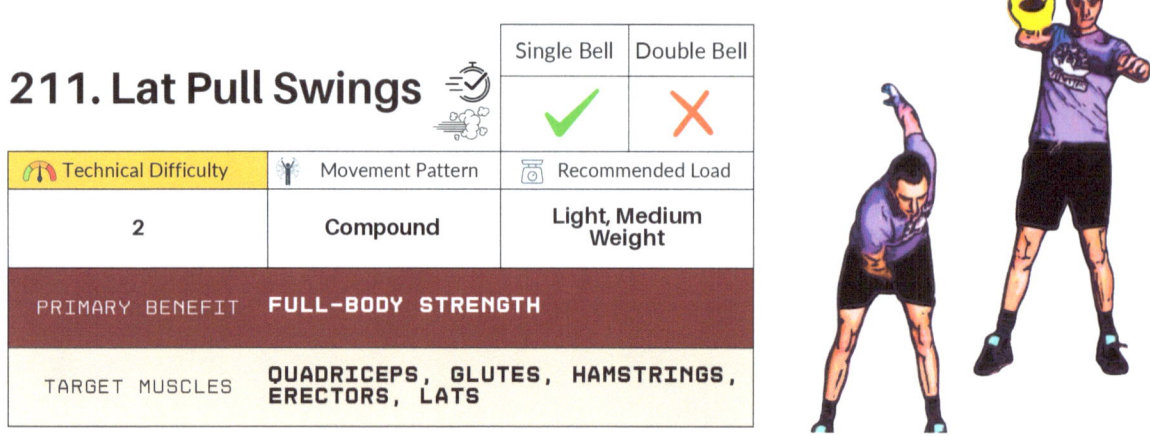

Swing the kettlebell with a straighter arm and rotate the torso toward the kettlebell during the downswing. As the bell rises, counter-rotate the torso and pull the shoulder back to accelerate the kettlebell. Focus on squeezing the lats. This move adds rotational tension and increases lat and oblique involvement compared to traditional swings.

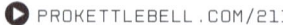

PROKETTLEBELL.COM/211

212. Rotational (Golf) Swings

	Single Bell	Double Bell
	✓	✗

Technical Difficulty	Movement Pattern	Recommended Load
2	Compound	Light, Medium Weight

PRIMARY BENEFIT	FULL-BODY, CORE AND ROTATIONAL STRENGTH
TARGET MUSCLES	QUADRICEPS, GLUTES, HAMSTRINGS, ABS, OBLIQUES, ERECTORS, LATS

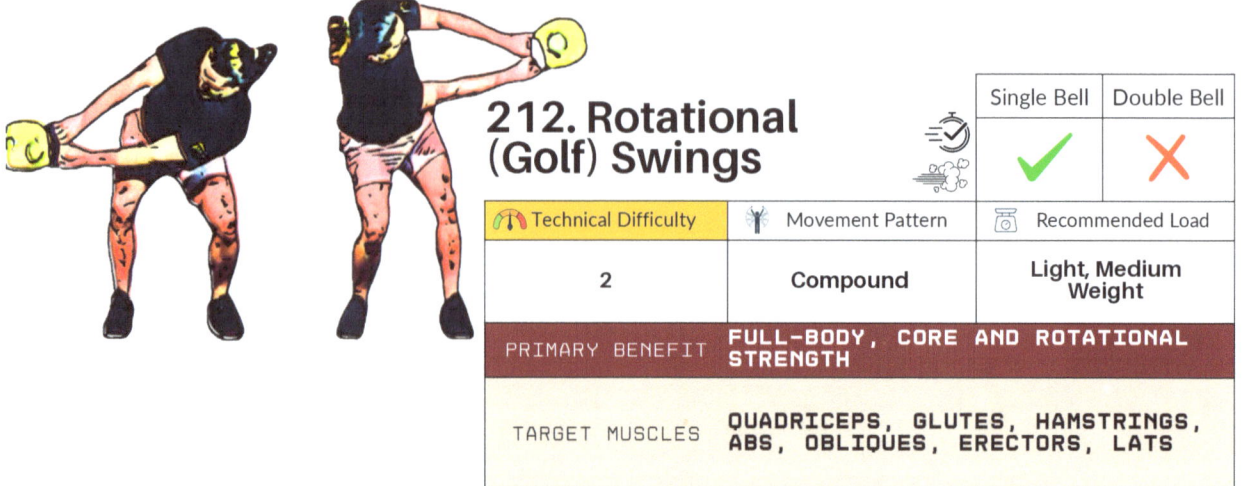

("Golf Swings") Place the kettlebell just in front of your toes. With bent knees, hips back, and a flat lumbar spine, hike the kettlebell laterally from side to side, rotating the trunk and hips (similar to a golf swing), moving the right pocket to the left as you twist and vice versa. Keep the chest up and the lumbar spine flat. Use a lighter kettlebell than usual and let your gaze follow the bell to maintain coordination and control.

PROKETTLEBELL.COM/212

213. Scoop Swings

PROKETTLEBELL.COM/213

	Single Bell	Double Bell
	✓	✓

Technical Difficulty	Movement Pattern	Recommended Load
2	Compound	Medium, Heavy Weight

PRIMARY BENEFIT	LEG AND POSTERIOR STRENGTH
TARGET MUSCLES	QUADRICEPS, GLUTES, HAMSTRINGS, ERECTORS, LATS

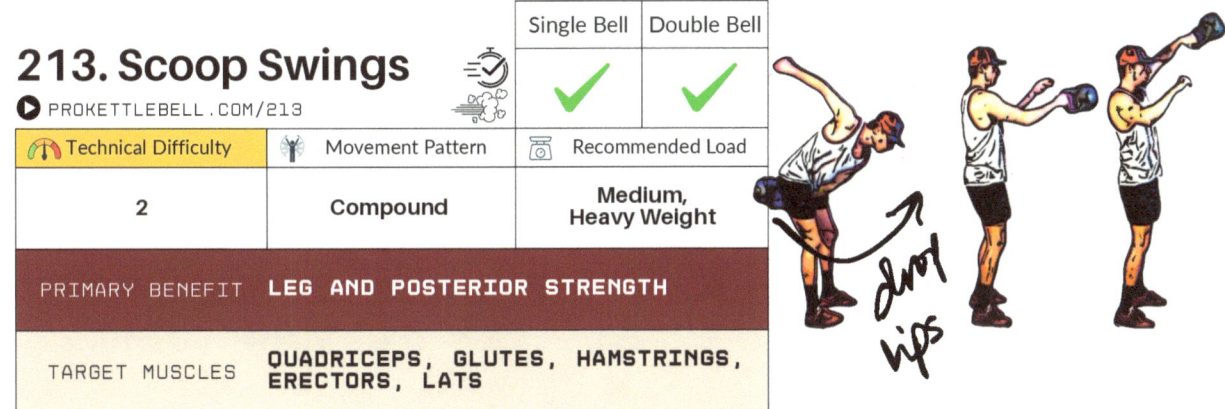

drop hips

Start in your single arm swing stance. As the kettlebell transitions out of the backswing, drop your hips low to scoop, creating a J-shaped swing arc. This move emphasizes vertical lift and recruits more from your quads. Maintain standard swing form, especially arm-body contact and hip engagement. You can adjust stance or add flair once comfortable, including flips or extended float time.

214. Single Kettlebell Inside Swing

	Single Bell	Double Bell
	✓	✗

Technical Difficulty	Movement Pattern	Recommended Load
2	Compound	Medium, Heavy Weight

PRIMARY BENEFIT	LEG, CORE STRENGTH AND CARDIO
TARGET MUSCLES	GLUTES, QUADRICEPS, HAMSTRINGS, ERECTORS, OBLIQUES

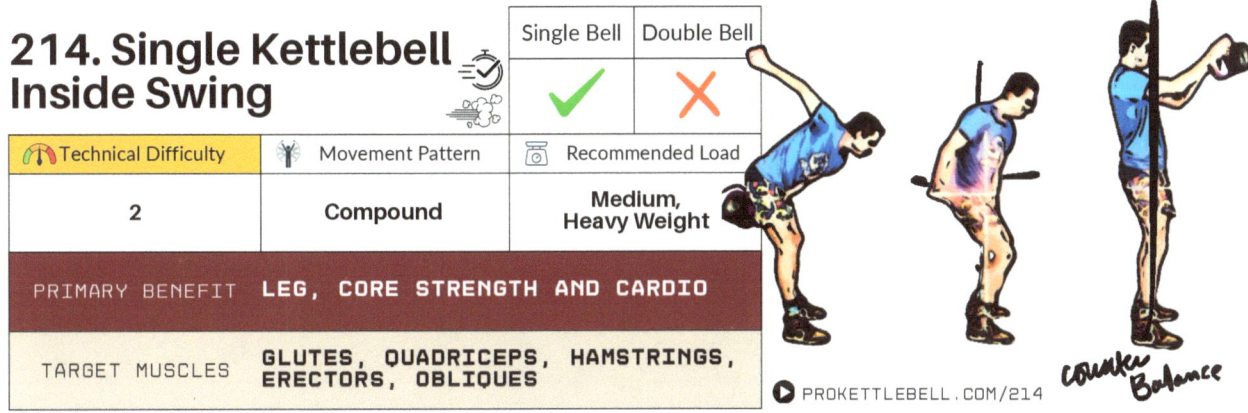

counter balance

PROKETTLEBELL.COM/214

Start with a single kettlebell placed directly in front of you. Hike it between your legs and swing it through the center of the body, hinging forward only after the arm contacts the torso. Keep the kettlebell high between the legs, never allowing it to drop below the knees. Keep weight in the heels and squeeze the glutes as you drive the kettlebell upward. The free arm stays relaxed, shadowing the movement. Maintain a neutral lumbar spine and bring the hips fully forward as you stand tall at the top of each repetition.

215. Double Swings, Outside & Inside

	Single Bell	Double Bell
	✗	✓

Technical Difficulty	Movement Pattern	Recommended Load
2	Compound	Medium, Heavy Weight

PRIMARY BENEFIT	FULL-BODY STRENGTH AND CONDITIONING
TARGET MUSCLES	QUADRICEPS, GLUTES, HAMSTRINGS, ERECTORS

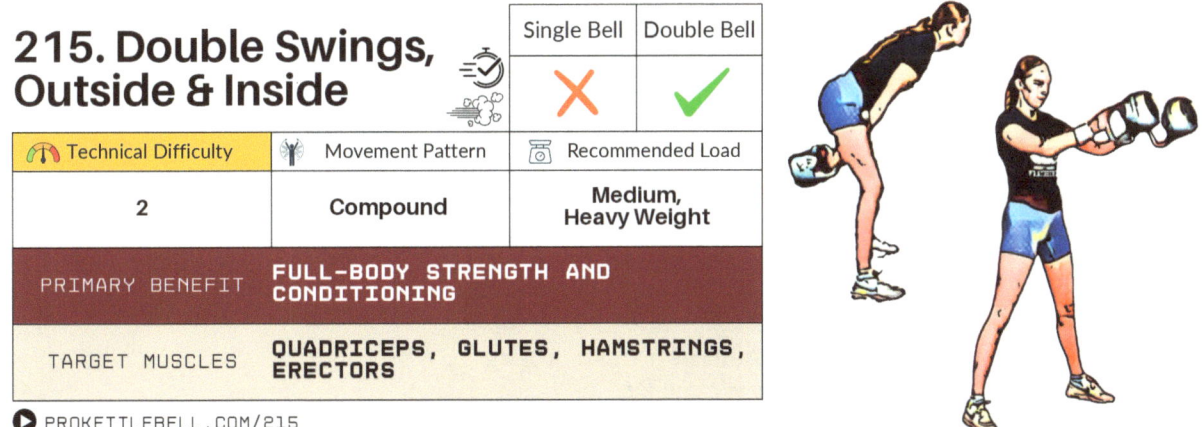

PROKETTLEBELL.COM/215

While single-arm swings use a shoulder-width (or slightly wider), often asymmetrical stance, double swings require symmetry and stance adjustments. For double inside swings (bells traveling between the legs), use a wider-than-normal stance, but only as wide as necessary. For outside swings (bells moving simultaneously outside the body), keep the feet closer together to allow hip clearance, carefully avoiding contact with the hips or knees. Both variations build strength and coordination and allow increased volume using two light to medium kettlebells.

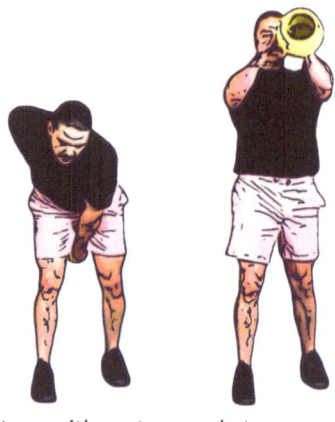

216. Single-Arm Staggered Swing

	Single Bell	Double Bell
	✓	✗

Technical Difficulty	Movement Pattern	Recommended Load
2	Compound	Medium, Heavy Weight

PRIMARY BENEFIT	ANTI-ROTATIONAL CORE STRENGTH
TARGET MUSCLES	QUADRICEPS, GLUTES, HAMSTRINGS, ERECTORS, LATS

Set up with a staggered stance opposite your usual side (left-hand swing, right foot forward). Swing the kettlebell backward, high between the legs (always maintaining arm-body contact when the bell is beneath your hips) and initiate the upswing with glute engagement and heel-drive through the back leg. The staggered stance challenges balance and corrects imbalances common in traditional single arm swings. The free arm may shadow the kettlebell to assist with momentum and rhythm. ▶ PROKETTLEBELL.COM/216

217. Stop Swing
▶ PROKETTLEBELL.COM/217

	Single Bell	Double Bell
	✓	✗

Technical Difficulty	Movement Pattern	Recommended Load
2	Compound	Medium, Heavy Weight

PRIMARY BENEFIT	POSTERIOR STRENGTH AND EXPLOSIVENESS
TARGET MUSCLES	GLUTES, QUADRICEPS, HAMSTRINGS, LATS

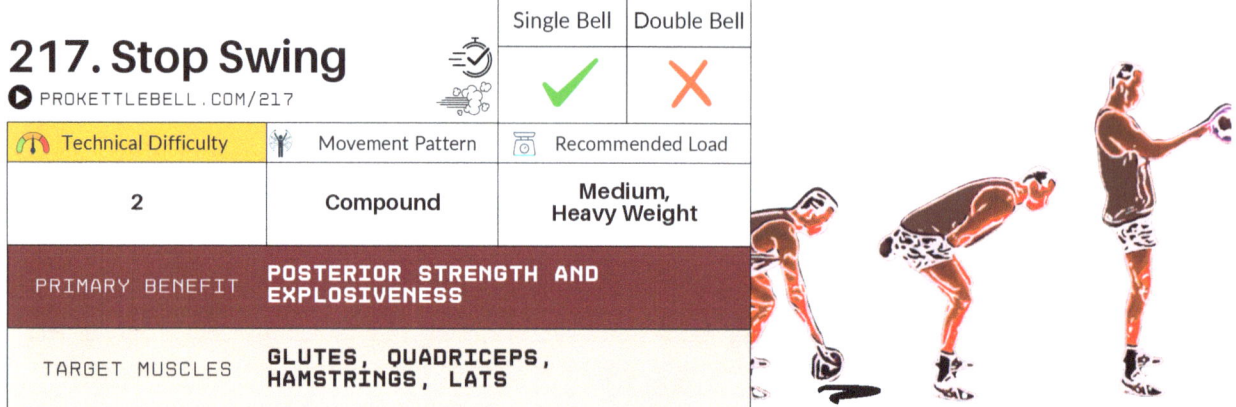

With both hands on the handle, hike the kettlebell back and swing it up to chest or shoulder height. On the subsequent backswing, drop your hips, keep your weight back, and maintain a flat lumbar spine as you guide the bell back to the ground in front of you. Unlike continuous swings, breaking the momentum after each rep increases engagement of the lats, glutes, and hamstrings. Use a slightly wider stance to allow a clean pass between the legs while preserving lumbar integrity.

218. Step-Out Stop Swings

	Single Bell	Double Bell
	✓	✗

Technical Difficulty	Movement Pattern	Recommended Load
2	Compound	Light, Medium Weight

PRIMARY BENEFIT	POSTERIOR CHAIN STRENGTH AND CONDITIONING W/LATERAL COMPONENT
TARGET MUSCLES	QUADRICEPS, GLUTES, QUADRICEPS, HAMSTRINGS, ERECTORS, LATS

▶ PROKETTLEBELL.COM/218

Hike the kettlebell as in a traditional two-hand swing, using a slightly wider stance. As the bell floats upward, step laterally—bring the left foot in, then step the right foot out wide—timing the step during the float. Stand tall at the apex before guiding the bell into the downswing. Park the bell between reps. This can be done traveling in one direction for multiple reps or in place, alternating steps side to side each rep.

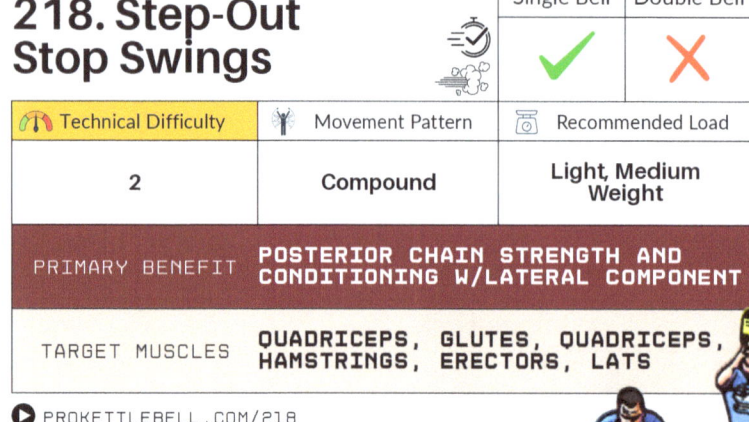

219. Swing + High Knee

	Single Bell	Double Bell
	✓	✗

Technical Difficulty	Movement Pattern	Recommended Load
2	Compound	Light, Medium Weight

PRIMARY BENEFIT	LOWER BODY, CORE STRENGTH AND CONDITIONING
TARGET MUSCLES	GLUTES, QUADRICEPS, HAMSTRINGS, ERECTORS

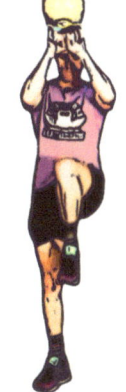

▶ PROKETTLEBELL.COM/219

Set up for a two-hand swing with the kettlebell 12–18 inches in front of you. As the bell swings up to chest height, lift one knee high. As the bell descends into the backswing, return your foot to the floor. You can alternate knees or focus on one side at a time. Maintain all swing non-negotiables including counterbalance and arm-body contact. This variation enhances glute engagement for that desirable kettlebooty, and coordination.

220. Swinging Bottoms-Up Lunge

	Single Bell	Double Bell
	✓	✗

Technical Difficulty	Movement Pattern	Recommended Load
2	Compound	Light, Medium, Heavy Weight

PRIMARY BENEFIT	LOWER BODY STRENGTH
TARGET MUSCLES	QUADRICEPS, GLUTES, HAMSTRINGS, ERECTORS, LATS, BICEPS

▶ PROKETTLEBELL.COM/220

Swing a kettlebell on the outside of your hip and freeze it in the bottoms-up position, with the bell vertical and stacked over your wrist and elbow. Lunge forward using the same leg as the kettlebell arm, then return to standing. Repeat on one side or alternate. Use a light kettlebell to test control prior to moving up in weight. For an extra challenge, begin the lunge during the swing rather than after.

221. Backward Gunslingers

	Single Bell	Double Bell
	✓	✗

Technical Difficulty	Movement Pattern	Recommended Load
3	Compound	Medium Weight

PRIMARY BENEFIT	FULL-BODY STRENGTH
TARGET MUSCLES	QUADRICEPS, GLUTES, HAMSTRINGS, LATS, ERECTORS, BICEPS

▶ PROKETTLEBELL.COM/221

Set up with your feet close together and the kettlebell outside one foot. Perform a single outside swing and as it reaches hip height, row it back like holstering a pistol. At full row, let it drop behind you, turn your palm, switch hands, and repeat on the other side. Focus on coordination, shoulder mobility, and maintaining strong form throughout. The backward row adds bicep and lat activation along with swing fundamentals.

SWINGS

222. Side-Hop Swing

PROKETTLEBELL.COM/222

	Single Bell	Double Bell
	✓	✗

Technical Difficulty	Movement Pattern	Recommended Load
3	Compound	Light, Medium, Heavy Weight

PRIMARY BENEFIT	FULL-BODY STRENGTH, COORDINATION AND CARDIO
TARGET MUSCLES	QUADRICEPS, GLUTES, HAMSTRINGS, ERECTORS, LATS

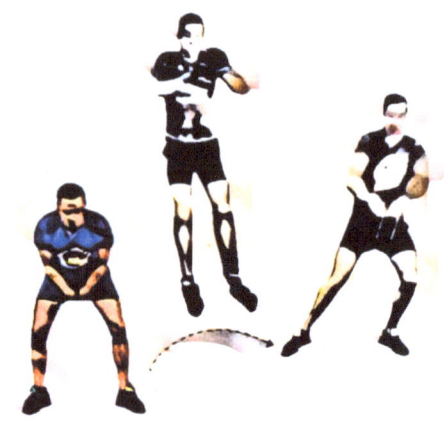

Set up for a two-hand swing. As the kettlebell floats upward, use that moment to move sideways, exchanging foot positions mid-air if traveling laterally. Maintain proper swing mechanics, especially counterbalancing and arm-body contact. The lateral movement should occur while the kettlebell is weightless to maintain stability. This variation adds a cardio and agility element while improving lateral coordination and leg drive.

223. Squat Swing

PROKETTLEBELL.COM/223

	Single Bell	Double Bell
	✓	✓

Technical Difficulty	Movement Pattern	Recommended Load
3	Compound	Light, Medium, Heavy Weight

PRIMARY BENEFIT	FULL-BODY STRENGTH WITH MORE EMPHASIS ON THE LEGS
TARGET MUSCLES	QUADRICEPS, GLUTES, HAMSTRINGS, ERECTORS

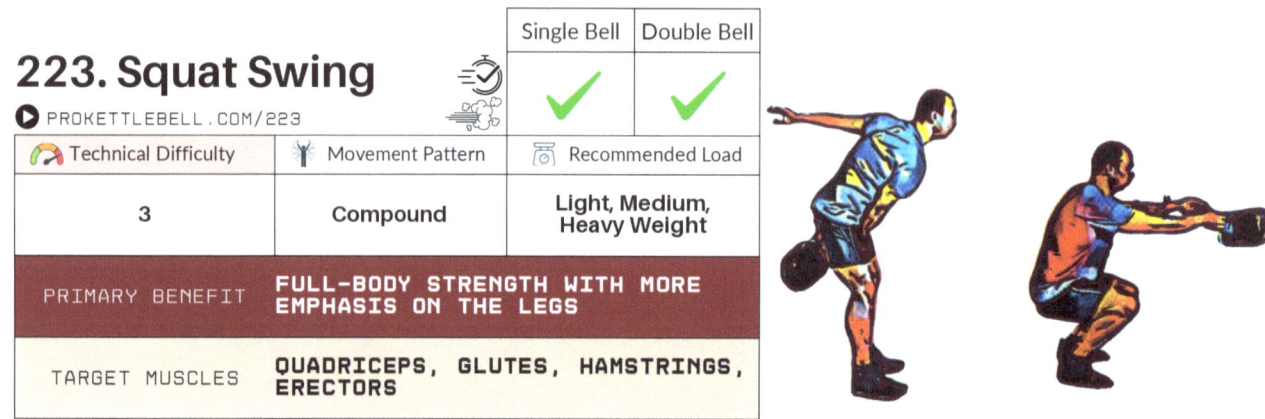

Swing the kettlebell. As the bell rises, squat, reaching the bottom of the squat as the kettlebell reaches the apex of the swing. *Do not begin the squat until the bell is weightless and flying upward.* Timing is critical. As the bell begins to descend, stand up quickly so you are fully upright before it passes your knees on the backswing, maintaining arm-body contact throughout the load phase. If needed, regress to a front-raise squat to build the strength, speed, and coordination required. Perform with one arm or two hands on one bell.

224. Walking Swings, Two-Hand

	Single Bell	Double Bell
	✓	✗

Technical Difficulty	Movement Pattern	Recommended Load
3	Compound	Light, Medium, Heavy Weight

PRIMARY BENEFIT	POSTERIOR AND QUAD STRENGTH
TARGET MUSCLES	QUADRICEPS, GLUTES, HAMSTRINGS, ERECTORS, LATS

PROKETTLEBELL.COM/224

Begin with the kettlebell on the ground 12-18 inches in front of you. Perform a regular two-hand swing, and as the kettlebell floats upward, step forward. Take one step per swing, when the bell is rising. You can walk by alternating legs or repeating on one leg at a time. Maintain all swing fundamentals including arm-body contact and proper counterbalance. The added movement engages your core and increases overall coordination.

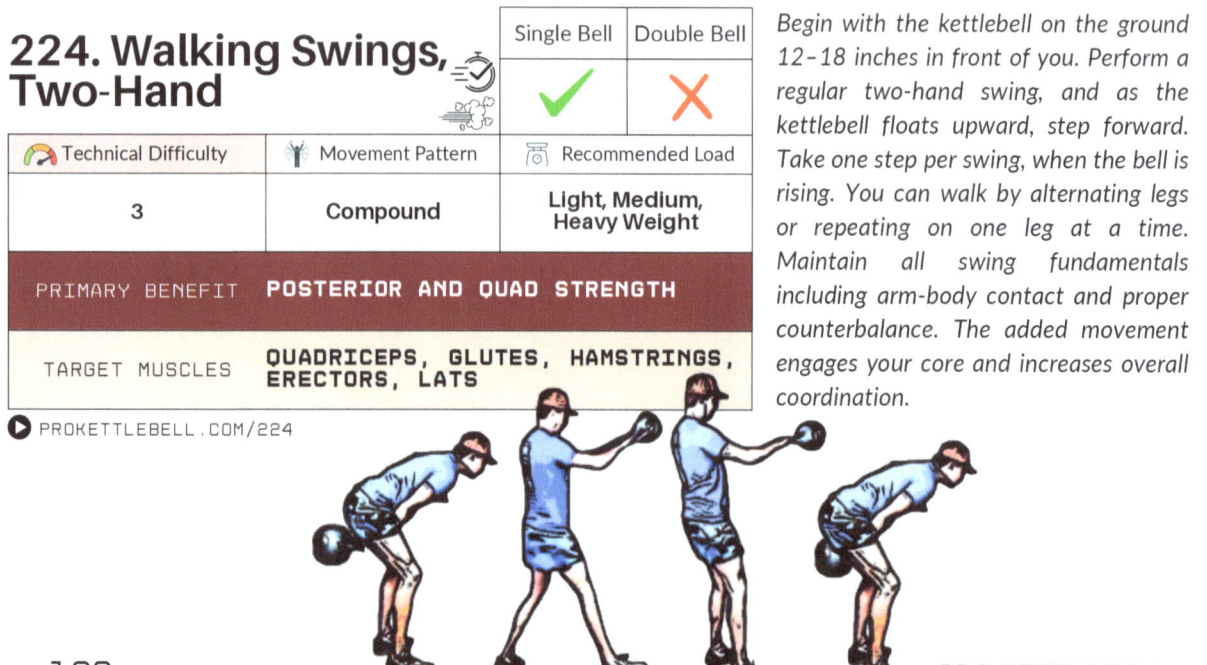

225. Fireman Clean

	Single Bell	Double Bell
	✓	✗

Technical Difficulty	Movement Pattern	Recommended Load
1	Compound	Heavy Weight

PRIMARY BENEFIT — ARM AND POSTERIOR STRENGTHS

TARGET MUSCLES — GLUTES, HAMSTRINGS, ERECTORS, BICEPS

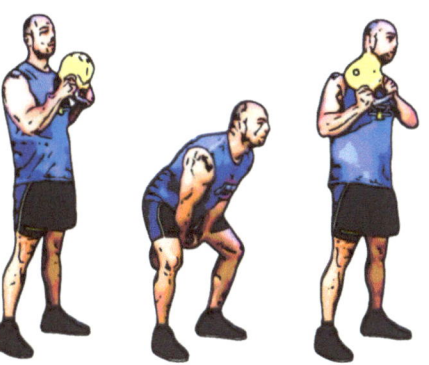

Hold the kettlebell bottom-side down by the horns. Use a swing-like ballistic motion to clean the kettlebell over each shoulder. Keep your arms tight to the ribs throughout the movement. Maintain a high swing path between the legs and avoid hitting your collarbone as you bring the bell over the shoulder. This clean develops explosive power in the legs, back, and biceps while reinforcing arm-body contact. ▶ PROKETTLEBELL.COM/225

226. Horn Clean

	Single Bell	Double Bell
	✓	✗

Technical Difficulty	Movement Pattern	Recommended Load
1	Compound	Medium, Heavy Weight

PRIMARY BENEFIT — POWER, TIMING AND COORDINATION

TARGET MUSCLES — GLUTES, HAMSTRINGS, QUADRICEPS, TRAPS, BICEPS, ERECTORS

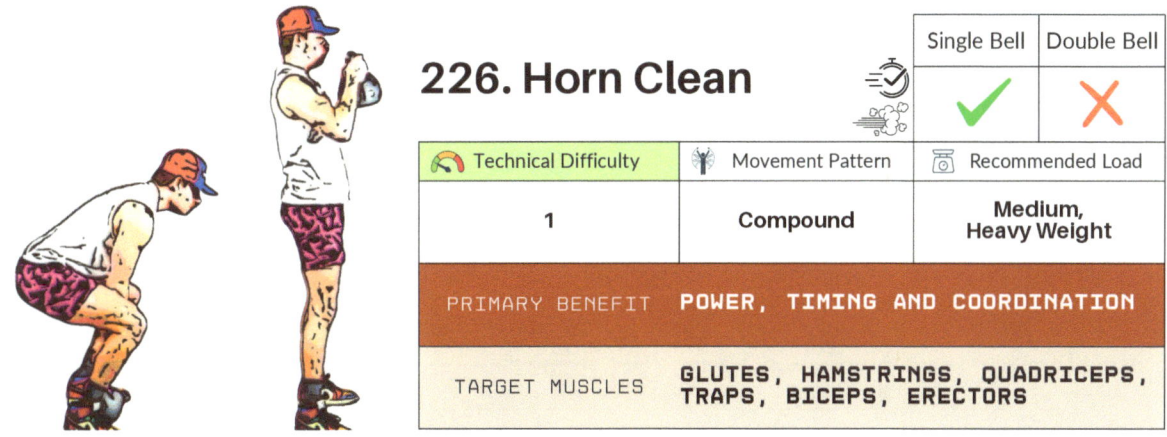

Stand over the kettlebell with the handle aligned across the balls of your feet. Drive through your hips and glutes, keeping arms straight. As the bell rises, shrug to create lift and catch it by the horns in front of your chest. Drop it close to the body and repeat. The bell should move in a straight line, staying tight to your frame. Maintain a flat back, upright chest, and explosive lower-body engagement. ▶ PROKETTLEBELL.COM/226

227. Horn Clean > Walkout Push-Up

	Single Bell	Double Bell
	✓	✗

Technical Difficulty	Movement Pattern	Recommended Load
1	Compound	Medium, Heavy Weight

▶ PROKETTLEBELL.COM/227

PRIMARY BENEFIT — FULL-BODY STRENGTH

TARGET MUSCLES — QUADRICEPS, GLUTES, HAMSTRINGS, ERECTORS, TRAPS, BICEPS, PECS, DELTOIDS, TRICEPS

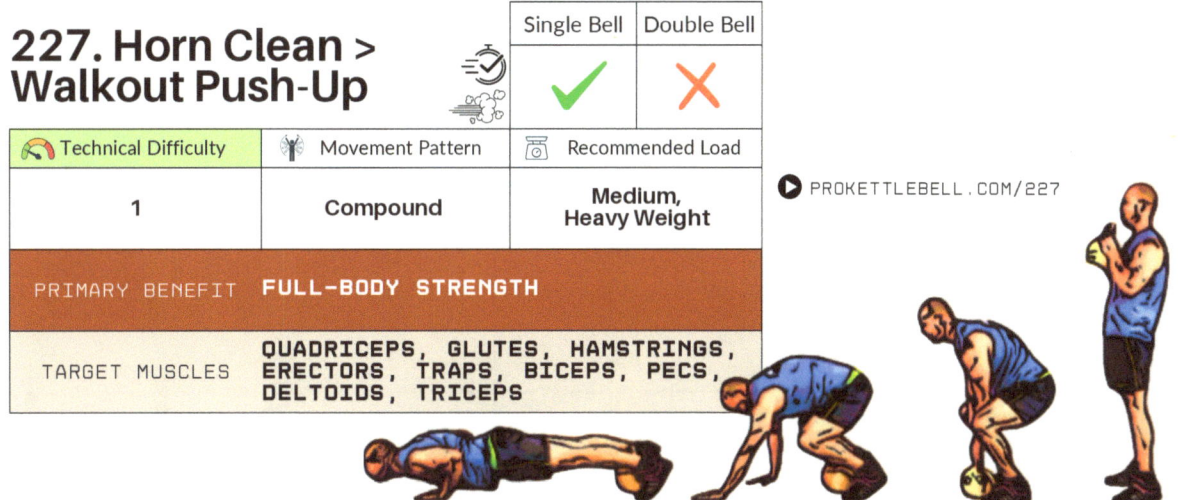

Start with a horn clean, catching the kettlebell by the horns. After lowering it between your feet, walk your hands out to a push-up position and complete a push-up. Walk your hands back to your feet and repeat the sequence. The movement integrates lower-body power, upper-body strength, and core stability in a continuous, full-body flow.

CLEANS

228. Horn Clean + Press

	Single Bell	Double Bell
	✓	✗

Technical Difficulty	Movement Pattern	Recommended Load
1	Compound	Medium, Heavy Weight

PRIMARY BENEFIT: FULL-BODY STRENGTH AND POWER

TARGET MUSCLES: QUADRICEPS, GLUTES, HAMSTRINGS, ERECTORS, DELTOIDS, TRICEPS

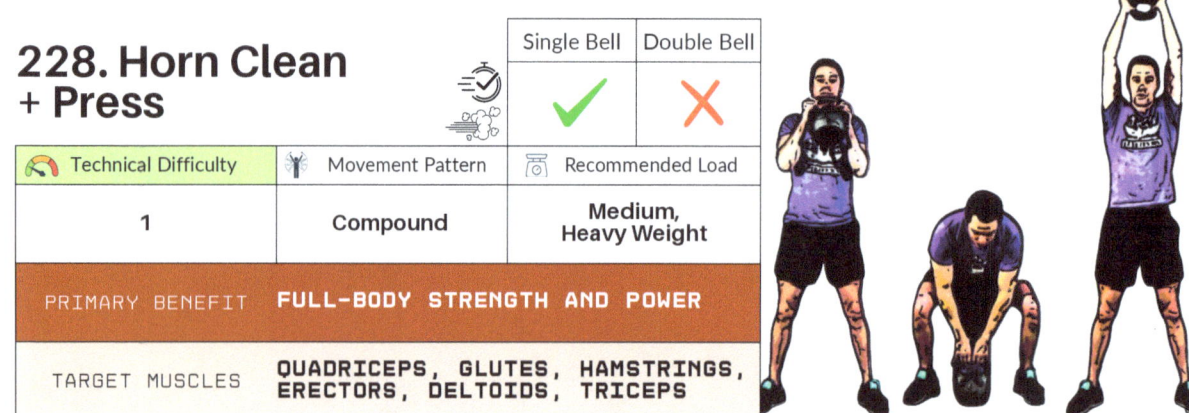

Perform a horn clean, catching the bell by the horns, then transition into a two-handed overhead press. Press until your arms are locked out overhead, then return the bell to the rack, then to the floor. The bell should move in a straight path. If the weight is heavy, you can modify by using a push press. This combo strengthens the legs, posterior chain, shoulders, and arms, integrating clean explosiveness with pressing control. ▶ PROKETTLEBELL.COM/228

229. Horn Clean + Squat Pulse

	Single Bell	Double Bell
	✓	✗

Technical Difficulty	Movement Pattern	Recommended Load
1	Compound	Medium, Heavy Weight

PRIMARY BENEFIT: FULL-BODY STRENGTH AND POWER

TARGET MUSCLES: QUADRICEPS, GLUTES, HAMSTRINGS, ERECTORS, LATS, DELTOIDS, BICEPS

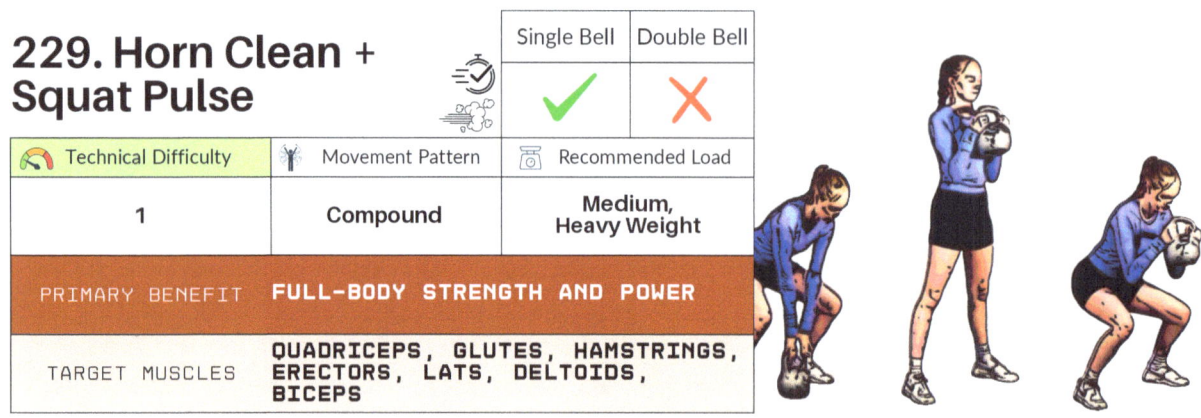

Start with the kettlebell behind the toes and perform a horn clean, catching it by the horns. Once in the rack, drop into a squat and perform a controlled pulse at the bottom for your desired count. Keep the lumbar flat, knees tracking toes, and the bell close to your centerline. This movement emphasizes lower-body endurance and strength by increasing time under tension, especially in the quads and glutes. ▶ PROKETTLEBELL.COM/229

230. Sledgehammer Cleans

	Single Bell	Double Bell
	✓	✗

Technical Difficulty	Movement Pattern	Recommended Load
1	Compound	Heavy Weight

PRIMARY BENEFIT: BICEPS AND POSTERIOR STRENGTH

TARGET MUSCLES: QUADRICEPS, GLUTES, HAMSTRINGS, ERECTORS, BICEPS

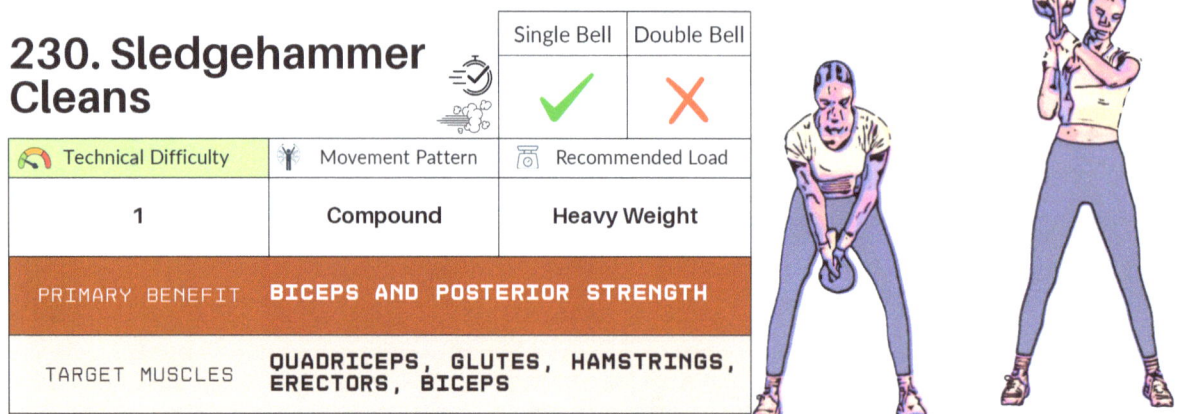

Hold the kettlebell like a sledgehammer, with hands stacked or using a golfer's grip for better control. Start with the bell between your legs and clean it over one shoulder in a swinging motion. Keep your arms close to your ribs and use your body weight to counterbalance. Alternate shoulders each rep, keeping control of the bell at the top. This exercise develops biceps and posterior chain explosiveness. ▶ PROKETTLEBELL.COM/230

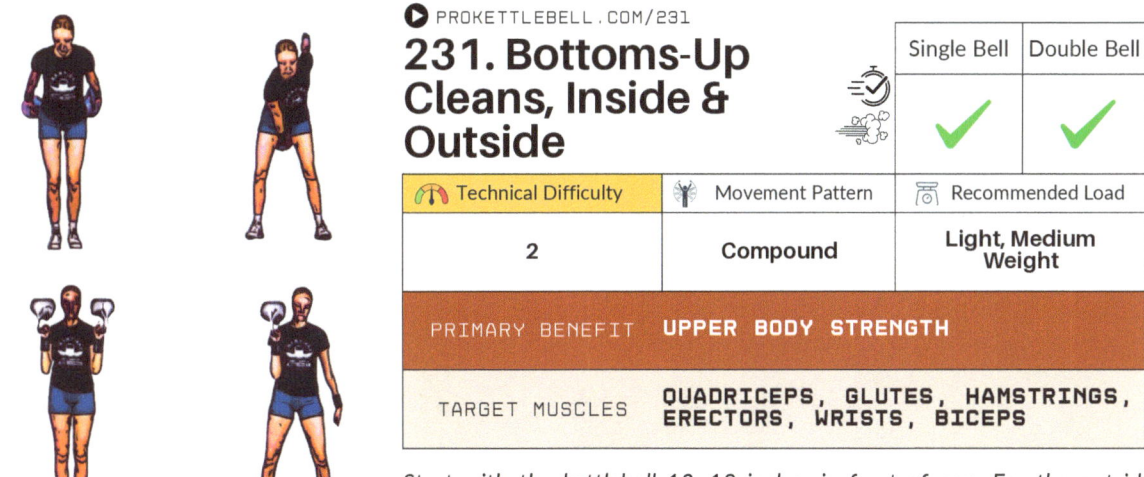

▶ PROKETTLEBELL.COM/231

231. Bottoms-Up Cleans, Inside & Outside

	Single Bell	Double Bell
	✓	✓

Technical Difficulty	Movement Pattern	Recommended Load
2	Compound	Light, Medium Weight

PRIMARY BENEFIT	UPPER BODY STRENGTH
TARGET MUSCLES	QUADRICEPS, GLUTES, HAMSTRINGS, ERECTORS, WRISTS, BICEPS

Start with the kettlebell 12–18 inches in front of you. For the outside version, stand with feet close together and hike the bell back like you're sitting into a chair. Clean the bell and catch it bottom side up, fixating it briefly in a balanced position. For the single version, take a wider stance to pass the kettlebell cleanly between your legs, then perform the same movement. This exercise emphasizes wrist, elbow, and shoulder stability, and grip strength through the bottoms-up hold.

232. Cleans, One-Arm

	Single Bell	Double Bell
	✓	✗

▶ PROKETTLEBELL.COM/232

Technical Difficulty	Movement Pattern	Recommended Load
2	Compound	Medium, Heavy Weight

PRIMARY BENEFIT	POSTERIOR STRENGTH AND EXPLOSIVENESS
TARGET MUSCLES	GLUTES, HAMSTRINGS, HIPS, ERECTORS, BICEPS, LATS

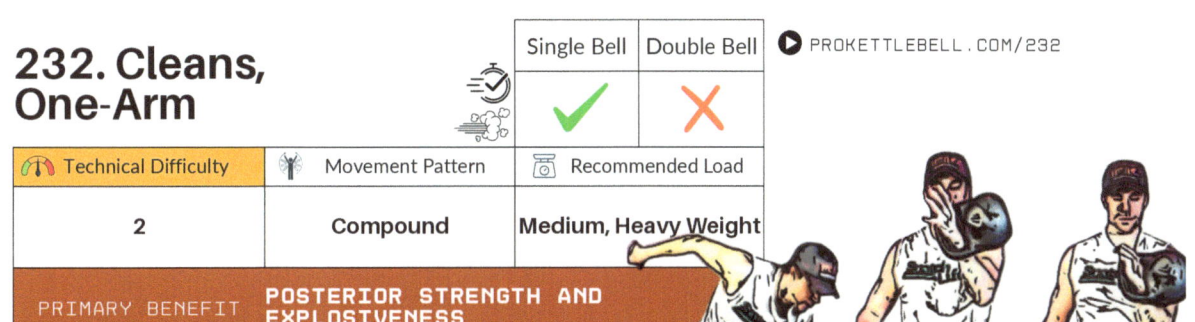

Begin by mastering a C-shaped swing kept close to the body with a vertically oriented handle. As the bell approaches chest height, release the fingertips and spear the palm through the window. From this "false" or "Olympic" grip, guide the elbow to the trunk and settle the bell into the rack position. Keep the bell within your frame and maintain strong arm-to-body contact. To descend, turn the palms up and let the handle roll back to the fingertips as you guide the bell into the backswing. Repeat. Maintain a flat back and generate drive from the hips and legs.

233. Cleans, Two-Arm

	Single Bell	Double Bell
	✗	✓

▶ PROKETTLEBELL.COM/233

Technical Difficulty	Movement Pattern	Recommended Load
2	Compound	Light, Medium, Heavy Weight

PRIMARY BENEFIT	POSTERIOR STRENGTH AND POWER
TARGET MUSCLES	QUADRICEPS, GLUTES, HAMSTRINGS, ERECTORS, LATS, BICEPS

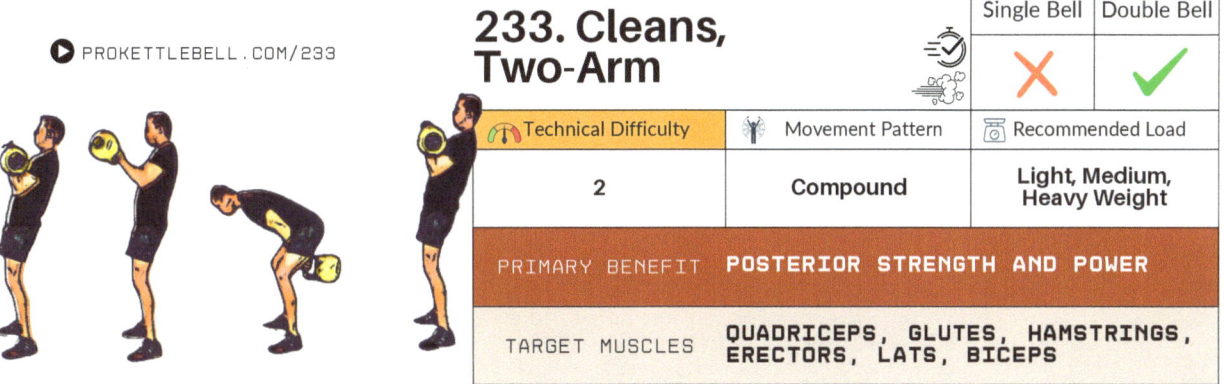

Start with two kettlebells positioned 12–18 inches in front of you and take a wider stance to accommodate both bells. Hike them back, then swing them upward, keeping the bells close to the body. As they approach chest height, release the handles and push the palms deeply through the windows. Lower the elbows toward the hips and guide the bells to the rack position. Keep the fingertips open to avoid pinching the fingers between handles as they land.

Start with a single kettlebell and perform an alternating swing followed by a clean. After cleaning into the left hand, step the right leg back diagonally into a curtsy squat, loading the front leg. Repeat by switching sides. The emphasis is on keeping the weight in the front leg, maintaining a secure rack position, a flat lumbar, and upright chest throughout the movement. This combination builds leg and core strength while adding bicep engagement during the clean.

234. Curtsy Cleans

PROKETTLEBELL.COM/234

	Single Bell	Double Bell
	✓	✗

Technical Difficulty	Movement Pattern	Recommended Load
2	Squat	Medium, Heavy Weight

PRIMARY BENEFIT	LOWER BODY STRENGTH
TARGET MUSCLES	QUADRICEPS, GLUTES, HAMSTRINGS, ERECTORS, OBLIQUES, DELTOIDS, BICEPS

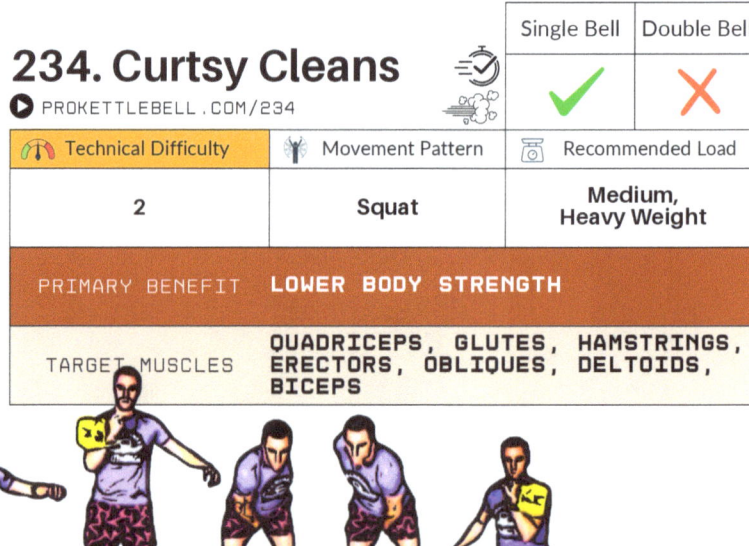

235. Dead Clean + High Knee

PROKETTLEBELL.COM/235

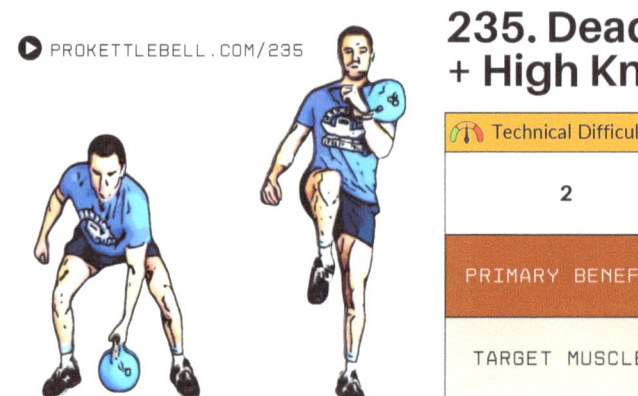

	Single Bell	Double Bell
	✓	✗

Technical Difficulty	Movement Pattern	Recommended Load
2	Compound	Heavy Weight

PRIMARY BENEFIT	FULL-BODY STRENGTH AND CONDITIONING
TARGET MUSCLES	QUADRICEPS, GLUTES, HAMSTRINGS, ERECTORS, LATS, BICEPS

Begin with a light to medium kettlebell positioned directly beneath your center of mass. Squat to initiate the dead clean, using mostly legs and maintaining a flat lumbar. As you drive the kettlebell into the rack, raise the opposite knee high, pausing briefly in that position. Lower both the bell and knee back to the starting point to reset for the next repetition. This movement builds coordination, leg strength, and balance simultaneously.

236. Dead Clean, One-Arm

PROKETTLEBELL.COM/236

	Single Bell	Double Bell
	✓	✓

Technical Difficulty	Movement Pattern	Recommended Load
2	Compound	Medium, Heavy Weight

PRIMARY BENEFIT	LEGS, CORE AND ARM EXPLOSIVENESS
TARGET MUSCLES	HIPS, GLUTES, QUADRICEPS, HAMSTRINGS, ERECTORS, TRAPS, BICEPS

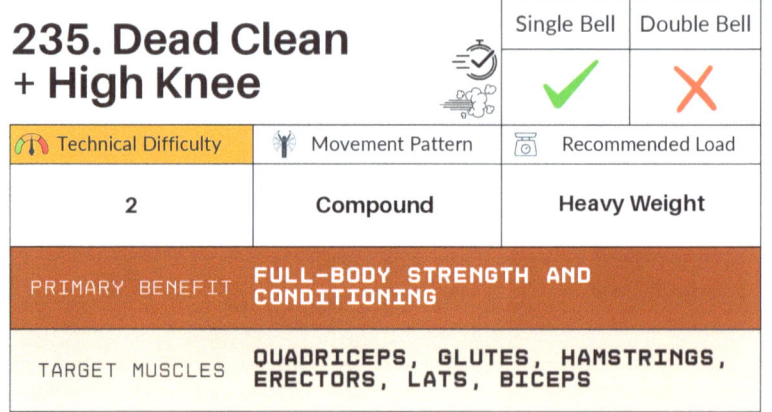

Stand directly over the kettlebell with feet slightly wider than shoulder-width. Push the hips back and keep the arm straight. Drive through the heels using the lower body, then shrug and pull the bell. As it approaches chest height, release the fingertips and spear the palm through the window to catch the bell in the rack position. Lower the bell vertically (do not swing), allowing the handle to fall into the fingertips to reduce friction on the palm. Repeat.

237. Gorilla Cleans

PROKETTLEBELL.COM/237

	Single Bell	Double Bell
	✗	✓

Technical Difficulty	Movement Pattern	Recommended Load
2	Compound	Light, Medium, Heavy Weight

PRIMARY BENEFIT: POSTERIOR STRENGTH AND EXPLOSIVENESS

TARGET MUSCLES: GLUTES, HAMSTRINGS, HIPS, ERECTORS, DELTOIDS, TRICEPS

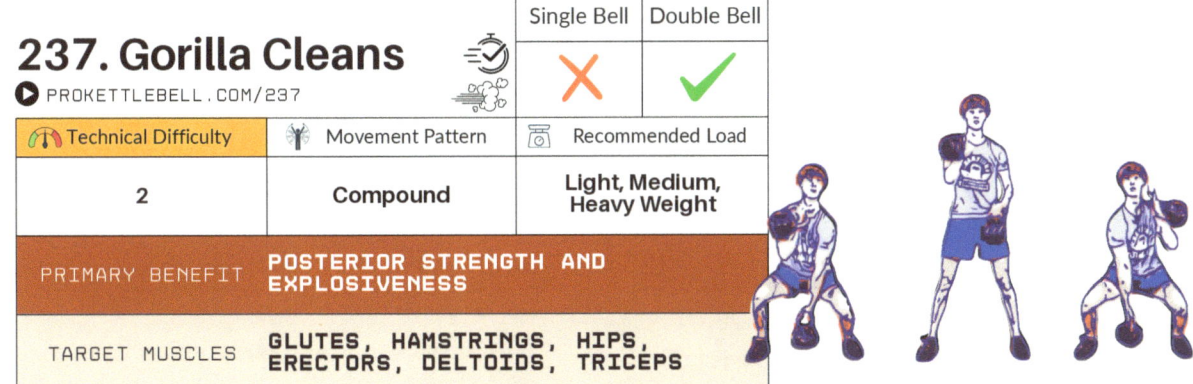

Begin in a wide stance with kettlebells in rack position. Drop one kettlebell while explosively cleaning the other, alternating sides with each rep. The bells should move vertically like elevator cables under your center of mass. Keep your chest up and lumbar flat, mimicking a "gorilla" stance. Emphasize rapid hand insertion and constant leg drive. This powerful bilateral movement targets the legs, erectors, and arms with coordination and tempo.

238. Horn Clean + Tip Toe Squat

	Single Bell	Double Bell
	✗	✓

Technical Difficulty	Movement Pattern	Recommended Load
2	Compound	Medium, Heavy Weight

PRIMARY BENEFIT: LEG AND FOOT STRENGTH/STABILITY

TARGET MUSCLES: CALVES, HAMSTRINGS, QUADRICEPS, GLUTES, ERECTORS, TRAPS, BICEPS

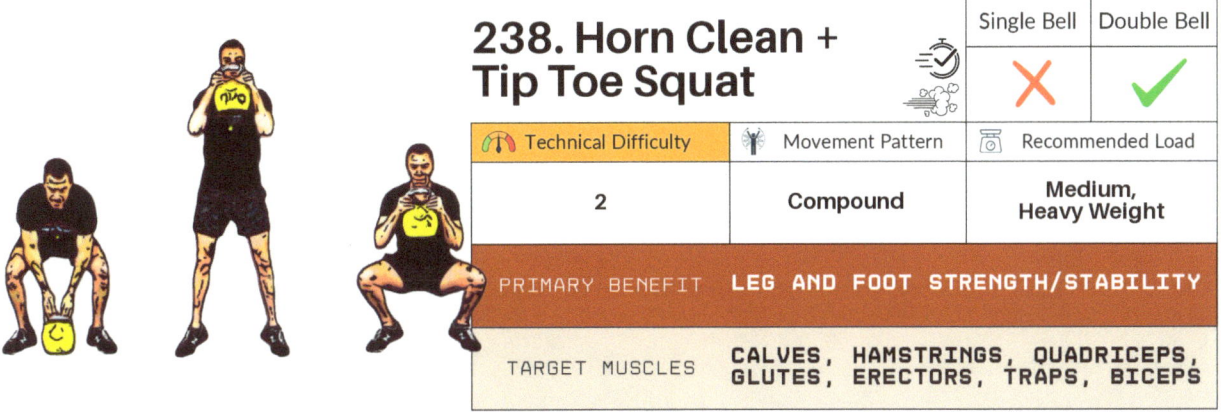

Perform a horn clean explosively, catching the kettlebell while on your tiptoes. From there, execute a squat while maintaining heel elevation. Keep your chest up, knees tracking toes, and the bell close to your body. After the squat, drop your heels and return the kettlebell to the starting position. This challenges balance and ankle mobility while strengthening the calves, feet, and hip flexors.

PROKETTLEBELL.COM/238

239. Horn Clean Squat Jack

	Single Bell	Double Bell
	✓	✗

Technical Difficulty	Movement Pattern	Recommended Load
2	Compound	Medium Weight

PRIMARY BENEFIT: FULL-BODY STRENGTH AND CONDITIONING

TARGET MUSCLES: QUADRICEPS, GLUTES, HAMSTRINGS, ERECTORS, LATS, BICEPS

PROKETTLEBELL.COM/239

Begin in a squat with a kettlebell between the feet, hooking the handle with your fingertips. Throw the bell upward and jump as it clears the knees. Catch the bell on its sides and land in a narrow squat, keeping it close to the centerline. Jump the feet back out to a wide stance while transitioning your hold back to the fingertip hook and guide the kettlebell back to the ground between the feet. Repeat. This movement combines explosive power with lower-body endurance and challenges full-body coordination.

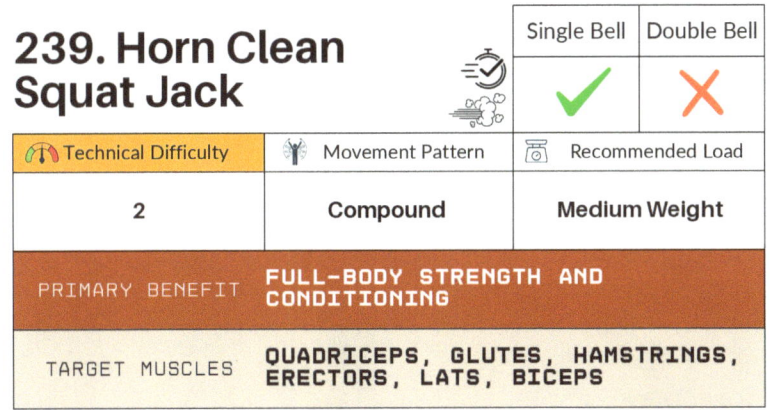

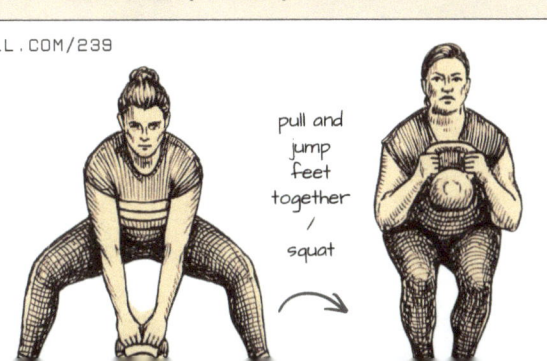

pull and jump feet together / squat

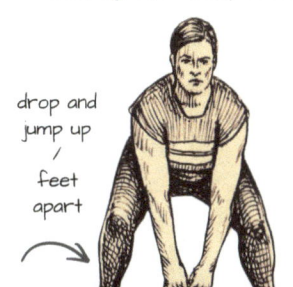

drop and jump up / feet apart

CLEANS

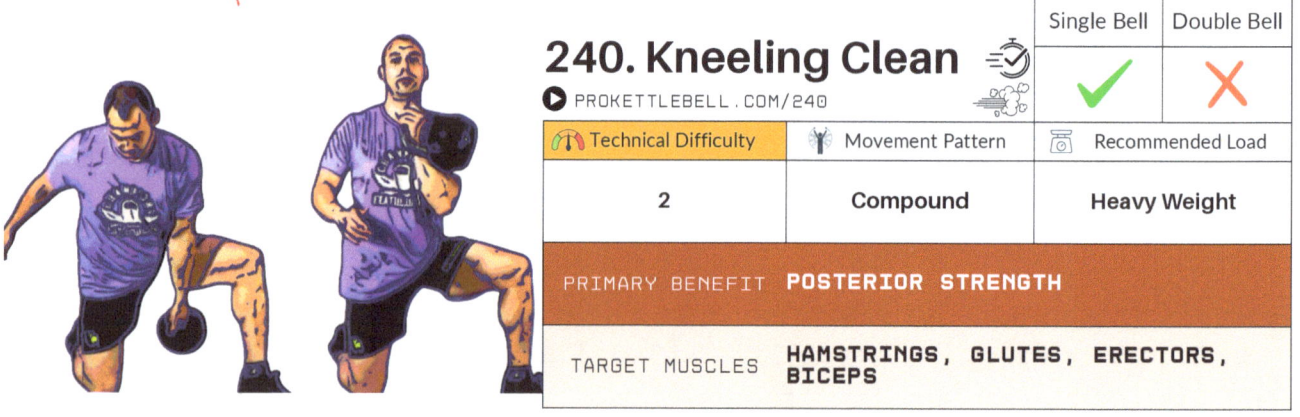

240. Kneeling Clean

PROKETTLEBELL.COM/240

	Single Bell	Double Bell
	✓	✗

Technical Difficulty	Movement Pattern	Recommended Load
2	Compound	Heavy Weight

PRIMARY BENEFIT — POSTERIOR STRENGTH

TARGET MUSCLES — HAMSTRINGS, GLUTES, ERECTORS, BICEPS

In a kneeling stance with one leg up, perform a clean using the hand on the same side as the forward leg. Drive with your hips and glutes to bring the kettlebell into the rack position. Let go momentarily to insert your hand fully into the window. Maintain an upright posture and consider using a pad for knee support. This variation focuses on hip and bicep strength with reduced lower-body assistance.

241. Kneeling Outside Cleans

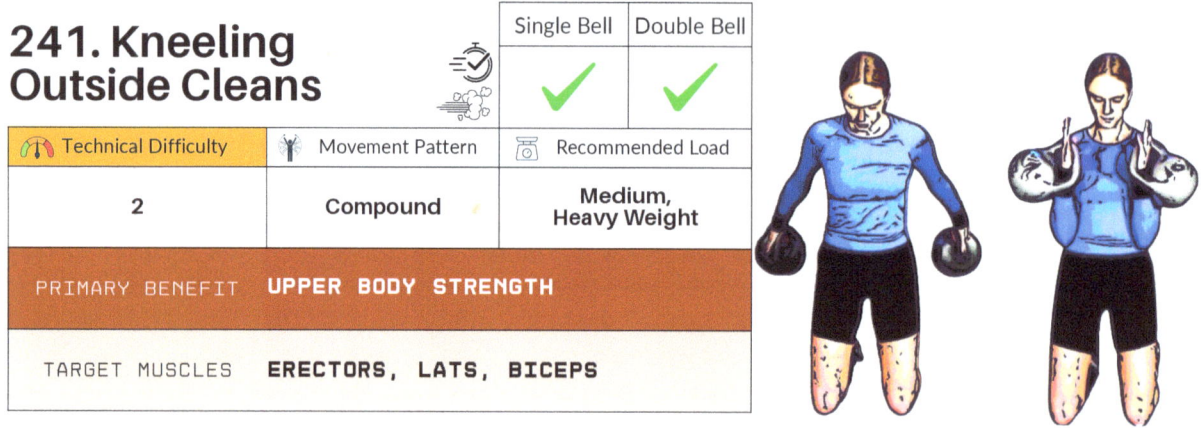

	Single Bell	Double Bell
	✓	✓

Technical Difficulty	Movement Pattern	Recommended Load
2	Compound	Medium, Heavy Weight

PRIMARY BENEFIT — UPPER BODY STRENGTH

TARGET MUSCLES — ERECTORS, LATS, BICEPS

Kneel upright with kettlebells placed just outside your knees. Hike them back slightly, then clean them to the outside, catching them in rack position. Keep your torso upright and avoid sitting on your heels. Without the aid of standing leverage, this version emphasizes upper-body strength, particularly the biceps and shoulders, as you fixate the bells into position.

PROKETTLEBELL.COM/241

242. Outside Clean + French Press

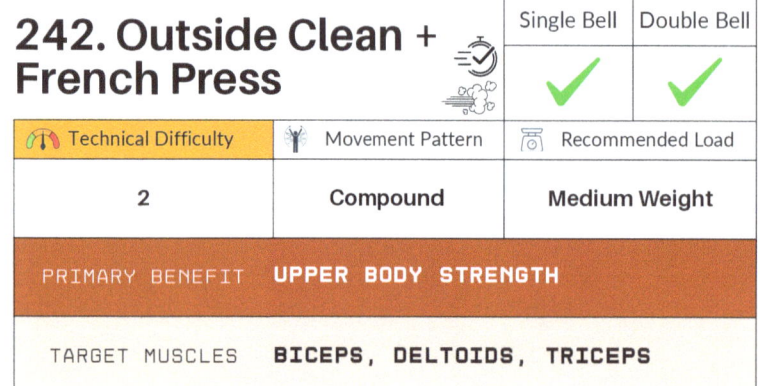
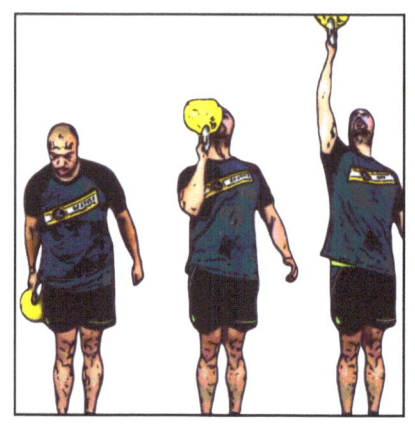

	Single Bell	Double Bell
	✓	✓

Technical Difficulty	Movement Pattern	Recommended Load
2	Compound	Medium Weight

PRIMARY BENEFIT — UPPER BODY STRENGTH

TARGET MUSCLES — BICEPS, DELTOIDS, TRICEPS

Start with your feet close together and the kettlebell 12–18 inches in front. Perform an outside bottoms-up clean, then immediately press it overhead in a French press style. Lower back to the upside-down rack and repeat. Holding the bell near the horn improves control, while a centered grip increases difficulty. This targets wrist, shoulder, and core stability through the press and clean combination.

PROKETTLEBELL.COM/242

243. Outside Swing +Clean

	Single Bell	Double Bell
	✓	✓

Technical Difficulty	Movement Pattern	Recommended Load
2	Compound	Medium, Heavy Weight

PRIMARY BENEFIT	FULL-BODY STRENGTH
TARGET MUSCLES	QUADRICEPS, GLUTES, HAMSTRINGS, LATS, ERECTORS, BICEPS, OBLIQUES

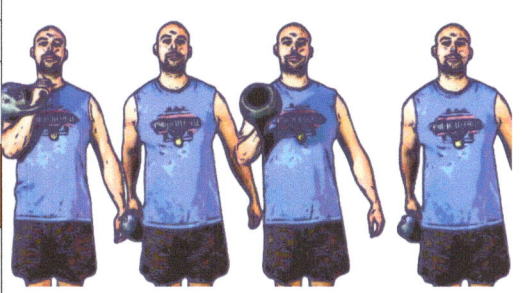

Combine an outside swing with an outside clean. Stand with your feet closer together and swing the kettlebell on the outside of your leg. At the top of the swing, insert your hand and guide the bell into the rack. With the offset load, the movement challenges core and unilateral stability more than a standard swing or clean, so use a lighter kettlebell for control and safety. ▶ PROKETTLEBELL.COM/243

244. Reverse Lunge Cleans

	Single Bell	Double Bell
	✓	✓

Technical Difficulty	Movement Pattern	Recommended Load
2	Lunge + Hinge	Light, Medium, Heavy Weight

PRIMARY BENEFIT	FULL-BODY STRENGTH
TARGET MUSCLES	QUADRICEPS, GLUTES, HAMSTRINGS, ERECTORS, LATS, BICEPS

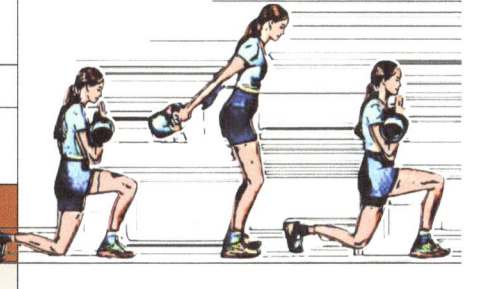

▶ PROKETTLEBELL.COM/244

Reverse lunges paired with inside or outside cleans ("inside" = between your legs, "outside" = feet together, swing outside your hip). In either case, as the bell rises, step into a reverse lunge with the same or opposite leg and catch the bell in the rack position on the descent. Keep the bell in the rack as you return to standing and repeat. A double-bell variation can be used for added resistance. Maintain an upright posture, knees tracking over the toes, and strong core engagement. Try a single speed-switch clean variation for a coordination challenge by switching hands mid-clean before stepping into the lunge.

▶ PROKETTLEBELL.COM/245

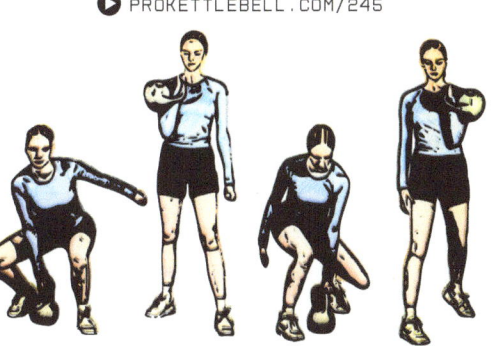

245. Split Lunge Dead Clean

	Single Bell	Double Bell
	✓	✗

Technical Difficulty	Movement Pattern	Recommended Load
2	Compound	Medium, Heavy Weight

PRIMARY BENEFIT	FULL-BODY STRENGTH AND POWER
TARGET MUSCLES	QUADRICEPS, GLUTES, HAMSTRINGS, ERECTORS, BICEPS, CALVES, HIP FLEXORS

Straddle the kettlebell in a split stance with one leg forward and one back. Grasp the bell with the hand on the back-leg side. Drive through both legs with a flat back and clean the bell into the rack position. Return the bell to the floor, release it, and perform a split lunge jump to switch legs. Land softly and repeat on the opposite side.
This power-focused movement develops lower-body explosiveness and coordination.

CLEANS

246. Split Stance Dead Clean

	Single Bell	Double Bell
	✓	✗

Technical Difficulty	Movement Pattern	Recommended Load
2	Compound	Medium, Heavy Weight

PRIMARY BENEFIT	FULL-BODY STRENGTH (CORE EMPHASIS)
TARGET MUSCLES	QUADRICEPS, GLUTES, HAMSTRINGS, ERECTORS, OBLIQUES, LATS, BICEPS

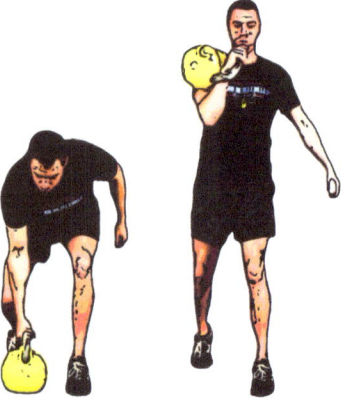

Set up in a split stance with the front leg aligned with the kettlebell. Use the opposite-side arm to grab the handle. Drive through both legs while keeping your lumbar flat and torso upright. As the bell rises, shrug and pull, inserting your hand deeply into the window to finish in the rack. Lower the bell to the floor and reset. These asymmetrical clean build cross-body strength and stability. ▶ PROKETTLEBELL.COM/246

247. Stop Clean

	Single Bell	Double Bell
	✓	✓

Technical Difficulty	Movement Pattern	Recommended Load
2	Compound	Medium, Heavy Weight

PRIMARY BENEFIT	POSTERIOR STRENGTH AND POWER
TARGET MUSCLES	QUADRICEPS, GLUTES, HAMSTRINGS, ERECTORS, LATS, BICEPS

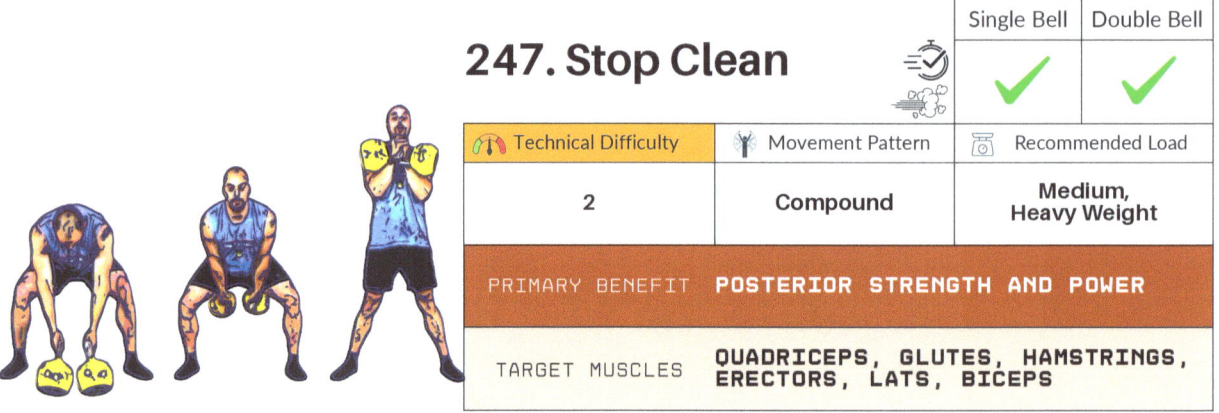

Place two kettlebells about 18 inches in front of you. Hinge at the hips with a flat back and hike the bells back, then clean them into the rack. After each backswing, park them in the same starting position to reset. This forces you to overcome inertia on every rep, increasing the demand on your lats, hips, and glutes. Use good form and take your time between reps for optimal power generation. ▶ PROKETTLEBELL.COM/247

248. Walking Hang Cleans

	Single Bell	Double Bell
	✓	✗

Technical Difficulty	Movement Pattern	Recommended Load
2	Compound	Light, Medium, Heavy Weight

PRIMARY BENEFIT	FULL-BODY STRENGTH, POWER AND CONDITIONING
TARGET MUSCLES	ERECTORS, QUADRICEPS, GLUTES, HAMSTRINGS, BICEPS

▶ PROKETTLEBELL.COM/248

Begin with the kettlebell in the rack position. Step forward with the opposite leg and drop the kettlebell, letting it hover above the ground with a straight arm as the step is completed. Drive through both feet and pull the kettlebell upward as you take a full step forward with your back leg. As you land the step, you'll catch the bell in the rack again. Continue the pattern for multiple reps prior to mirroring on the opposite side.

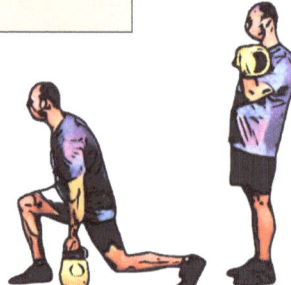

249. Figure-8 Clean

	Single Bell	Double Bell
	✓	✗

Technical Difficulty	Movement Pattern	Recommended Load
3	Compound	Light, Medium, Heavy Weight

PRIMARY BENEFIT	FULL-BODY STRENGTH AND COORDINATION
TARGET MUSCLES	QUADRICEPS, GLUTES, HAMSTRINGS, ERECTORS, OBLIQUES, LATS, BICEPS

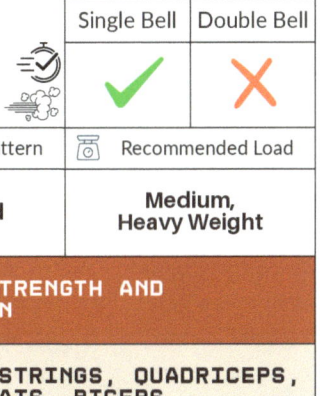

From an athletic stance, pass the kettlebell high between the legs from front to back, catching it behind the body with the opposite hand. Loop the bell around the body and repeat the figure-8t a second time. After the second pass, use a cross-body toss to switch hands and catch the kettlebell in the rack position on the opposite side (speed-switch). Repeat. This complex demands rhythm, timing, and precise hand insertion while integrating lower body, core, and upper body engagement.

▶ PROKETTLEBELL.COM/249

Begin with a single-arm swing. After the backswing, drive the bell upward and toss it across the centerline, catching it with the opposite hand in a speed-switch clean to the rack position. From the rack, reset into another one-arm swing and repeat the speed-switch clean. Keep the swing path close to the body. This dynamic complex builds coordination, timing, and full-body conditioning by combining swing power with clean precision.

250. Speed-Switch Swing n' Clean

	Single Bell	Double Bell
	✓	✗

Technical Difficulty	Movement Pattern	Recommended Load
3	Compound	Medium, Heavy Weight

PRIMARY BENEFIT	POSTERIOR STRENGTH AND COORDINATION
TARGET MUSCLES	GLUTES, HAMSTRINGS, QUADRICEPS, ERECTORS, LATS, BICEPS

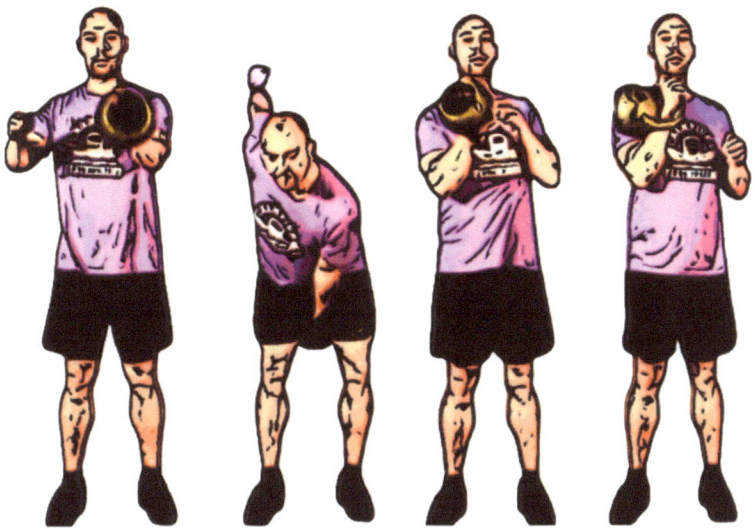

▶ PROKETTLEBELL.COM/250

CLEANS

251. Assisted Hang Snatch

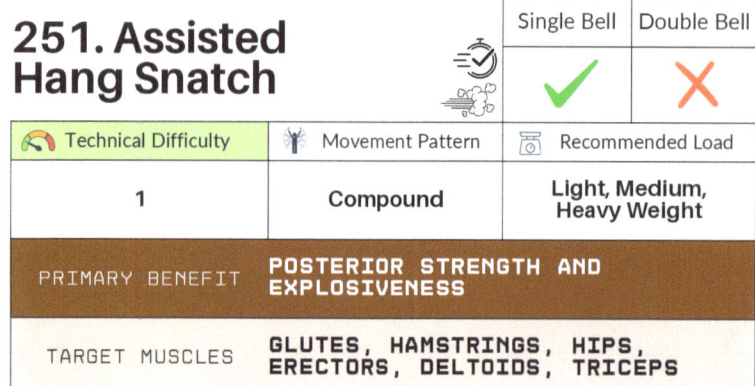
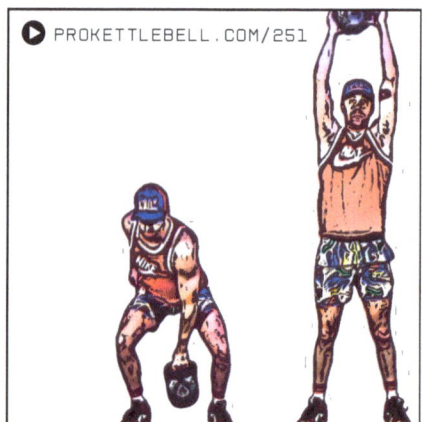

	Single Bell	Double Bell
	✓	✗

Technical Difficulty	Movement Pattern	Recommended Load
1	Compound	Light, Medium, Heavy Weight

PRIMARY BENEFIT	POSTERIOR STRENGTH AND EXPLOSIVENESS
TARGET MUSCLES	GLUTES, HAMSTRINGS, HIPS, ERECTORS, DELTOIDS, TRICEPS

Begin with a light to medium kettlebell hanging between your legs. Initiate the lift using about 70% legs, 20% back, and 10% arms. As the bell rises to chest height, assist it with your free hand to guide it into an overhead position. This version omits the complex hand insertion of a regular snatch, making it beginner-friendly. Bring the bell back to the chest and drop it close to your body for the next rep. Keep the bell traveling vertically and under your center of mass.

252. Bottoms-Up Snatch

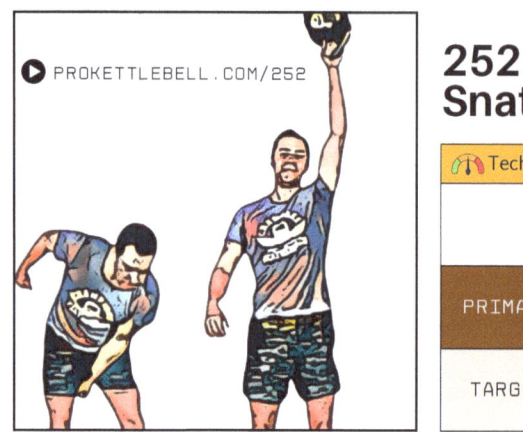
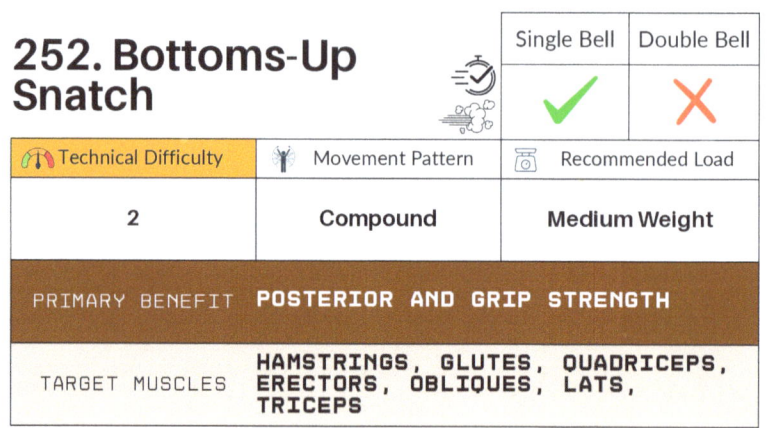

	Single Bell	Double Bell
	✓	✗

Technical Difficulty	Movement Pattern	Recommended Load
2	Compound	Medium Weight

PRIMARY BENEFIT	POSTERIOR AND GRIP STRENGTH
TARGET MUSCLES	HAMSTRINGS, GLUTES, QUADRICEPS, ERECTORS, OBLIQUES, LATS, TRICEPS

Begin in your swing/snatch stance with the kettlebell about 12–18 inches in front. Gripping near the horn with thumb and index finger for better control, hike it back, swing it forward with a J-shaped trajectory and press the kettlebell into a bottoms-up lockout position where the bell is vertical and the handle points down. This variation reduces the need for traditional hand insertion and emphasizes forearm, grip strength, and control. Drop it back down with proper arm-body contact and balance.

253. Double Hand-Insertion Drill

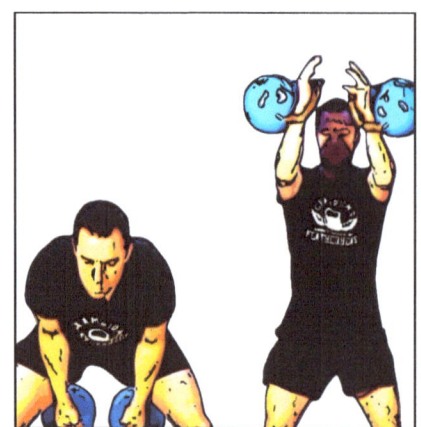
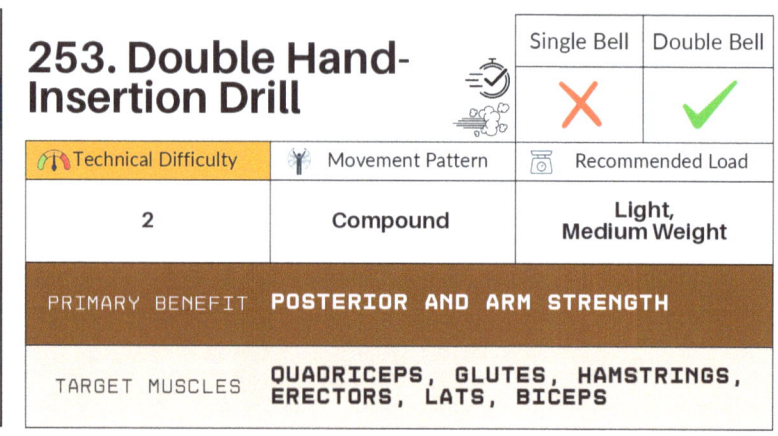

	Single Bell	Double Bell
	✗	✓

Technical Difficulty	Movement Pattern	Recommended Load
2	Compound	Light, Medium Weight

PRIMARY BENEFIT	POSTERIOR AND ARM STRENGTH
TARGET MUSCLES	QUADRICEPS, GLUTES, HAMSTRINGS, ERECTORS, LATS, BICEPS

Prepare to perform a double clean. Hike the bells back. On the upswing, quickly insert your hands through the window of each bell as they rise. Squeeze your lats and briefly freeze the bells with elbows at 90 degrees and full hand insertion before dropping them back down. You can vary the height—low, medium, or high—to get comfortable inserting your hands at different points. PROKETTLEBELL.COM/253

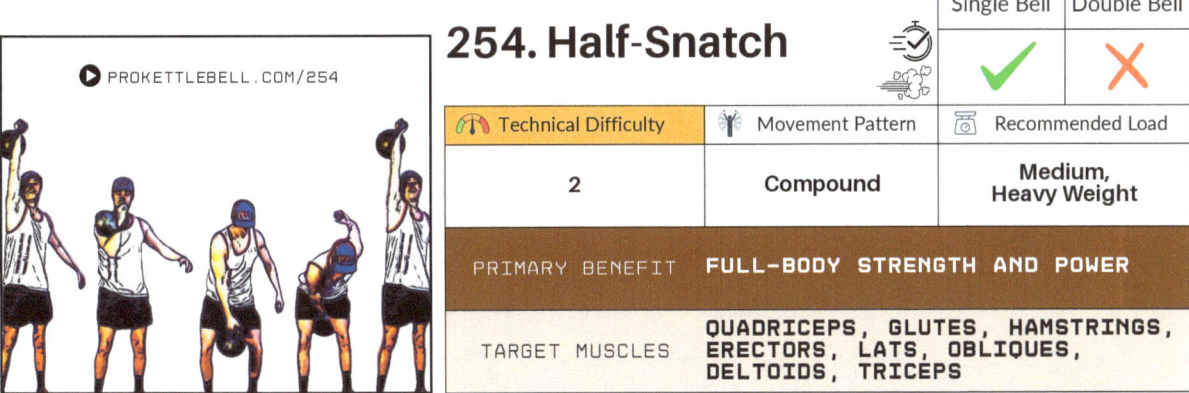

254. Half-Snatch

	Single Bell	Double Bell
	✓	✗

Technical Difficulty	Movement Pattern	Recommended Load
2	Compound	Medium, Heavy Weight

PRIMARY BENEFIT	FULL-BODY STRENGTH AND POWER
TARGET MUSCLES	QUADRICEPS, GLUTES, HAMSTRINGS, ERECTORS, LATS, OBLIQUES, DELTOIDS, TRICEPS

Mastered the swing and clean? It's time to snatch! Powerfully swing a kettlebell with a "J-shaped" trajectory so it's traveling close to you. As the bell reaches chest height, quickly let go of the handle, push your whole palm through the window, and guide it to a stop directly over your shoulder with a straight arm and bicep near your cheek. Initiate the backswing by turning your palm upward and letting the handle fall into your fingertips as you shift your weight slightly back, letting the bell fall close to your body. Repeat. Snatching uses power from your entire body, especially the legs and posterior chain.

255. Lo/Hi Swing-to-Snatch

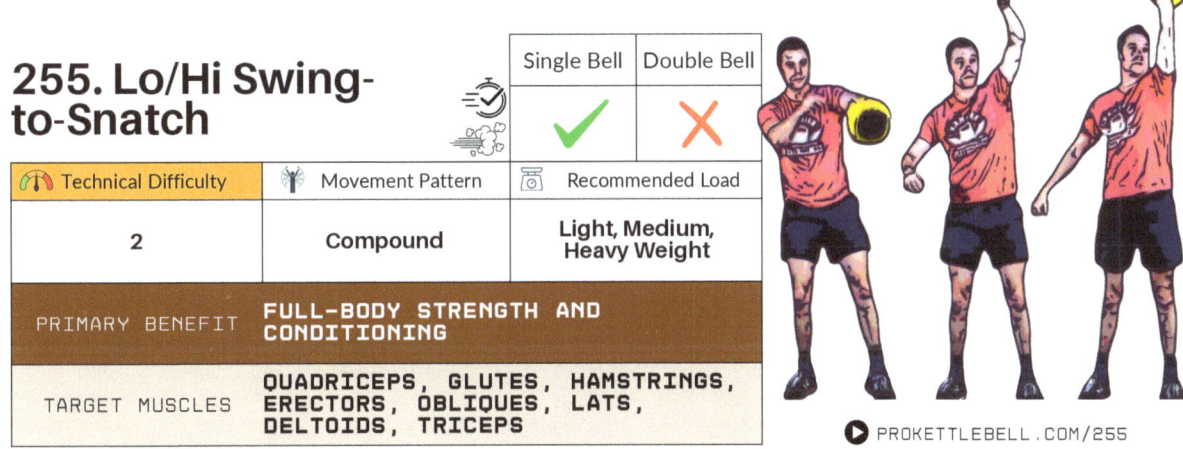

	Single Bell	Double Bell
	✓	✗

Technical Difficulty	Movement Pattern	Recommended Load
2	Compound	Light, Medium, Heavy Weight

PRIMARY BENEFIT	FULL-BODY STRENGTH AND CONDITIONING
TARGET MUSCLES	QUADRICEPS, GLUTES, HAMSTRINGS, ERECTORS, OBLIQUES, LATS, DELTOIDS, TRICEPS

A series of low swing, high swing, and snatch, this sequence builds power from the floor up, teaching proper timing and increasing posterior chain activation. Focus on generating power through your whole body—not just the hips. Use fast hand insertion and secure fixation over your shoulder. Each phase should be smooth and controlled, reinforcing good swing mechanics before the final snatch.

256. Reverse Lunge Snatch

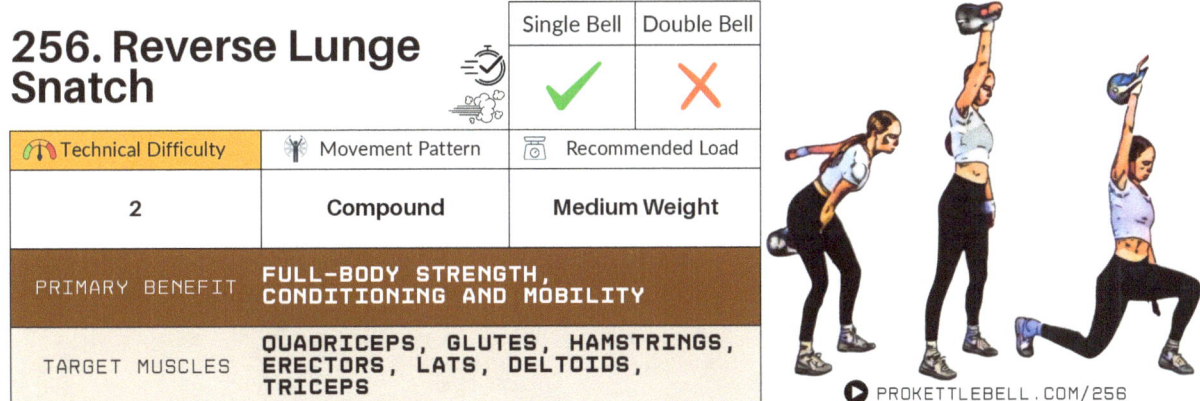

	Single Bell	Double Bell
	✓	✗

Technical Difficulty	Movement Pattern	Recommended Load
2	Compound	Medium Weight

PRIMARY BENEFIT	FULL-BODY STRENGTH, CONDITIONING AND MOBILITY
TARGET MUSCLES	QUADRICEPS, GLUTES, HAMSTRINGS, ERECTORS, LATS, DELTOIDS, TRICEPS

Perform a snatch and fixate the kettlebell overhead. Step back into a reverse lunge with the leg on the same side as the kettlebell, then return to standing. You may alternate legs each repetition. Keep the bell stacked over the shoulder and maintain alignment through the ankle, knee, and hip. Begin by segmenting the snatch and lunge. For added challenge, initiate the lunge mid-snatch and catch the bell overhead as you land.

SNATCHES

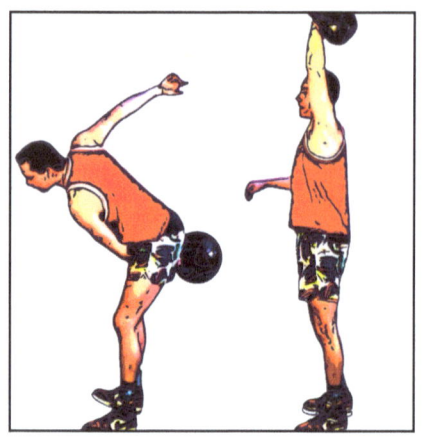

257. Snatch

▶ PROKETTLEBELL.COM/257

	Single Bell	Double Bell
	✓	✗

Technical Difficulty	Movement Pattern	Recommended Load
2	Compound	Light, Medium, Heavy Weight

PRIMARY BENEFIT	FULL-BODY STRENGTH, POWER AND ENDURANCE
TARGET MUSCLES	QUADRICEPS, GLUTES, HAMSTRINGS, ERECTORS, LATS, OBLIQUES, DELTOIDS, TRICEPS

Mastered the swing and clean? It's time to snatch! Set the kettlebell 12-18 inches in front of you. Hike it back and swing it up, keeping a "J-shaped" trajectory so the bell is traveling close to you. As the kettlebell reaches chest height, quickly let to of the handle and push your whole palm through the window. Guide the kettlebell into a stop directly over your shoulder, with a straight arm and bicep near your cheek. To drop the kettlebell in the backswing, turn your palm upward and let the the handle fall into your fingertips as you counterbalance by shifting weight slightly back, letting the bell fall close to your body. Repeat. Snatching uses power from your entire body, especially the legs and posterior chain.

258. Stop Snatch

	Single Bell	Double Bell
	✓	✓

Technical Difficulty	Movement Pattern	Recommended Load
2	Compound	Medium Weight

PRIMARY BENEFIT	CORE AND POSTERIOR STRENGTH
TARGET MUSCLES	QUADRICEPS, GLUTES, HAMSTRINGS, ERECTORS, LATS, DELTOIDS, TRICEPS

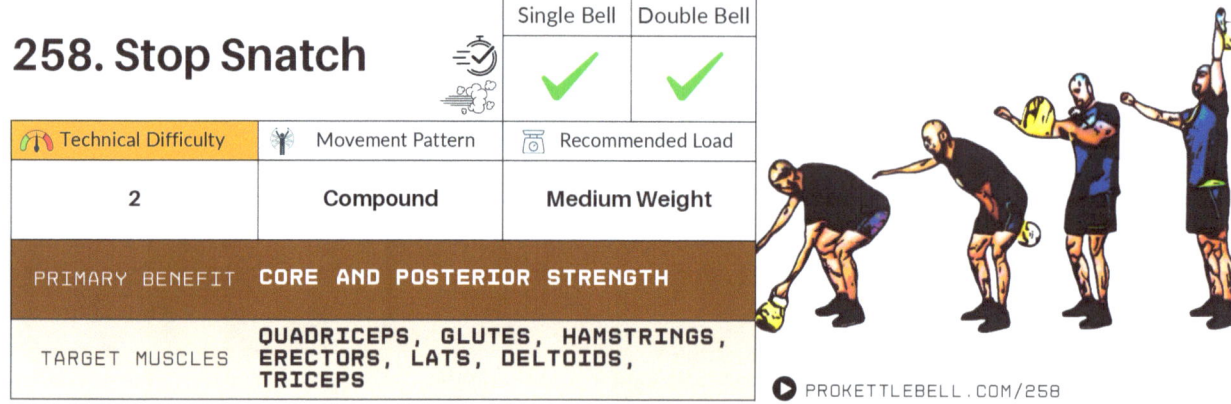

▶ PROKETTLEBELL.COM/258

Park the kettlebell about 12-18 inches in front of you. From an athletic stance, hike it back, swing, and snatch it overhead with a quick hand insertion. Lock it out, drop it into the backswing, then park it on the ground each time, fully resetting. This eliminates momentum between reps, increasing engagement of the lats, glutes, and hamstrings. Focus on a powerful hike and stable overhead fixation. Each rep starts fresh, enhancing strength and technique.

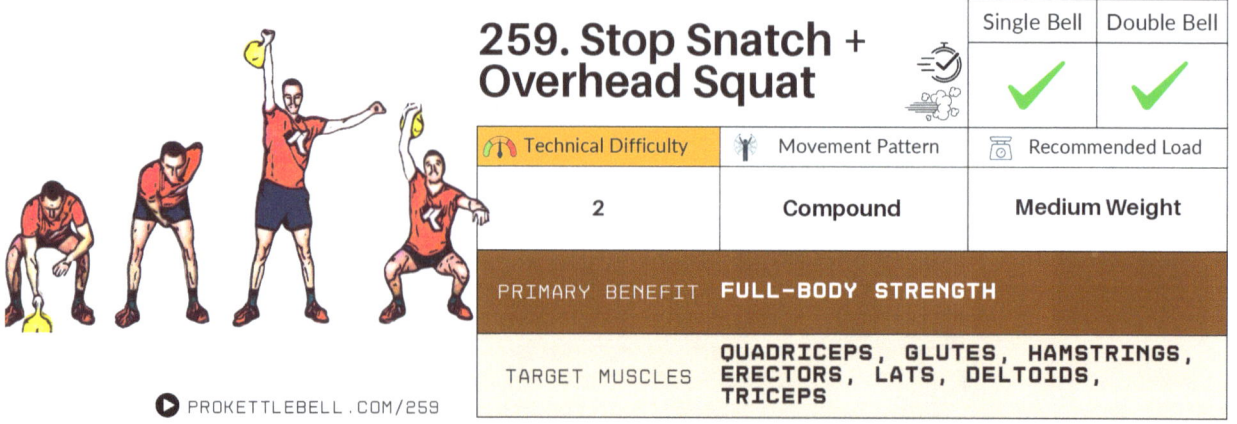

259. Stop Snatch + Overhead Squat

	Single Bell	Double Bell
	✓	✓

Technical Difficulty	Movement Pattern	Recommended Load
2	Compound	Medium Weight

PRIMARY BENEFIT	FULL-BODY STRENGTH
TARGET MUSCLES	QUADRICEPS, GLUTES, HAMSTRINGS, ERECTORS, LATS, DELTOIDS, TRICEPS

▶ PROKETTLEBELL.COM/259

Use a light kettlebell that allows for a deep, stable overhead squat. Perform a snatch and lock the bell overhead. Descend into an overhead squat with heels grounded and knees tracking the toes, keeping the bell stacked over the shoulder. Stand back up, then drop the bell into a backswing and return it to the ground. Repeat on both sides. Only squat as deep as proper form allows. This complex blends explosive power with mobility and balance.

260. Alternating Snatch

	Single Bell	Double Bell
	✓	✗

Technical Difficulty	Movement Pattern	Recommended Load
3	Compound	Medium Weight

PRIMARY BENEFIT	FULL-BODY STRENGTH AND CONDITIONING
TARGET MUSCLES	QUADRICEPS, GLUTES, HAMSTRINGS, OBLIQUES, ERECTORS, LATS, SHOULDERS, TRICEPS

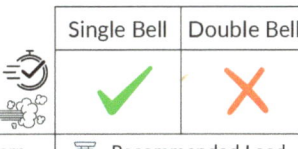

▶ PROKETTLEBELL.COM/260

Start with the kettlebell in front of you in your swing/snatch stance. Perform a single-arm snatch and fixate the bell overhead, stacked over the shoulder and center of mass. Drop it into a backswing, then swing to waist height, switch hands, complete another backswing, and snatch with the opposite hand. This movement builds coordination and allows higher volume through hand switching. Maintain strong arm-to-body connection and effective counterbalance for stability and safety.

261. Speed-Switch Snatch

	Single Bell	Double Bell
	✓	✗

Technical Difficulty	Movement Pattern	Recommended Load
3	Compound	Medium Weight

PRIMARY BENEFIT	FULL-BODY STRENGTH, POWER AND COORDINATION
TARGET MUSCLES	QUADRICEPS, GLUTES, HAMSTRINGS, ERECTORS, LATS, OBLIQUES, DELTOIDS, TRICEPS

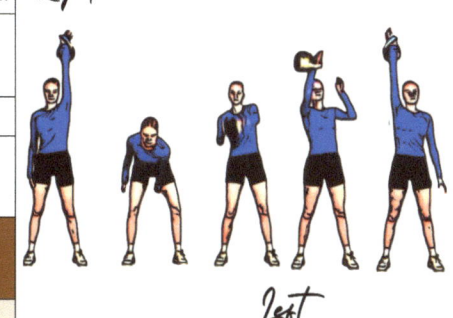

▶ PROKETTLEBELL.COM/233

Start a snatch, but as the bell swings up, guide it slightly across your body. At chest height, let go of it and grab it with the opposite hand to complete the lockout overhead on the non-starting side. Drop it into a backswing, and repeat the speed-switch to the snatch on the opposite arm with the next rep. This movement builds speed, timing, and grip coordination. Counterbalance during the swing and maintain arm-body contact during the weight-bearing phase to stay safe and controlled.

262. Curtsy Snatch

	Single Bell	Double Bell
	✓	✗

Technical Difficulty	Movement Pattern	Recommended Load
3	Compound	Medium Weight

PRIMARY BENEFIT	FULL-BODY STRENGTH AND MOBILITY
TARGET MUSCLES	QUADRICEPS, GLUTES, HAMSTRINGS, ERECTORS, LATS, DELTOIDS, TRICEPS, OBLIQUES, HIP STABILIZERS

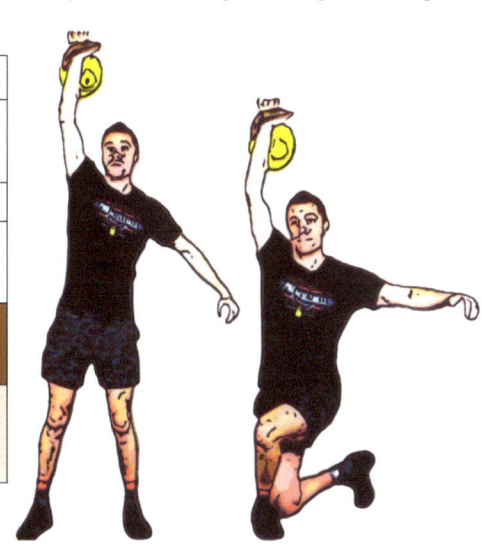

▶ PROKETTLEBELL.COM/262

Perform a snatch to get the kettlebell overhead and fixated. Then, step the same-side leg diagonally behind you into a curtsy lunge. The front leg remains loaded with heel down, torso upright. Return to start, snatch again, and repeat. Try beginning the lunge mid-snatch for added challenge. Perform equal reps on each side.

263. Double Half-Snatch

	Single Bell	Double Bell
	✗	✓

Technical Difficulty	Movement Pattern	Recommended Load
3	Compound	Medium Weight

PRIMARY BENEFIT	FULL-BODY STRENGTH AND POWER
TARGET MUSCLES	QUADRICEPS, GLUTES, HAMSTRINGS, ERECTORS, LATS, DELTOIDS, TRICEPS

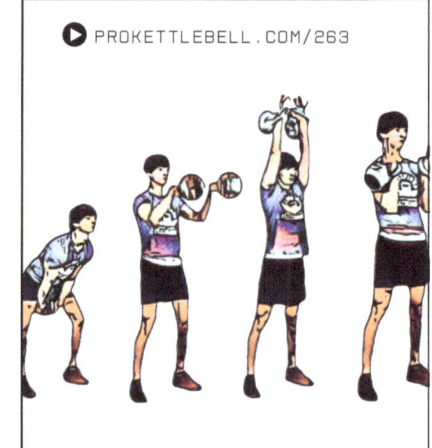

With two kettlebells set 12-18 inches in front, stand in an athletic stance and hike them back. Swing both bells up and insert your hands quickly through the windows as they rise, locking them out overhead and finding fixation. Instead of dropping them down into another swing, lower them into the rack position. From there, initiate a backswing followed by the next double snatch. This method requires more power from the legs and posterior chain as it lacks stored momentum from an overhead drop.

264. Double Snatch

PROKETTLEBELL.COM/264

	Single Bell	Double Bell
	✗	✓

Technical Difficulty	Movement Pattern	Recommended Load
3	Compound	Medium Weight

PRIMARY BENEFIT	FULL-BODY STRENGTH AND CONDITIONING
TARGET MUSCLES	QUADRICEPS, GLUTES, HAMSTRINGS, ERECTORS, LATS, DELTOIDS, TRICEPS

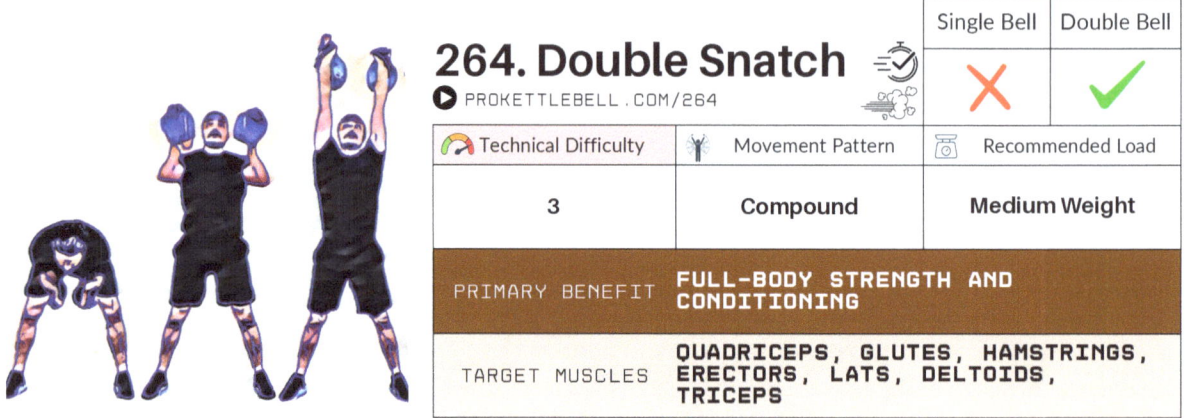

Begin with two kettlebells positioned 12-18 inches in front of you. Take a wide stance to allow space between the legs. Hike the bells back and swing them upward, releasing the grip and driving the hands fully through the windows as the bells rise. Lock both bells overhead with the arms stacked over the shoulders. Unlike a single snatch, the double snatch mandates a vertical, parallel backswing path to prevent the bells from colliding. Adjust the path to parallel as soon as possible upon dropping from overhead. This movement demands precise technique, timing, and effective counterbalancing.

265. Figure-8 Half Snatch

	Single Bell	Double Bell
	✓	✗

Technical Difficulty	Movement Pattern	Recommended Load
3	Compound	Medium Weight

PRIMARY BENEFIT	POSTERIOR STRENGTH AND COORDINATION
TARGET MUSCLES	QUADRICEPS, GLUTES, HAMSTRINGS, ERECTORS, LATS, DELTOIDS, BICEPS

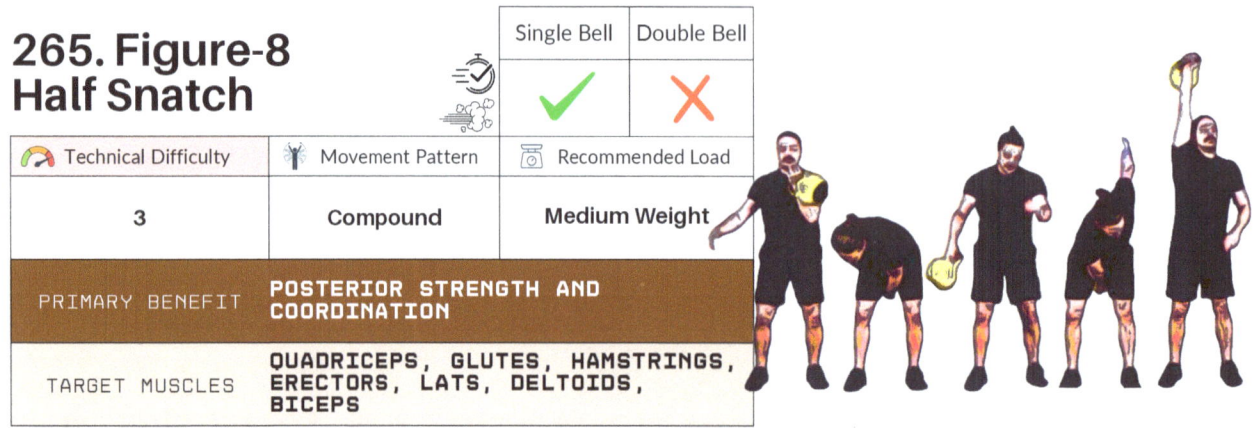

Step 1: From a single bell rack position, perform the first half of a figure-8 (pass front to back between your legs with a hand-switch behind the knee). Step 2: Once the bell is in front of you again, pull it into a backswing. Step 3: From the backswing, perform a full snatch. Reset: Bring it down to the rack position. Repeat and begin the next rep with a figure-8 loop the other direction. A great challenge for coordination and control. PROKETTLEBELL.COM/265

266. Figure-8 Snatch

	Single Bell	Double Bell
	✓	✗

Technical Difficulty	Movement Pattern	Recommended Load
3	Compound	Medium Weight

PRIMARY BENEFIT	FULL-BODY STRENGTH, POWER AND COORDINATION
TARGET MUSCLES	GLUTES, QUADRICEPS, HAMSTRINGS, ERECTORS, OBLIQUES, LATS, DELTOIDS, TRICEPS

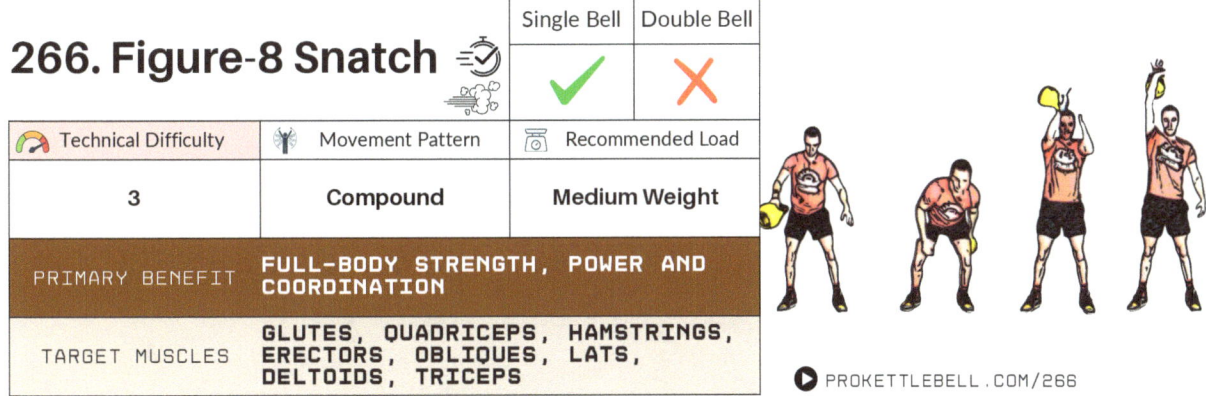

PROKETTLEBELL.COM/266

A full figure-8, culminating with a speed-switch snatch. Using a wider stance, swing the kettlebell in a figure-eight pattern—front to back. As the bell completes the second loop, perform a speed switch at chest-height and complete the snatch with the opposite hand. Return to the start and repeat. This advanced move requires good timing, balance, and full-body control, so ensure you're proficient in each individual component first.

267. Stop Swing Switch-Snatch

	Single Bell	Double Bell
	✓	✗

Technical Difficulty	Movement Pattern	Recommended Load
3	Compound	Medium Weight

PRIMARY BENEFIT	FULL-BODY STRENGTH AND CONDITIONING
TARGET MUSCLES	QUADRICEPS, GLUTES, HAMSTRINGS, ERECTORS, LATS, OBLIQUES, DELTOIDS, TRICEPS

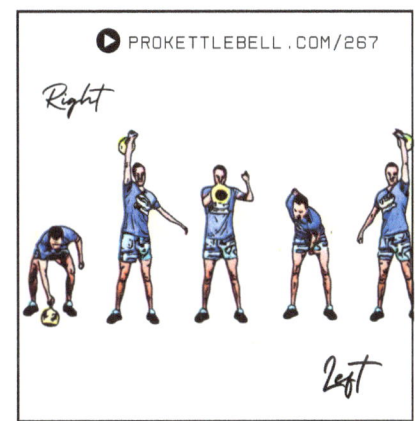

PROKETTLEBELL.COM/267

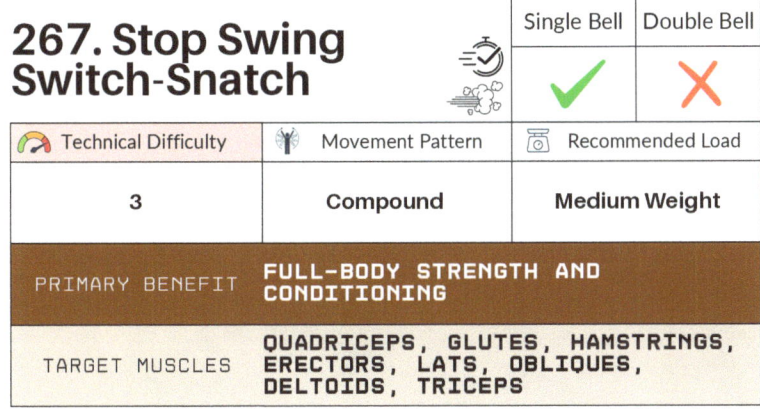

Park the kettlebell 12-18 inches in front. Hike it back, swing, and switch hands mid-swing, finishing the snatch with the new hand. Perform a backswing out of the drop from overhead, park it again on the ground and repeat. Because you're switching hands each time, grip fatigue is reduced, allowing for more volume. Focus on fast, clean hand insertion and keeping your weight counterbalanced with a flat back when you start and finish each rep.

268. Survival Snatch (Hang Snatch)

PROKETTLEBELL.COM/268

	Single Bell	Double Bell
	✓	✗

Technical Difficulty	Movement Pattern	Recommended Load
3	Compound	Medium Weight

PRIMARY BENEFIT	POSTERIOR STRENGTH
TARGET MUSCLES	QUADRICEPS, GLUTES, HAMSTRINGS, ERECTORS, LATS, DELTOIDS, TRICEPS

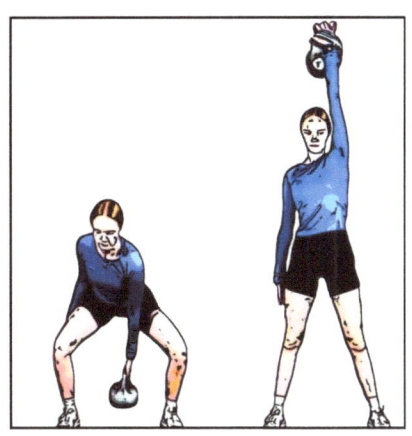

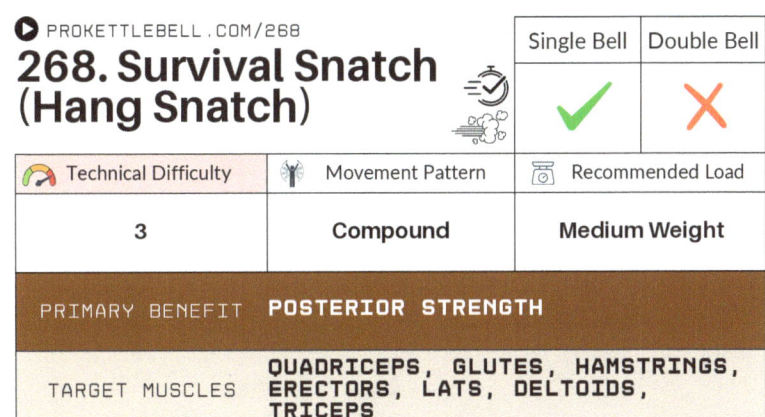

Start with a snatch. For the drop, let the kettlebell fall vertically in front of you, aiming between your feet, rather than arcing into a backswing. Bend your legs, catch it softly and let it hover above the ground. Explosively straighten your legs and pull, driving the kettlebell upward and into another overhead lockout. This technique saves grip strength and focuses on leg and vertical power.

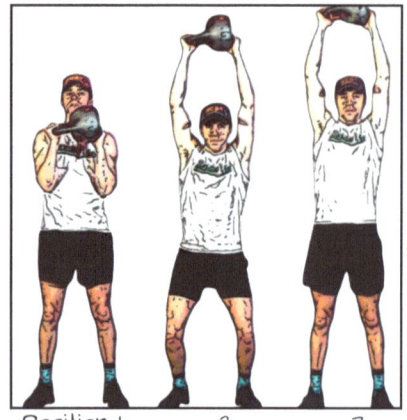

Position 1   2   3

269. 3-Position Drill
PROKETTLEBELL.COM/269

	Single Bell	Double Bell
	✓	✗

Technical Difficulty	Movement Pattern	Recommended Load
2	Compound	Light, Medium Weight

PRIMARY BENEFIT	FULL-BODY STRENGTH AND EXPLOSIVENESS
TARGET MUSCLES	CALVES, QUADRICEPS, GLUTES, ERECTORS, LATS, DELTOIDS, TRICEPS

Begin holding a kettlebell in a sideways rack (position one). Freeze, ensuring elbow-hip connection and the kettlebells aligned over your hips and knees, weights between your heels and toes. Next, hop and drop into position two: the undersquat, keeping the kettlebell over your center of mass. Pause before standing up into the final lockout, arms as straight as possible overhead (position three). After holding the lockout, return the kettlebell to the rack and repeat. Each position should remain still to build static strength and reinforce alignment. Often performed with doubles, five-ten seconds per position is common practice.

270. Jerk, Two-Hand

	Single Bell	Double Bell
	✓	✗

Technical Difficulty	Movement Pattern	Recommended Load
2	Compound	Heavy Weight

PRIMARY BENEFIT	FULL-BODY STRENGTH AND EXPLOSIVENESS
TARGET MUSCLES	CALVES, QUADRICEPS, GLUTES, ERECTORS, LATS, DELTOIDS, TRICEPS

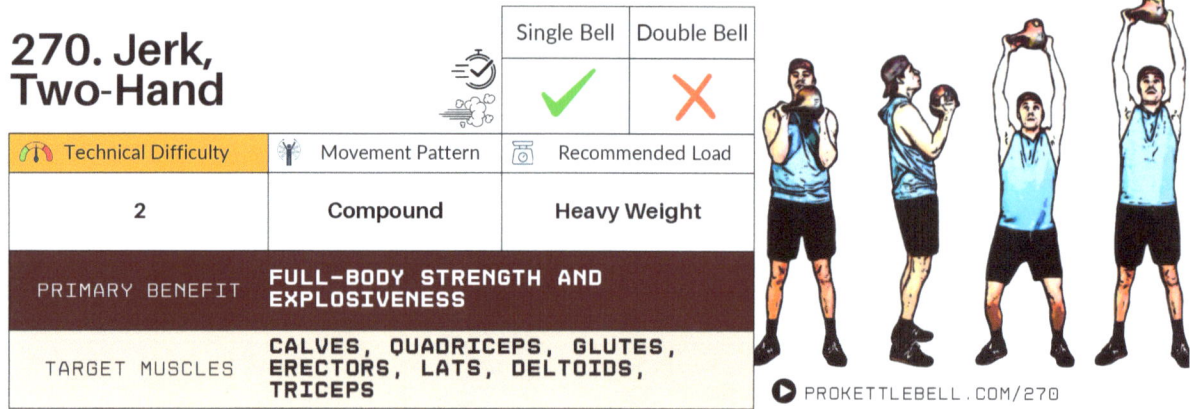

PROKETTLEBELL.COM/270

Begin the two-hand jerk by positioning one hand on the handle and the other on the base of a single kettlebell held sideways in the rack. From here, perform a semi-squat and then explosively jump into the undersquat while keeping the kettlebell aligned overhead. After catching it, stand tall into a full lockout, ensuring straight knees and elbows. Return to the rack to reset. Maintain arm-body contact during the lift and prioritize balance, alignment, and controlled lockout before initiating the next rep.

271. Bumps
PROKETTLEBELL.COM/271

	Single Bell	Double Bell
	✓	✓

Technical Difficulty	Movement Pattern	Recommended Load
3	Compound	Light, Medium Weight

PRIMARY BENEFIT	FULL-BODY POWER
TARGET MUSCLES	CALVES, QUADRICEPS, GLUTES, HAMSTRINGS, ERECTORS

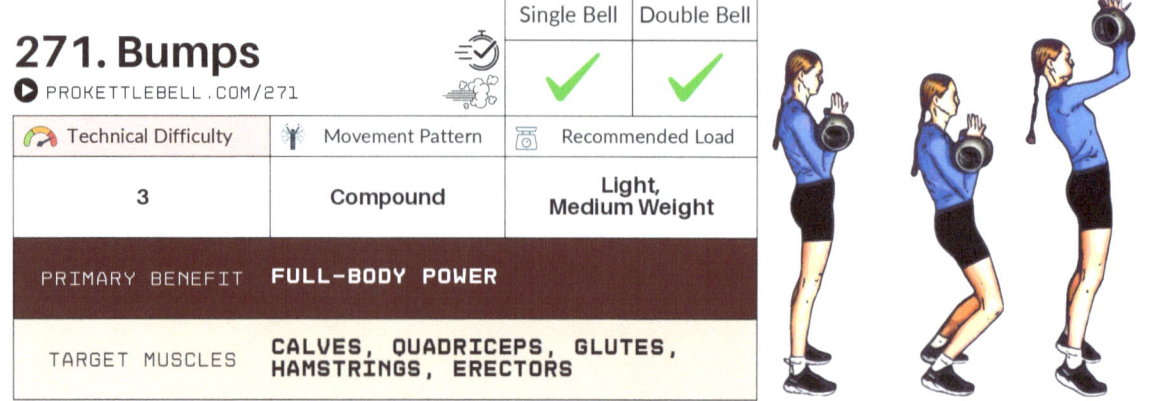

Begin bumps by cleaning two kettlebells into the rack position with elbows resting on your iliac crest and the bells aligned over your feet. From here, execute a rapid semi-squat followed by an explosive upward movement using your ankles, knees, and hips in a triple extension. This action causes the kettlebells to rise slightly above forehead height. Maintain a straight path for the bells directly over your hips. As they descend, absorb the weight by reconnecting your elbows to your hips, maintaining control and alignment throughout.

272. Double 3-Position Drill

PROKETTLEBELL.COM/272

	Single Bell	Double Bell
	✗	✓

Technical Difficulty	Movement Pattern	Recommended Load
3	Compound	Light, Medium Weight

PRIMARY BENEFIT	FULL-BODY STRENGTH
TARGET MUSCLES	QUADRICEPS, GLUTES, HAMSTRINGS, ERECTORS, LATS, DELTOIDS, TRICEPS

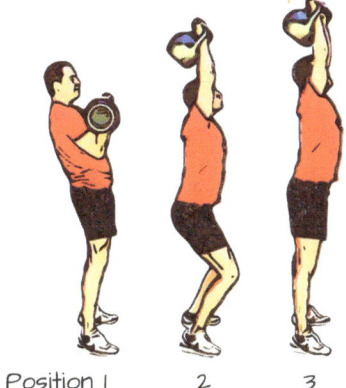

Position 1   2   3

Begin the double kettlebell three-position drill by cleaning both bells into the rack. Hold still for a few controlled breaths with heels grounded. Then, perform a small jump to drop into the undersquat, catching the bells overhead with locked arms and legs, keeping them balanced over your base. After a brief hold, stand into full overhead lockout, pause, then return to the rack. This drill sharpens mobility, balance, and posture through each phase of the jerk. Five-ten seconds per position is common practice.

273. Jerk, One-Arm

	Single Bell	Double Bell
	✓	✗

Technical Difficulty	Movement Pattern	Recommended Load
3	Compound	Heavy Weight

PRIMARY BENEFIT	FULL-BODY STRENGTH AND EXPLOSIVENESS
TARGET MUSCLES	CALVES, QUADRICEPS, GLUTES, ERECTORS, LATS, DELTOIDS, TRICEPS

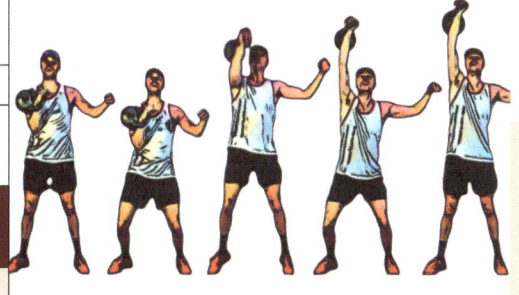

PROKETTLEBELL.COM/273

Clean a single kettlebell into the rack position, with your legs absorbing the load. Initiate the movement by dipping into a shallow semi-squat (the first dip), then spring on to your toes, using the momentum and power to launch the kettlebell upward. As the bell reaches its apex, drop underneath it into a quick undersquat to receive it overhead with a locked elbow. Stand up fully with your knees and elbow locked to achieve fixation. Return to the rack and repeat for reps.

274. Jerk, Two-Arm

PROKETTLEBELL.COM/274

	Single Bell	Double Bell
	✗	✓

Technical Difficulty	Movement Pattern	Recommended Load
3	Compound	Medium, Heavy Weight

PRIMARY BENEFIT	FULL-BODY STRENGTH AND POWER
TARGET MUSCLES	CALVES, QUADRICEPS, GLUTES, HAMSTRINGS, ERECTORS, LATS, DELTOIDS, TRICEPS

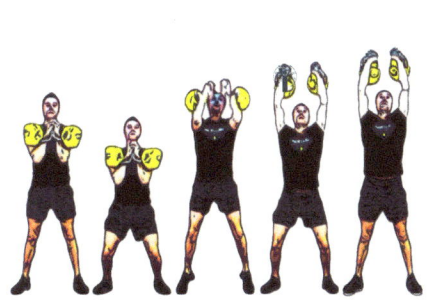

The double kettlebell jerk builds on the single-arm pattern, requiring symmetrical coordination, greater core stability, and increased power output—while reinforcing key principles like a vertical drive path, precise timing, and sharp overhead fixation. Begin by cleaning both kettlebells into the rack position, ensuring firm elbow-to-hip connection and vertical stacking over your center mass. From here, perform the same movement phases as the single-arm jerk: dip into a shallow semi-squat to load, then explode upward with triple extension, springing onto your toes. As the bells rise, quickly land beneath them in an undersquat to catch with locked elbows. Once stabilized, stand fully to fixation, with hips, knees, and arms extended. Return the bells to the rack, straighten your legs, and repeat.

JERKS

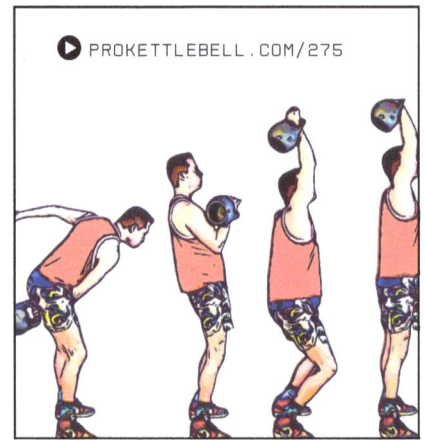

275. Long Cycle (Clean + Jerk)

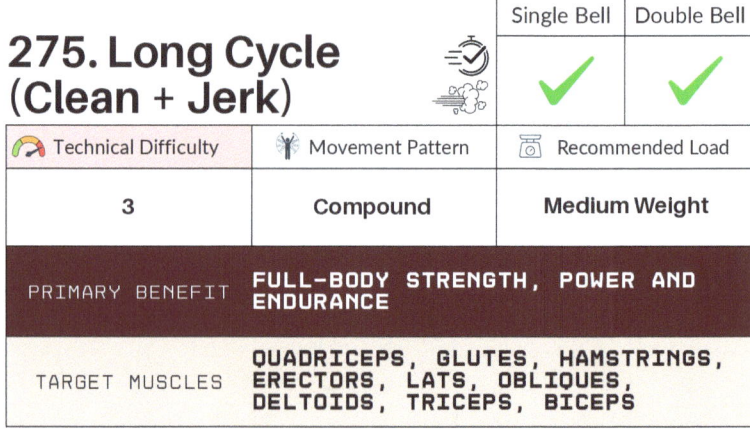

	Single Bell	Double Bell
	✓	✓

Technical Difficulty	Movement Pattern	Recommended Load
3	Compound	Medium Weight

PRIMARY BENEFIT	FULL-BODY STRENGTH, POWER AND ENDURANCE
TARGET MUSCLES	QUADRICEPS, GLUTES, HAMSTRINGS, ERECTORS, LATS, OBLIQUES, DELTOIDS, TRICEPS, BICEPS

Long cycle is a clean followed by a jerk. Rinse and repeat! To perform one or two-arm long cycle, execute a clean to bring the kettlebell(s) to the rack position. Straighten your legs and follow immediately with a jerk, driving the bell upward and dropping into the undersquat before standing tall with straight arms to complete the repetition. Return the bells to the rack and immediately begin another clean to repeat the cycle. Ensure each phase is distinct and that the kettlebell remains over your center mass throughout for stability and safety.

276. Speed-Switch Long Cycle

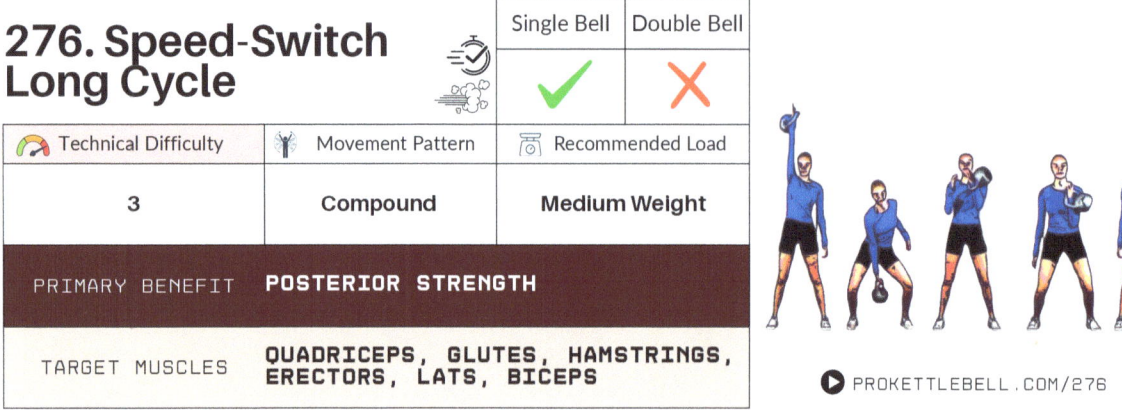

	Single Bell	Double Bell
	✓	✗

Technical Difficulty	Movement Pattern	Recommended Load
3	Compound	Medium Weight

PRIMARY BENEFIT	POSTERIOR STRENGTH
TARGET MUSCLES	QUADRICEPS, GLUTES, HAMSTRINGS, ERECTORS, LATS, BICEPS

Begin with a single kettlebell in the rack position. Quickly drive into a jerk, locking the kettlebell overhead before returning to the rack. After the rep, drop the kettlebell into a backswing. On the upswing, propel the bell across your center line and switch hands (the "speed-switch," landing in the rack position on the opposite side, where you'll begin the next jerk. This exercise builds technique and conditioning through increased volume provided by frequent hand transitions.

277. Split Jerk

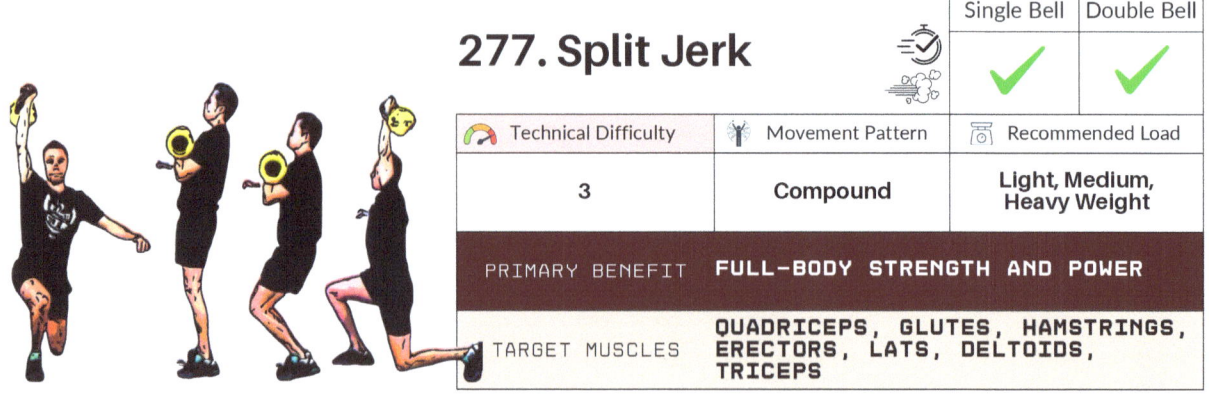

	Single Bell	Double Bell
	✓	✓

Technical Difficulty	Movement Pattern	Recommended Load
3	Compound	Light, Medium, Heavy Weight

PRIMARY BENEFIT	FULL-BODY STRENGTH AND POWER
TARGET MUSCLES	QUADRICEPS, GLUTES, HAMSTRINGS, ERECTORS, LATS, DELTOIDS, TRICEPS

To perform the single kettlebell split jerk, clean the bell into the rack and stand tall with feet together. Load your legs with a semi-squat and explode through the triple extension into a split lunge jump as the kettlebell extends into lockout. Land softly with the kettlebell stacked over your center line. Once stable, stand tall with a locked-out arm, bring your feet together and return the bell to the rack. Alternate which leg is forward with each rep. Match repetitions on the other arm.

Full-Body & Compound Movements
Strength & Conditioning

---— Section Five ——---

Deadlifts
Plank Combinations
Thrusters & Getups
Walks/Carries

Strength & Conditioning

1. Deadlifts

21-Deadlifts	121
Ballistic Deadlift	121
Conventional Two-Hand Deadlift	121
Diagonal Deadlifts	122
Gurney Deadlifts	122
Jefferson Deadlift	122
Kickstand Deadlift	123
Racked Deadlift	123
Romanian Deadlifts	123
Romanian Suitcase Deadlift	124
Rotating Deadlift	124
Single-Leg Gurney Deadlift	124
Suitcase Deadlift	125
Sumo Deadlift	125
Tik-Tok Deadlifts	125
Double Deadlift + Renegade Row	126
Pendulum Deadlift	126

2. Compound Planks

Double Kettlebell Plank Jacks	127
Floor-to-Kettlebell Plank	127
KB Touch + Spiderman Plank	127
Plank Palm Taps	128
Plank Push n' Pull	128
Side Plank Pull-Unders	128
Lateral Kettlebell Plank Walks	129
Motorcycles	129
Bear Crawl Pull	129

3. Thrusters & Getups

Thruster	130
Bottoms-Up Thruster	130
Thruster Twist, Single	130
Thruster Twist, Bottoms Up	131
Thruster Twist, Double	131
Narrow/Wide Thrusters	131
Slingshot Thruster	132
Deck Squat Thruster	132
Goblet Toss Thruster	132
Two-Hand Anyhow	133
Surrenders	133
Double Overhead Surrenders	133
Handless Getup	134
Turkish Getup	135

4. Walks / Holds / Carries

Farmer Carry / Farmer Hold	136
Pull-Over March	136
Racked Waiter Carry	136
Walking One-Arm Waiter Carry	137
Bottoms-Up High Knees	137
Duck Walk	137

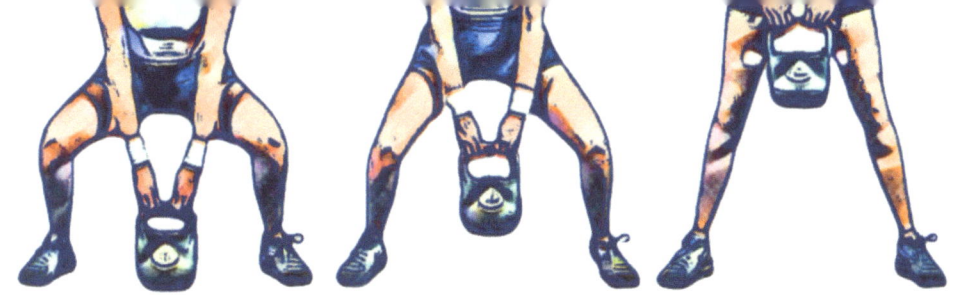

A spin-off of 21- curls (a series of 7 reps each of three different phases of the movement), 21s increase time under tension to maximize muscle engagement. Start with seven reps moving from the ground to halfway up, then seven from the top to halfway down, finishing with seven full-range reps. Throughout, maintain deadlift form: keep feet flat, hips back, lumbar flat, and knees tracking toes. Arms should remain straight, and the kettlebell close to the center of mass.

278. 21-Deadlifts

PROKETTLEBELL.COM/278

	Single Bell	Double Bell
	✓	✓

Technical Difficulty	Movement Pattern	Recommended Load
1	Hinge	Heavy Weight

PRIMARY BENEFIT	POSTERIOR STRENGTH AND HYPERTROPHY
TARGET MUSCLES	GLUTES, QUADRICEPS, HAMSTRINGS, ERECTORS

279. Ballistic Deadlift

PROKETTLEBELL.COM/279

	Single Bell	Double Bell
	✓	✓

Technical Difficulty	Movement Pattern	Recommended Load
1	Hinge	Medium Weight

PRIMARY BENEFIT	LOWER BODY EXPLOSIVENESS AND CORE STRENGTH
TARGET MUSCLES	QUADRICEPS, GLUTES, HAMSTRINGS, CALVES, ERECTORS, ABDOMINALS

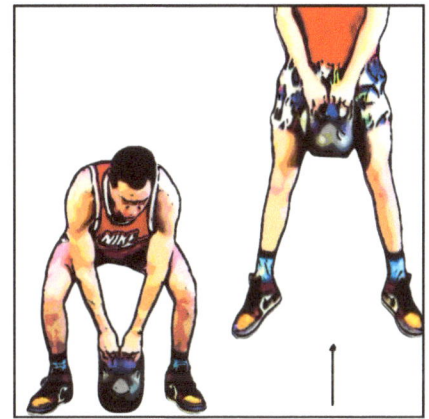

This is an explosive variation of the deadlift, adding a jump to intensify the movement. Begin with the kettlebell between your feet, centered under your body. With arms locked straight and tight to your torso, drive upward forcefully to jump while maintaining deadlift alignment. Return the kettlebell to the floor each rep. Rest as needed to maintain form. This powerful move trains speed and power while reinforcing proper deadlift mechanics.

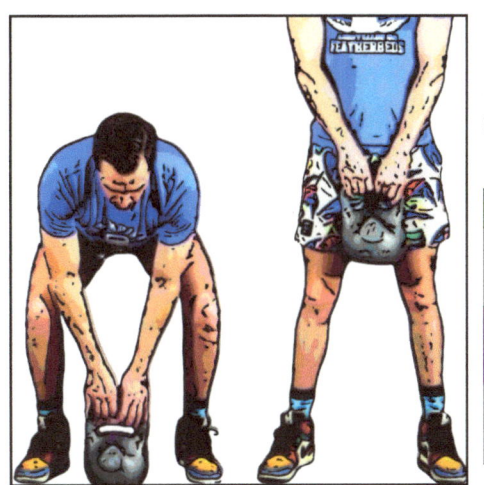

280. Conventional Two-Hand Deadlift

	Single Bell	Double Bell
	✓	✗

Technical Difficulty	Movement Pattern	Recommended Load
1	Hinge	Heavy Weight

PRIMARY BENEFIT	CORE AND BACK STRENGTH
TARGET MUSCLES	HAMSTRINGS, GLUTES, ERECTORS, TRAPS

PROKETTLEBELL.COM/280

Position the kettlebell between your heels and toes, directly under your center line. Sit your hips back with a flat lumbar, chest up, and arms straight. Drive through your legs to stand up, squeezing glutes and quads at the top. Unlike barbell deadlifts, your hands stay inside your legs. Always bring the bell back to the floor and keep it close to the body to protect your back. Customize stance width based on mobility.

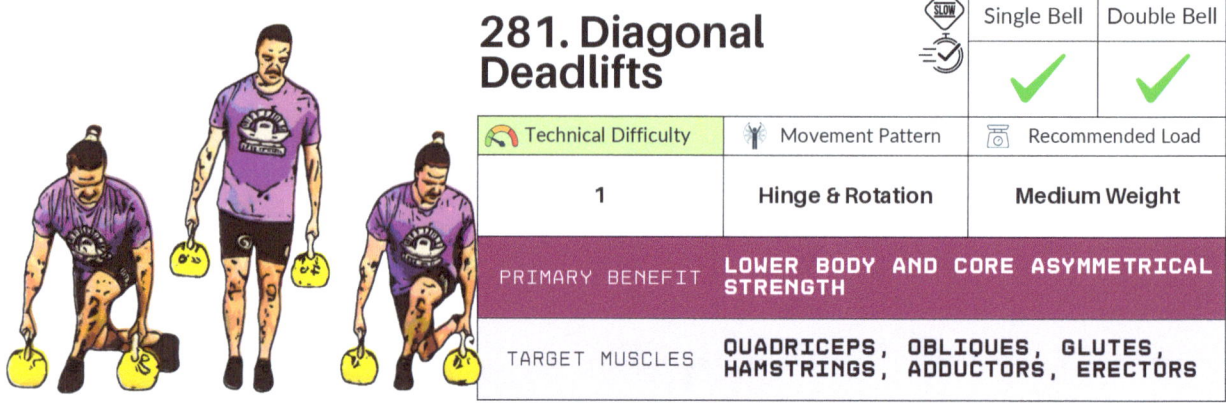

281. Diagonal Deadlifts

	Single Bell	Double Bell
SLOW	✓	✓

Technical Difficulty	Movement Pattern	Recommended Load
1	Hinge & Rotation	Medium Weight

PRIMARY BENEFIT	LOWER BODY AND CORE ASYMMETRICAL STRENGTH
TARGET MUSCLES	QUADRICEPS, OBLIQUES, GLUTES, HAMSTRINGS, ADDUCTORS, ERECTORS

Start with feet together and kettlebells at your sides. Step one foot diagonally backward into a curtsy squat and lower the bells to the floor. Lift the bells and return the back leg to feet together. Next, step diagonally forward with the opposite leg into a cross squat, lowering the kettlebells outside the front foot. Push through the front heel to lift the bells and return to the start. Maintain a flat back and upright chest, with arms straight throughout. The front leg bears the load and the knee must track the toes. ▶ PROKETTLEBELL.COM/281

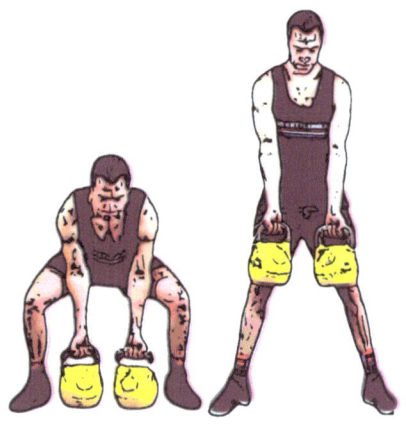

▶ PROKETTLEBELL.COM/282

282. Gurney Deadlifts

	Single Bell	Double Bell
SLOW	✗	✓

Technical Difficulty	Movement Pattern	Recommended Load
1	Hinge	Heavy Weight

PRIMARY BENEFIT	LOWER BODY, CORE STRENGTH AND MOBILITY
TARGET MUSCLES	QUADRICEPS, GLUTES, HAMSTRINGS, ERECTORS, LATS

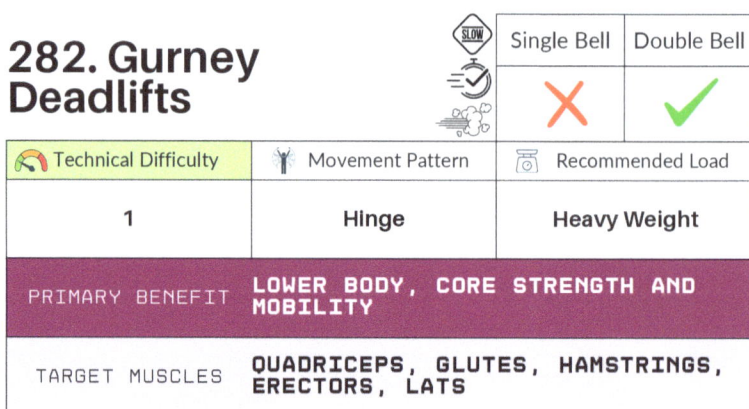

Using a gurney grip (palms forward), pick up two kettlebells either in a narrow suitcase or wider stance. Keep weights close to your center of mass and drive through your heels, maintaining a flat back and extended arms. This mimics lifting heavy objects like furniture. The forward-facing grip stretches the forearms and activates stabilizers, making this variation practical and effective for real-life lifting scenarios.

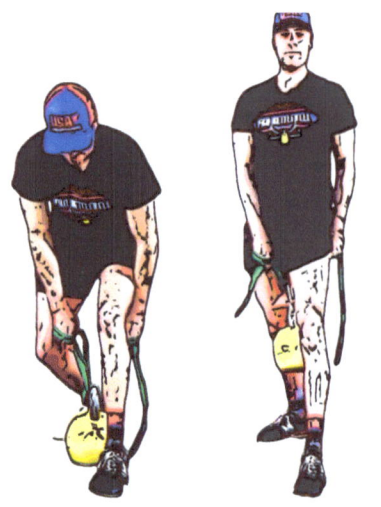

▶ PROKETTLEBELL.COM/283

283. Jefferson Deadlift

	Single Bell	Double Bell
SLOW	✓	✗

Technical Difficulty	Movement Pattern	Recommended Load
1	Hinge	Heavy Weight

PRIMARY BENEFIT	LEG AND CORE STRENGTH
TARGET MUSCLES	QUADRICEPS, GLUTES, HAMSTRINGS, OBLIQUES, ERECTORS, LATS, ARMS

Straddle a kettlebell threaded with a strap or towel. With one foot facing forward and the other at a 45° angle, grab the strap and stand up by driving through both legs evenly. Keep the kettlebell directly beneath you, arms straight, chest up, and back flat. This deadlift mimics real-world lifting asymmetry and challenges your coordination. You can add more kettlebells on the strap to increase load safely.

284. Kickstand Deadlift

	Single Bell	Double Bell
	✓	✓

Technical Difficulty	Movement Pattern	Recommended Load
1	Hinge	Medium, Heavy Weight

PRIMARY BENEFIT	LEG, BACK AND CORE STRENGTH
TARGET MUSCLES	HAMSTRINGS, GLUTES, QUADRICEPS ERECTORS

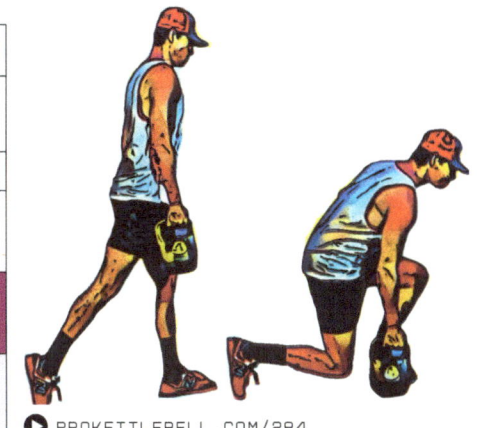

PROKETTLEBELL.COM/284

With the kettlebell beside your front foot, stagger your stance so the rear foot acts as a light stabilizer. Hinge at the hips, keeping your back flat and chest lifted as you raise and lower the kettlebell from the ground. The majority of the work is done by the front leg. Arms remain straight, and the kettlebell travels in a straight path. Adjust the rear foot's distance for balance, but always ensure alignment through the front foot, knee, and hip.

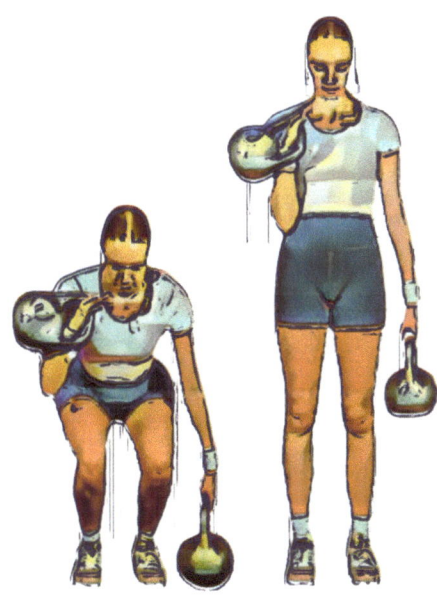

285. Racked Deadlift

	Single Bell	Double Bell
	✗	✓

Technical Difficulty	Movement Pattern	Recommended Load
1	Hinge	Medium, Heavy Weight

PRIMARY BENEFIT	ASYMMETRICAL FULL-BODY STRENGTH
TARGET MUSCLES	QUADRICEPS, GLUTES, HAMSTRINGS, ERECTORS, OBLIQUES, LATS, DELTOIDS, BICEPS

Start with one kettlebell racked at your chest and another on the floor. With the free arm, hinge down and lift the second kettlebell while keeping your spine neutral and chest upright. The racked bell stays tight to your frame, and the other arm moves straight down and up. This deadlift simulates real-life lifting where you're holding one object while picking up another, promoting core and unilateral strength.

PROKETTLEBELL.COM/285

286. Romanian Deadlift

	Single Bell	Double Bell
	✓	✗

Technical Difficulty	Movement Pattern	Recommended Load
1	Hinge	Heavy Weight

PRIMARY BENEFIT	POSTERIOR STRENGTH AND MOBILITY
TARGET MUSCLES	GLUTES, HAMSTRINGS, ERECTORS

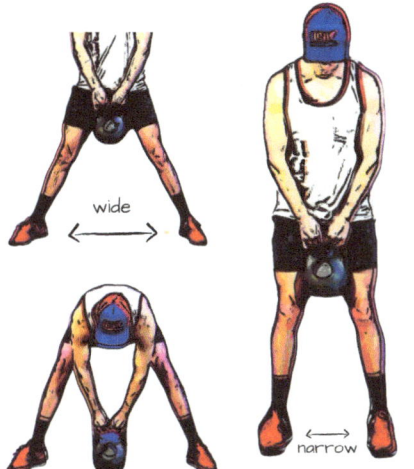

Keep your knees relatively straight while hinging at the hips. The kettlebell stays close to your center mass as you lower with a flat back and lifted chest. Focus on stretching the hamstrings and loading the glutes. Adjust your stance width and depth based on flexibility. This version limits knee bend, intensifying posterior chain engagement. Use platforms or boxes if needed to maintain form through limited mobility.

PROKETTLEBELL.COM/286

DEADLIFTS

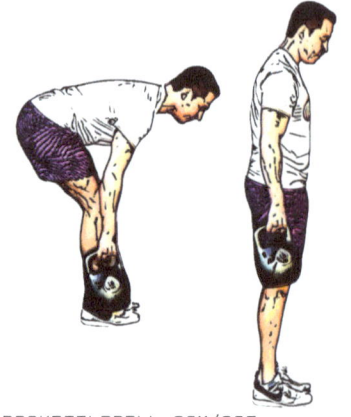

287. Romanian Suitcase Deadlift

	Single Bell	Double Bell
SLOW	✓	✓

Technical Difficulty	Movement Pattern	Recommended Load
1	Hinge	Heavy Weight

PRIMARY BENEFIT	POSTERIOR STRENGTH
TARGET MUSCLES	GLUTES, HAMSTRINGS

▶ PROKETTLEBELL.COM/287

Similar to the Romanian deadlift but performed with weights outside your legs in a suitcase grip. Feet are narrow, heels down, and knees aligned with toes. Lower as far as you can while keeping your back flat and chest high. Feel the hamstring stretch, then drive through your heels to rise. Arms stay straight, and the bell must remain between your heel and toe line. This builds strength with added lateral stability.

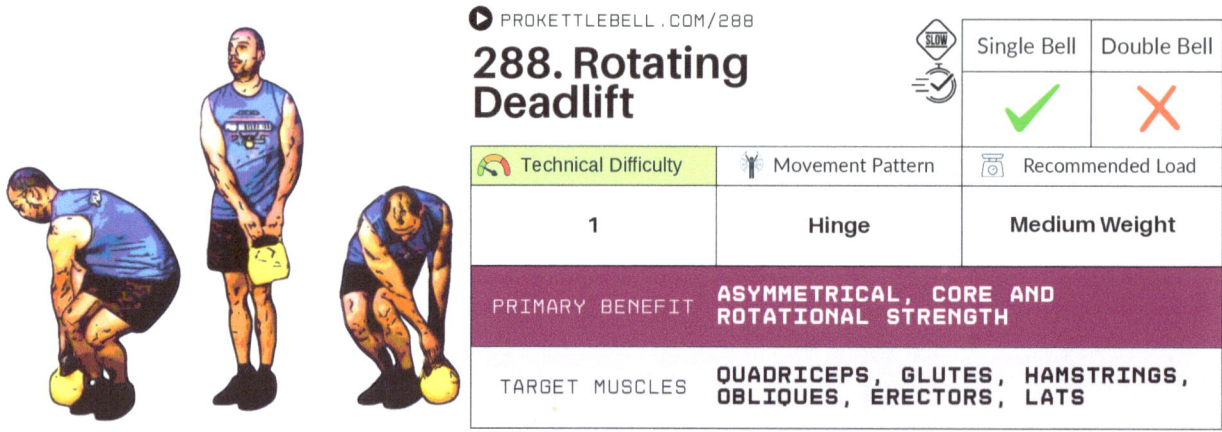

▶ PROKETTLEBELL.COM/288

288. Rotating Deadlift

	Single Bell	Double Bell
SLOW	✓	✗

Technical Difficulty	Movement Pattern	Recommended Load
1	Hinge	Medium Weight

PRIMARY BENEFIT	ASYMMETRICAL, CORE AND ROTATIONAL STRENGTH
TARGET MUSCLES	QUADRICEPS, GLUTES, HAMSTRINGS, OBLIQUES, ERECTORS, LATS

With the kettlebell set to one side, pick it up while keeping it close to your legs, then rotate and place it on the opposite side. Maintain a flat back, chest up, and straight arms throughout. This movement mimics real-life lifting at awkward angles and improves mobility and control through the trunk, knees, and hips. Start light to focus on precision and balance during the rotation phase.

289. Single-Leg Gurney Deadlift

	Single Bell	Double Bell
SLOW	✓	✗

Technical Difficulty	Movement Pattern	Recommended Load
1	Hinge	Medium, Heavy Weight

PRIMARY BENEFIT	LEG AND CORE STRENGTH
TARGET MUSCLES	QUADRICEPS, GLUTES, HAMSTRINGS, ERECTORS, LATS

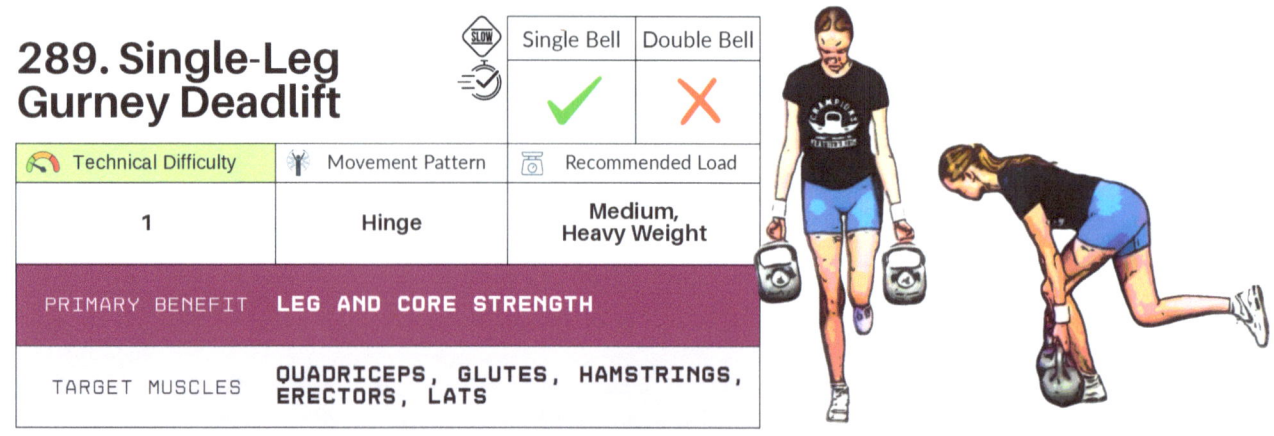

With palms forward in a gurney grip, hinge at the hips as one leg extends behind you for balance. The weight stays behind your toes, chest up, and back flat. This single-leg version targets stabilizers, glutes, and hamstrings while building balance and control. Arms remain straight, and the movement should be slow and controlled to prevent injury and reinforce symmetry.

▶ PROKETTLEBELL.COM/289

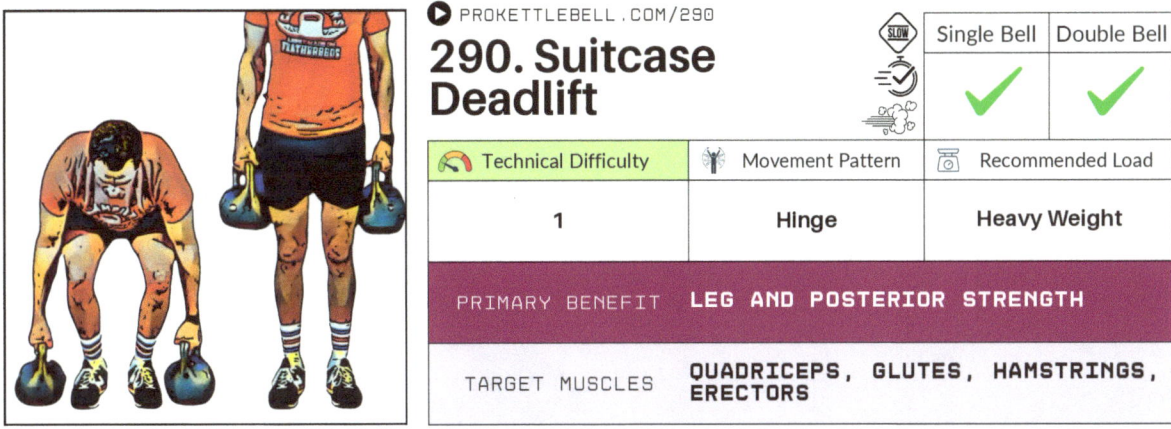

290. Suitcase Deadlift

PROKETTLEBELL.COM/290

	Single Bell	Double Bell
	✓	✓

Technical Difficulty	Movement Pattern	Recommended Load
1	Hinge	Heavy Weight

PRIMARY BENEFIT	LEG AND POSTERIOR STRENGTH
TARGET MUSCLES	QUADRICEPS, GLUTES, HAMSTRINGS, ERECTORS

Stand with a narrow stance and kettlebells outside your legs. Feet, knees, and hips are aligned, and heels stay flat. Hinge down to grab the bells, keeping the weight close to your center mass. Arms stay straight, and you lift by driving through your legs, not pulling with your arms. Return the bells to the ground each rep. This variation challenges lateral stability and simulates real-world asymmetrical lifting.

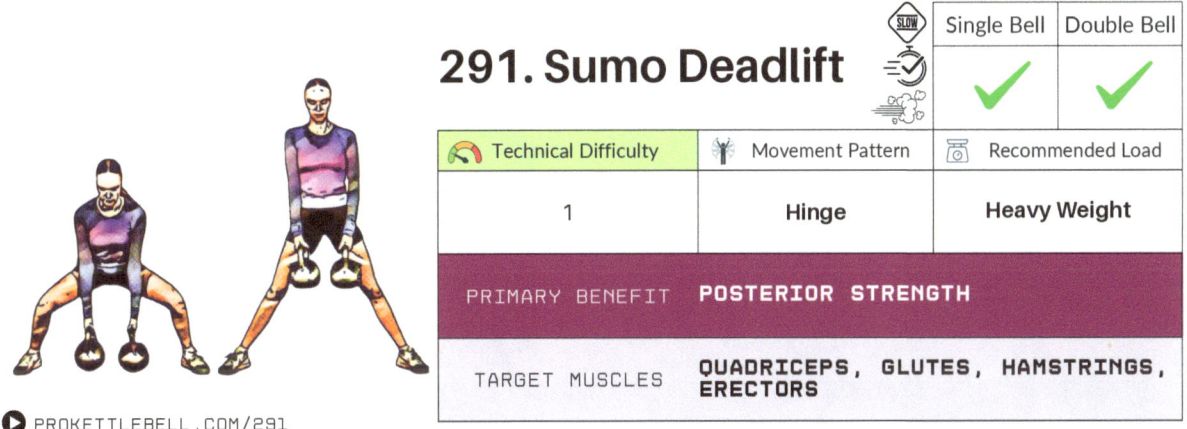

291. Sumo Deadlift

	Single Bell	Double Bell
	✓	✓

Technical Difficulty	Movement Pattern	Recommended Load
1	Hinge	Heavy Weight

PRIMARY BENEFIT	POSTERIOR STRENGTH
TARGET MUSCLES	QUADRICEPS, GLUTES, HAMSTRINGS, ERECTORS

PROKETTLEBELL.COM/291

Set your feet wide and point your toes slightly out. Place the kettlebells close under your body, behind your toes. Sit down with a flat back, chest lifted, and arms straight to grab the bells. Drive up by wedging your legs, finishing with hips forward and shoulders neutral. Return to the ground fully each rep. This version favors those with long limbs or limited mobility and emphasizes inner thigh and hip strength.

292. Tik-Tok Deadlifts

	Single Bell	Double Bell
	✓	✓

Technical Difficulty	Movement Pattern	Recommended Load
1	Hinge	Medium, Heavy Weight

PRIMARY BENEFIT	LEG AND CORE STRENGTH
TARGET MUSCLES	QUADRICEPS, GLUTES, HAMSTRINGS, ERECTORS, LATS

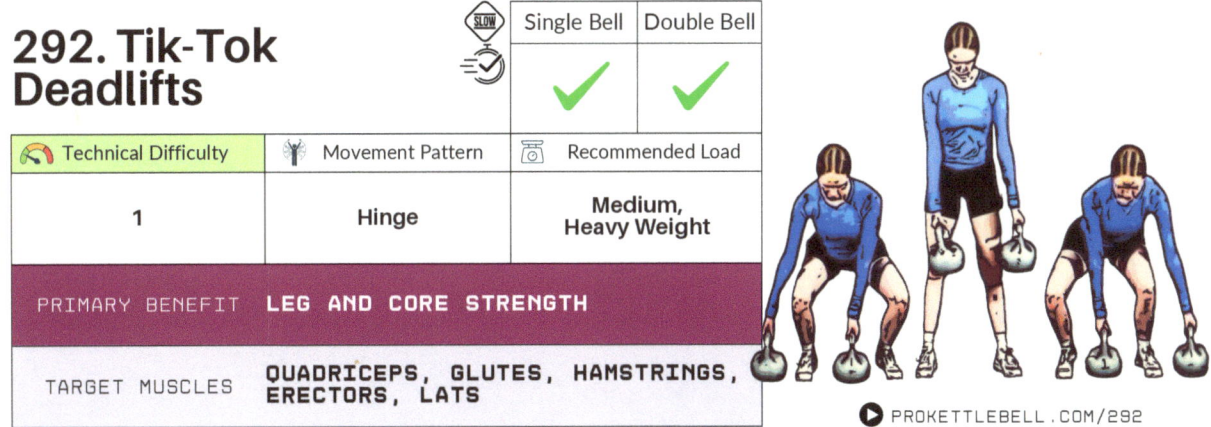

PROKETTLEBELL.COM/292

Stand asymmetrically with one foot inside and one outside a pair of kettlebells. Keeping your back flat, chest up, and arms straight, lift the kettlebells and swing them across your body to the other side. Alternate sides each rep. The bells should stay close to your legs and behind your toes at all times. This move trains real-world asymmetrical lifting strength and emphasizes control and alignment throughout.

DEADLIFTS

Begin with two kettlebells between your feet and perform a standard deadlift. Set them down and jump into a plank with wide feet for stability. Perform a row on each side, keeping elbows tight to your ribs. Return to standing and repeat. Maintain a flat back throughout and ensure kettlebells stay beneath your center mass. This combination builds both lower body and upper body strength in one fluid sequence.

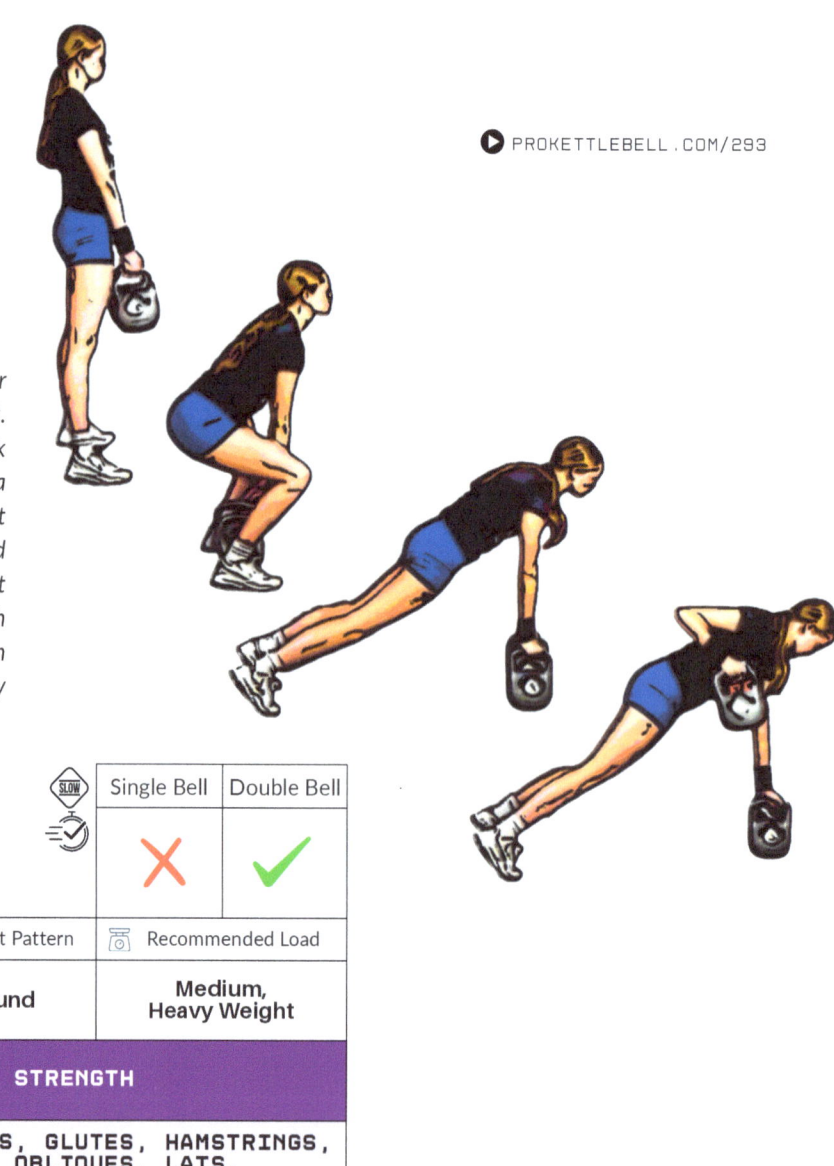

▶ PROKETTLEBELL.COM/293

293. Double Deadlift + Renegade Row

	Single Bell	Double Bell
SLOW	✗	✓

Technical Difficulty	Movement Pattern	Recommended Load
2	Compound	Medium, Heavy Weight

PRIMARY BENEFIT	FULL-BODY STRENGTH
TARGET MUSCLES	QUADRICEPS, GLUTES, HAMSTRINGS, ERECTORS, OBLIQUES, LATS, BICEPS

294. Pendulum Deadlift

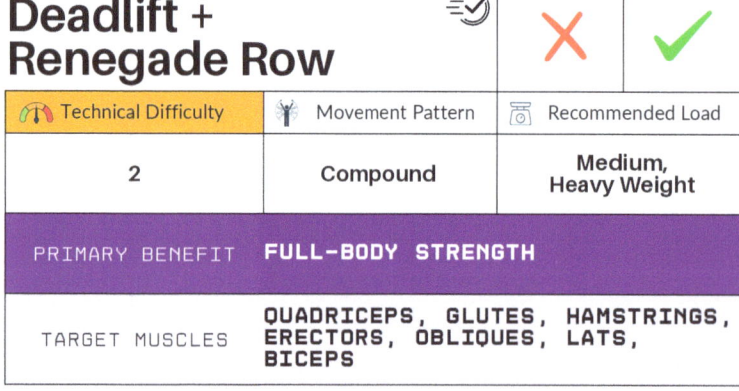

	Single Bell	Double Bell
SLOW	✓	✓

Technical Difficulty	Movement Pattern	Recommended Load
2	Hinge	Medium, Heavy Weight

PRIMARY BENEFIT	LOWER BODY AND CORE STRENGTH
TARGET MUSCLES	GLUTES, HAMSTRINGS, ABS, OBLIQUES, ERECTORS, LATS

Stand with feet together, holding a kettlebell in one hand. Hinge forward as the leg on the kettlebell side extends behind you. Maintain a flat lumbar and upright chest. This movement challenges your core, especially the obliques, as you resist rotation from the one-sided load. The planted leg does most of the work, targeting glutes and hamstrings while improving balance and anti-rotational strength. ▶ PROKETTLEBELL.COM/294

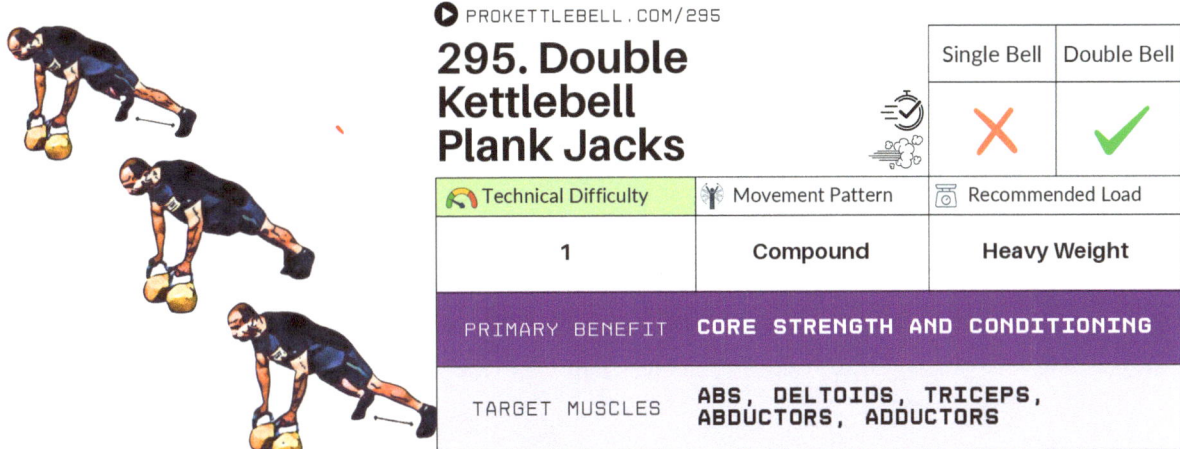

PROKETTLEBELL.COM/295

295. Double Kettlebell Plank Jacks

	Single Bell	Double Bell
	✗	✓

Technical Difficulty	Movement Pattern	Recommended Load
1	Compound	Heavy Weight

PRIMARY BENEFIT	CORE STRENGTH AND CONDITIONING
TARGET MUSCLES	ABS, DELTOIDS, TRICEPS, ABDUCTORS, ADDUCTORS

Start in a plank position with both hands gripping the handles of two kettlebells, which should be directly under your shoulders and about shoulder-width apart. Keep your body in a straight line from head to heels, avoiding a swayback or raised hips. From this position, jump your feet out wide and then back together, just like a jumping jack, while maintaining the strong plank. This move targets core strength and elevates your heart rate.

296. Floor-to-Kettlebell Plank

	Single Bell	Double Bell
	✗	✓

Technical Difficulty	Movement Pattern	Recommended Load
1	Compound	Heavy Weight

PRIMARY BENEFIT	UPPER BODY AND CORE STRENGTH
TARGET MUSCLES	ABS, OBLIQUES, ERECTORS, LATS, DELTOIDS, TRICEPS

PROKETTLEBELL.COM/296

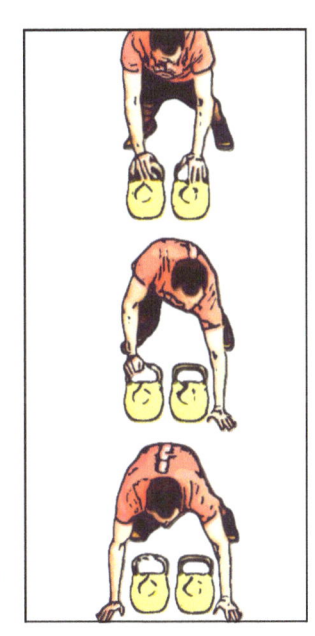

Begin with a pair of kettlebells on the ground, their handles parallel and stable. Plank on top of the kettlebells, keeping a flat back. Lower one hand to the floor, followed by the other, then return to the kettlebells one hand at a time. Alternate which hand leads. Keep the movement slow and controlled to maintain form and fully engage the abs, obliques, delts, pecs, and triceps.

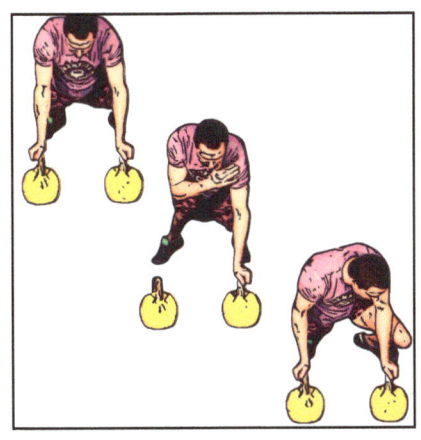

297. KB Touch + Spiderman Plank

	Single Bell	Double Bell
	✗	✓

Technical Difficulty	Movement Pattern	Recommended Load
1	Compound	Heavy Weight

PRIMARY BENEFIT	UPPER BODY AND CORE STRENGTH
TARGET MUSCLES	DELTOIDS, TRICEPS, ABS, OBLIQUES

Using two sturdy kettlebells, plank with hands gripping the handles and your body aligned. Touch your right hand to your left shoulder, then your left hand to your right shoulder, minimizing hip rotation. Then bring your right knee toward your right elbow, followed by the left knee to the left elbow. Continue this sequence with control. This move strengthens the core, delts, pecs, and obliques while testing balance and stability.

PROKETTLEBELL.COM/297

COMPOUND PLANKS

298. Plank Palm Taps

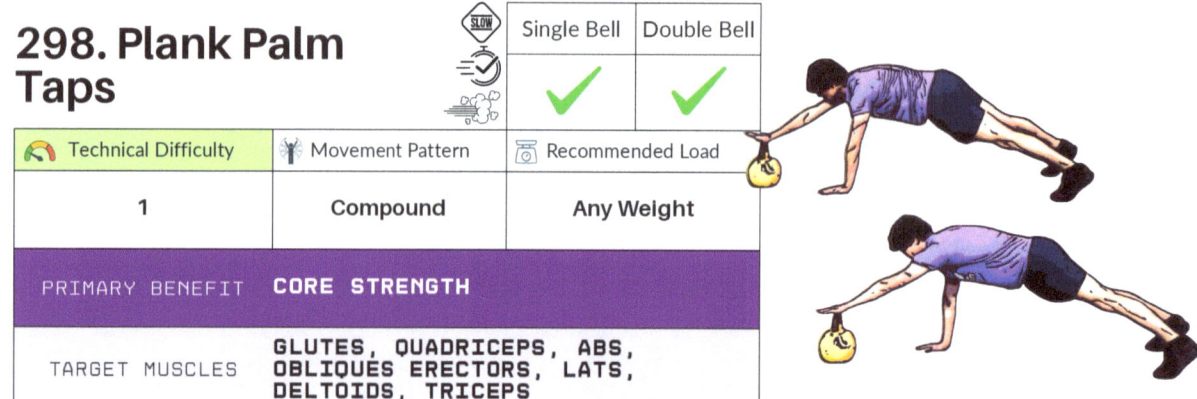

	Single Bell	Double Bell
	✓	✓

Technical Difficulty	Movement Pattern	Recommended Load
1	Compound	Any Weight

PRIMARY BENEFIT	CORE STRENGTH
TARGET MUSCLES	GLUTES, QUADRICEPS, ABS, OBLIQUES ERECTORS, LATS, DELTOIDS, TRICEPS

In a strong plank position with your hands beneath your shoulders and body aligned head to heel, reach forward to tap the top of a kettlebell with one palm, then alternate. You can modify by doing the movement from your knees. A wider foot stance helps with stability, while a narrower one increases difficulty. This move works the core, triceps, and deltoids, and reinforces plank form. ▶ PROKETTLEBELL.COM/298

299. Plank Push n' Pull

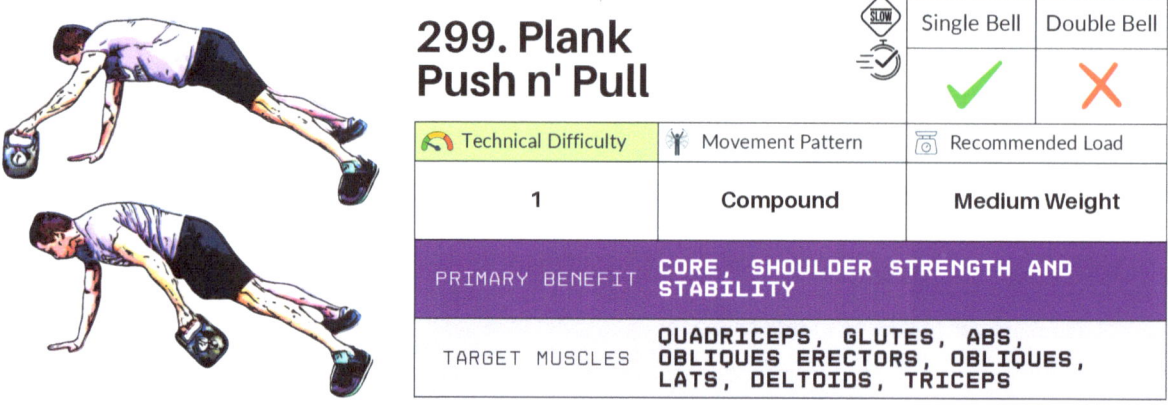

	Single Bell	Double Bell
	✓	✗

Technical Difficulty	Movement Pattern	Recommended Load
1	Compound	Medium Weight

PRIMARY BENEFIT	CORE, SHOULDER STRENGTH AND STABILITY
TARGET MUSCLES	QUADRICEPS, GLUTES, ABS, OBLIQUES ERECTORS, OBLIQUES, LATS, DELTOIDS, TRICEPS

Set a light kettlebell slightly ahead of your plank position. From a solid plank, reach with one arm to pull the kettlebell toward you, then push it forward again. Keep your hips steady by widening your feet. Use a lightweight since the movement extends outside your center of mass, putting pressure on shoulders, core, and glutes. You can modify by performing it on your knees or using a light object like a water bottle. ▶ PROKETTLEBELL.COM/299

300. Side Plank Pull-Unders

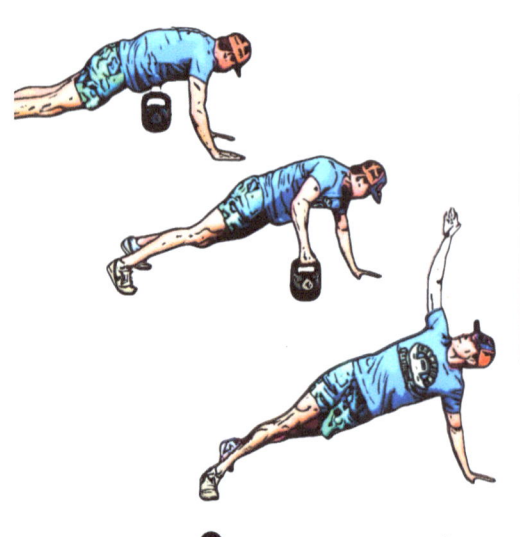

	Single Bell	Double Bell
	✓	✗

Technical Difficulty	Movement Pattern	Recommended Load
1	Compound	Medium Weight

PRIMARY BENEFIT	CORE STRENGTH
TARGET MUSCLES	ABS, OBLIQUES, ERECTORS, LATS, DELTOIDS, TRICEPS

▶ PROKETTLEBELL.COM/300

Start in a strong plank with a kettlebell positioned just outside your chest. Reach under your torso with one arm to pull the kettlebell across your body. After pulling, rotate into a side plank, raising the same arm to the sky. Lower back to plank and repeat, alternating sides. Keep your hips level until the kettlebell is stationary, then rotate. This controlled movement targets the abs, obliques, delts, and triceps.

301. Lateral Kettlebell Plank Walks

	Single Bell	Double Bell
	✗	✓

Technical Difficulty	Movement Pattern	Recommended Load
2	Compound	Heavy Weight

PRIMARY BENEFIT	ARM AND CORE STRENGTH
TARGET MUSCLES	ABS, ERECTORS, OBLIQUES, LATS, DELTOIDS, PECS, TRICEPS

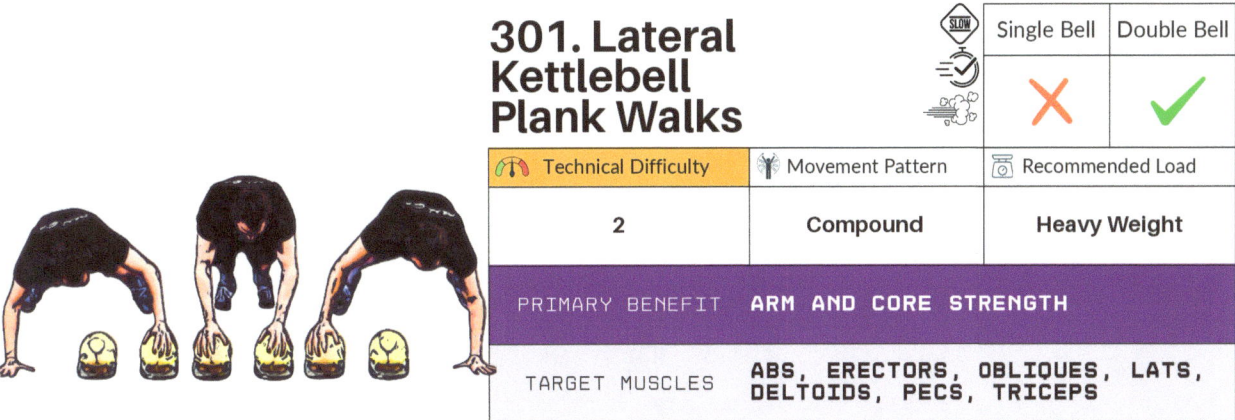

Place two kettlebells side by side, either with handles facing down for more surface area or upright for a challenge. Plank with each hand on a kettlebell, ensuring a straight line from wrists through shoulders to feet. Step your right hand and foot out, then bring them back, repeating on the left side. Move slowly and deliberately to maintain control. This exercise targets upper body stability and core strength. ▶ PROKETTLEBELL.COM/301

302. Motorcycles

	Single Bell	Double Bell
	✓	✗

Technical Difficulty	Movement Pattern	Recommended Load
2	Compound	Heavy Weight

PRIMARY BENEFIT	UPPER BODY AND CORE STRENGTH
TARGET MUSCLES	ABS, OBLIQUES, LATS, PECS, DELTOIDS, TRICEPS

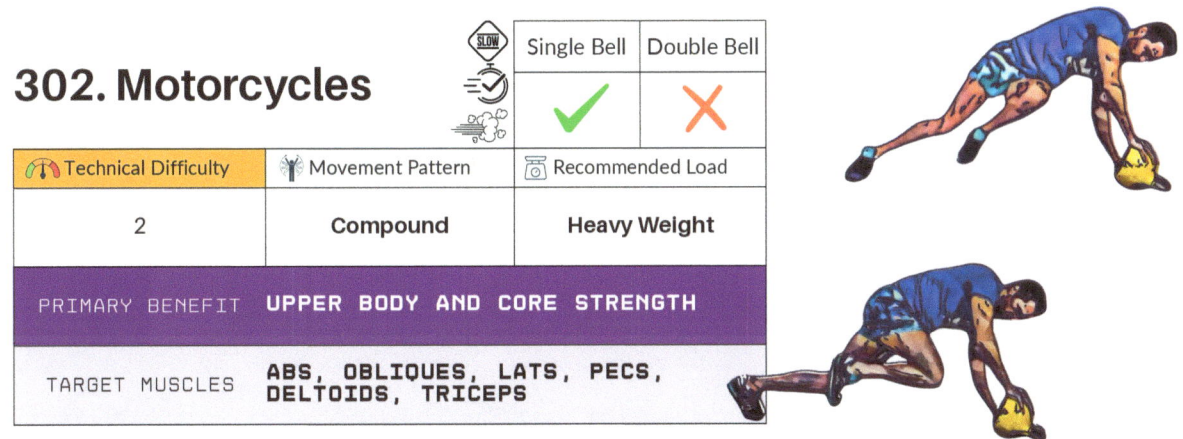

Start in a plank with one hand on top of a kettlebell. Rotate your hips about 45 degrees toward the kettlebell and begin mountain-climber-like leg motions. Keep your torso aligned and hips low, mimicking a sharp turn on a motorcycle. Hand placement on the kettlebell can vary for comfort. ▶ PROKETTLEBELL.COM/302

303. Bear Crawl Pull

	Single Bell	Double Bell
	✓	✗

Technical Difficulty	Movement Pattern	Recommended Load
2	Compound	Light Weight

PRIMARY BENEFIT	CORE STRENGTH AND MOBILITY
TARGET MUSCLES	QUADRICEPS, HAMSTRINGS, ABS, OBLIQUES, ERECTORS, DELTOIDS, TRICEPS

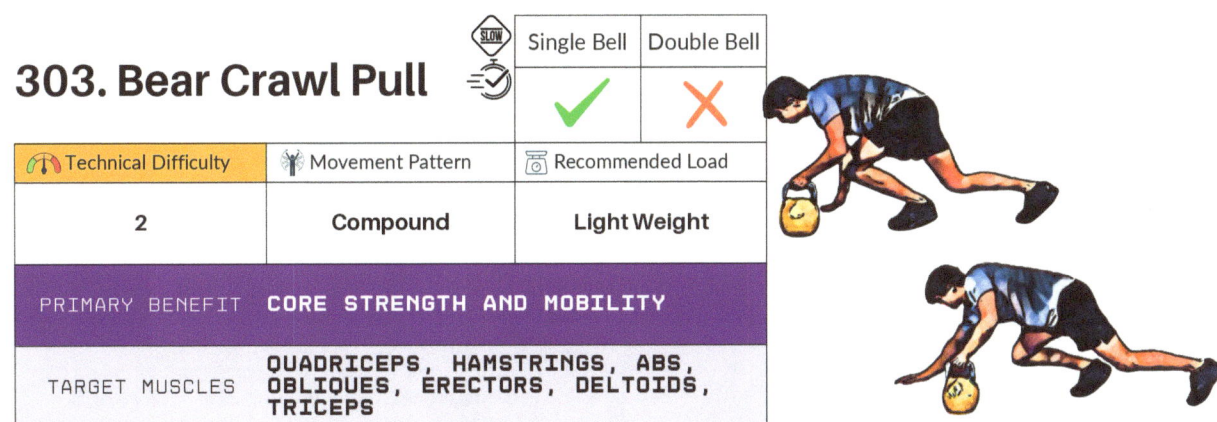

Begin in a bear crawl position with knees off the ground and a single kettlebell placed underneath your shoulder. Crawl forward while dragging the kettlebell with you, keeping your elbows close to your ribs. Maintain control and keep the weight close to your body. This full-body move was designed for first responders and develops core, shoulder, arm, and leg strength while elevating heart rate. ▶ PROKETTLEBELL.COM/303

COMPOUND PLANKS

304. Thruster

PROKETTLEBELL.COM/304

	Single Bell	Double Bell
	✓	✗

Technical Difficulty	Movement Pattern	Recommended Load
1	Compound	Medium, Heavy Weight

PRIMARY BENEFIT	LEGS, CORE, ARM STRENGTH AND CONDITIONING
TARGET MUSCLES	QUADRICEPS, GLUTES, HAMSTRING, CORE, SHOULDERS, TRICEPS

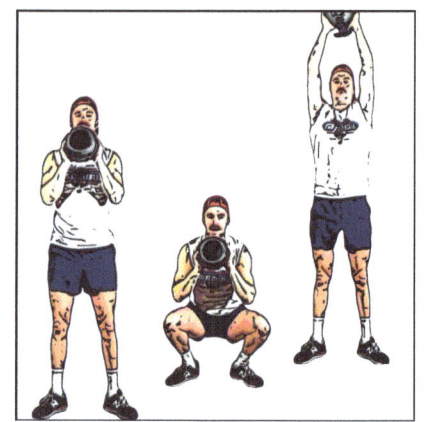

Stand in a squat stance with a kettlebell held in both hands at chest level. Drop into a full squat with good alignment—knees tracking toes, back flat, chest up. As you rise from the squat, drive the kettlebell straight overhead into a full lockout. Hold momentarily at the top for joint loading benefits. Bring the kettlebell(s) back to your chest and repeat. Perform with two-hands on one bell, or "single-arm," holding one or two kettlebells in the rack position.

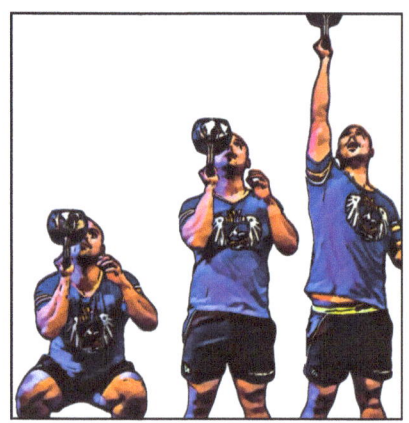

305. Bottoms-Up Thruster

	Single Bell	Double Bell
	✓	✗

Technical Difficulty	Movement Pattern	Recommended Load
1	Compound	Light, Medium Weight

PRIMARY BENEFIT	LEGS, CORE, ARM STRENGTH AND CONDITIONING
TARGET MUSCLES	QUADRICEPS, GLUTES, HAMSTRING, CORE, SHOULDERS, TRICEPS, BICEPS

Begin with the kettlebell in a bottoms-up rack position—held by the handle with the bottom of the bell facing upward and balanced near your chest. Stand with your feet shoulder-width apart. Lower into a squat, keeping your chest upright, back flat, and knees tracking your toes. As you drive up from the bottom of the squat, press the kettlebell overhead while maintaining the bottoms-up position. Lock out at the top with control to engage the shoulder and stabilize the wrist and grip. Lower the bells back to your chest and repeat. This variation challenges full-body power while heavily engaging wrist, forearm, and shoulder stability. ▶ PROKETTLEBELL.COM/305

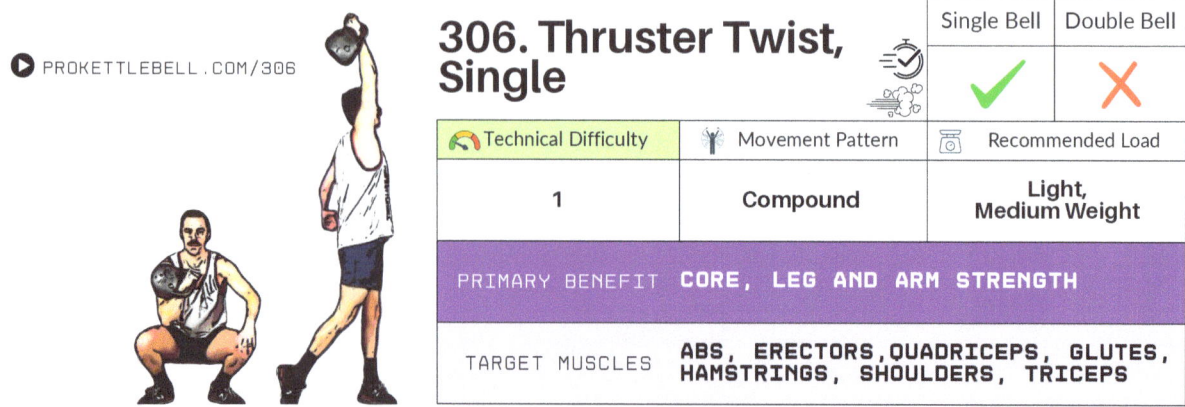

▶ PROKETTLEBELL.COM/306

306. Thruster Twist, Single

	Single Bell	Double Bell
	✓	✗

Technical Difficulty	Movement Pattern	Recommended Load
1	Compound	Light, Medium Weight

PRIMARY BENEFIT	CORE, LEG AND ARM STRENGTH
TARGET MUSCLES	ABS, ERECTORS, QUADRICEPS, GLUTES, HAMSTRINGS, SHOULDERS, TRICEPS

Hold the kettlebell in the rack position with one arm. Perform a squat with great form—chest up, hips back, heels down. As you rise, twist 90 degrees toward the opposite side and press the kettlebell overhead. For example, if the bell is in your right hand, twist left and press. Return to center and repeat. Let the heel of the pressing side lift slightly during the twist to prevent strain in your knees and hips while promoting proper trunk rotation.

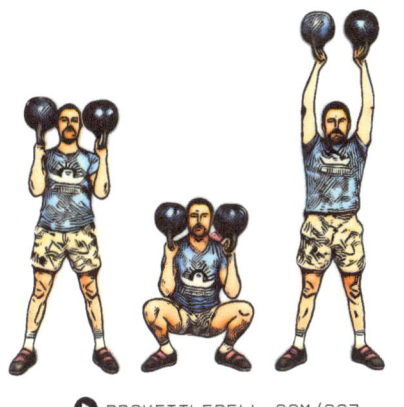

307. Thruster, Double Bottoms Up

	Single Bell	Double Bell
	✓	✓

Technical Difficulty	Movement Pattern	Recommended Load
2	Squat, Push Rotate	Light, Medium Weight

PRIMARY BENEFIT	FULL-BODY STRENGTH AND CONDITIONING
TARGET MUSCLES	QUADRICEPS, GLUTES, HAMSTRINGS, ERECTORS, OBLIQUES, LATS, DELTOIDS, TRICEPS

▶ PROKETTLEBELL.COM/307

Begin holding two kettlebells upside-down and balanced near your chest. Stand with your feet shoulder-width apart. Lower into a squat, keeping your chest upright, back flat, and knees tracking your toes. As you drive up from the bottom of the squat, press the kettlebells overhead while maintaining the bottoms-up position. Lock out at the top with control to engage the shoulder and stabilize the wrist and grip. Bring the bells back to the chest and repeat. Hold the handles near the corners for maximum control. For added challenge, hold the kettlebells in the center of the handles.

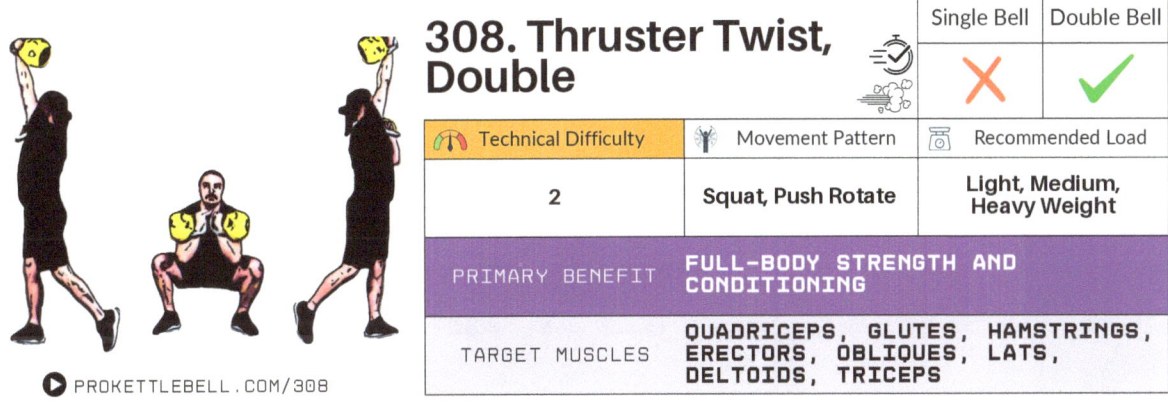

308. Thruster Twist, Double

	Single Bell	Double Bell
	✗	✓

Technical Difficulty	Movement Pattern	Recommended Load
2	Squat, Push Rotate	Light, Medium, Heavy Weight

PRIMARY BENEFIT	FULL-BODY STRENGTH AND CONDITIONING
TARGET MUSCLES	QUADRICEPS, GLUTES, HAMSTRINGS, ERECTORS, OBLIQUES, LATS, DELTOIDS, TRICEPS

▶ PROKETTLEBELL.COM/308

Clean two kettlebells into the rack position and assume a squat stance. Lower into a deep squat, then as you rise, twist to one side while pressing the opposite arm overhead. For example, twist left and press with the right arm. Return to center, squat again, and repeat the twist to the opposite side. Allow your back foot to pivot during the twist to avoid unnecessary strain on your knee. This move improves spinal mobility and coordination.

309. Narrow/Wide Thrusters

	Single Bell	Double Bell
	✗	✓

Technical Difficulty	Movement Pattern	Recommended Load
2	Compound	Medium Weight

PRIMARY BENEFIT	FULL-BODY STRENGTH AND CONDITIONING
TARGET MUSCLES	QUADRICEPS, GLUTES, HAMSTRINGS, ERECTORS, LATS, DELTOIDS, TRICEPS

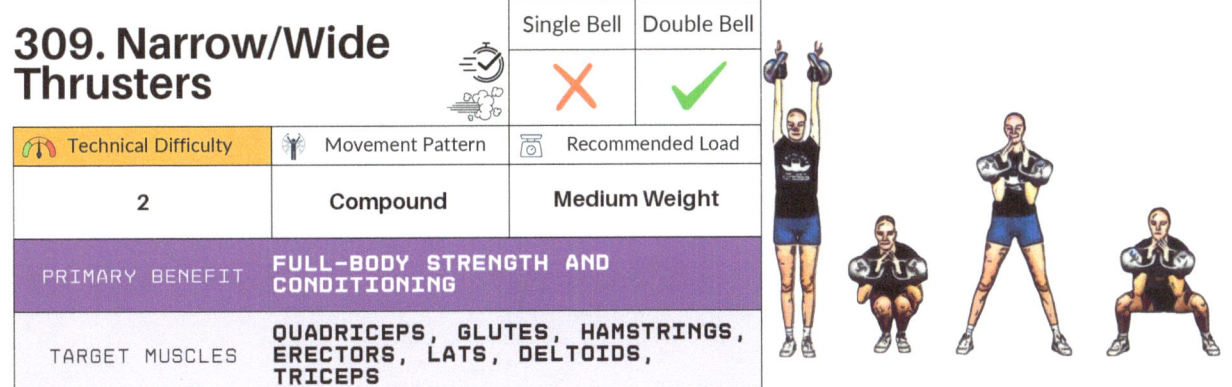

▶ PROKETTLEBELL.COM/309

Clean two kettlebells into the rack position. Begin with a narrow stance, ankles, knees, and hips aligned. Perform a narrow squat, press the bells overhead, and bring them back to rack. Step out to a wider stance and perform a wide squat and press. Continue alternating between narrow and wide squat thrusts. Keep your chest upright, lumbar flat, and knees tracking toes for every rep, with a strong overhead lockout to complete each movement.

310. Slingshot Thruster

	Single Bell	Double Bell
	✓	✗

Technical Difficulty	Movement Pattern	Recommended Load
2	Compound	Medium Weight

PRIMARY BENEFIT: CORE, LEG AND ARM STRENGTH

TARGET MUSCLES: ABS, ERECTORS, QUADS, GLUTES, HAMSTRINGS, SHOULDERS, TRICEPS

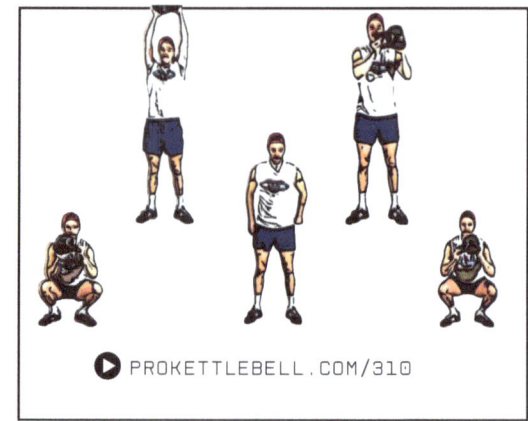

▶ PROKETTLEBELL.COM/310

Hold the kettlebell with both hands and begin a slingshot by swinging it behind your back and catching it in front with the opposite hand. From there, perform a deep squat with the bell close to your chest and press it overhead as you stand. Return the bell to the front and initiate another slingshot, switching hands. Alternate sides with each rep. Maintain squat form and finish each press with the bell directly overhead for maximal joint engagement.

311. Deck Squat Thruster

	Single Bell	Double Bell
	✓	✗

Technical Difficulty	Movement Pattern	Recommended Load
2	Compound	Medium, Heavy Weight

PRIMARY BENEFIT: CORE STRENGTH

TARGET MUSCLES: ABS, OBLIQUES, ERECTORS, LATS, DELTOIDS, TRICEPS

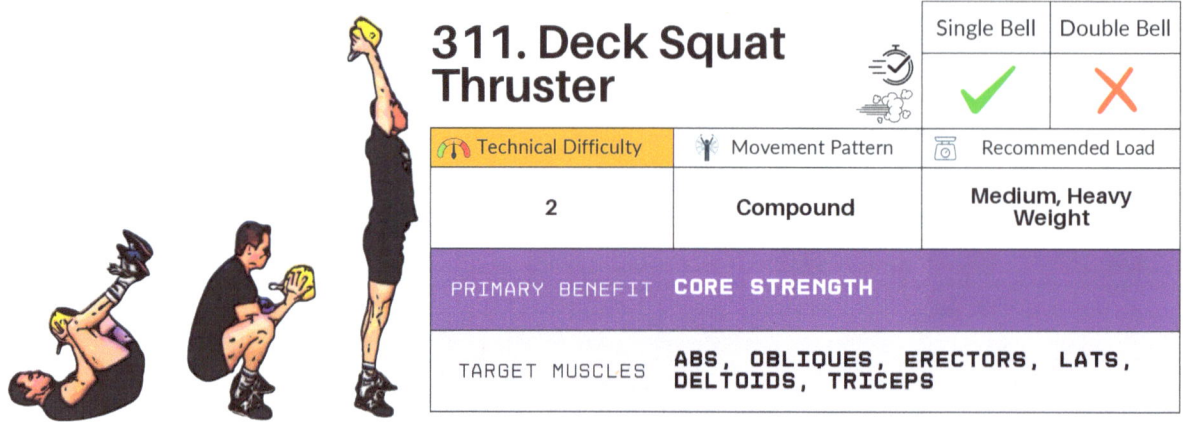

Hold the kettlebell at chest height, standing with feet shoulder-width apart. Sit all the way down into a deep squat, then roll back onto your shoulder blades without letting the kettlebell pull you out of position. Use momentum to roll forward and stand up smoothly, keeping the kettlebell close to your chest. As you reach full standing, press the kettlebell overhead into a locked-out position. Avoid rolling onto your neck and ensure you're fully stacked over your feet before pressing. ▶ PROKETTLEBELL.COM/311

312. Goblet Toss Thruster

	Single Bell	Double Bell
	✓	✗

Technical Difficulty	Movement Pattern	Recommended Load
3	Compound	Medium, Heavy Weight

PRIMARY BENEFIT: FULL-BODY STRENGTH AND CONDITIONING

TARGET MUSCLES: QUADRICEPS, GLUTES, HAMSTRINGS, ERECTORS, DELTOIDS, TRICEPS

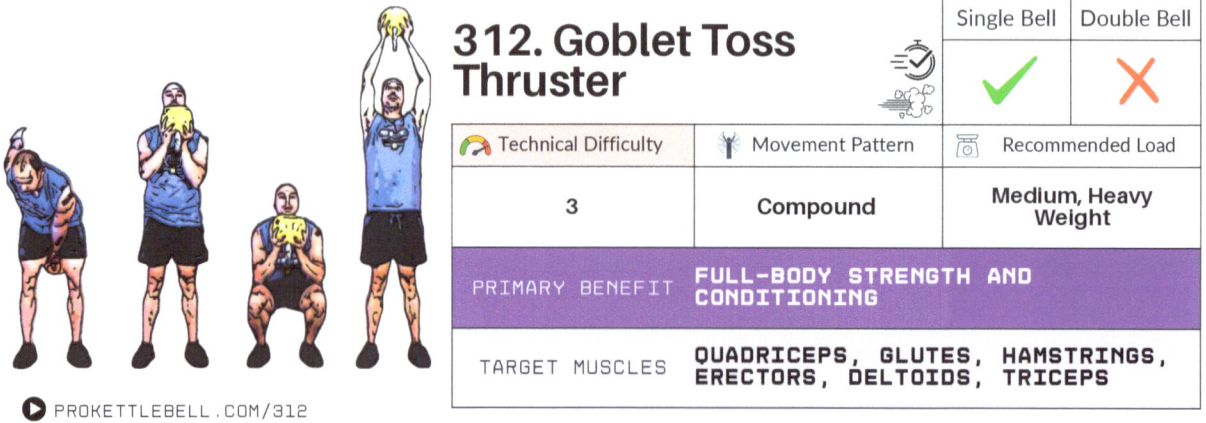

▶ PROKETTLEBELL.COM/312

Start with a wide enough stance to allow a kettlebell swing between your legs. Swing and catch the kettlebell bottom-up in a goblet position. Drop into a deep goblet squat, keeping the bell close. As you rise, press the kettlebell straight overhead into a lockout position. Control the kettlebell's momentum, ensuring your form remains intact throughout. This exercise combines strength and explosive power while engaging the full body.

313. Two-Hand Anyhow

	Single Bell	Double Bell
SLOW	✓	✗

Technical Difficulty	Movement Pattern	Recommended Load
3	Compound	Light, Medium Weight

PRIMARY BENEFIT	FULL-BODY STRENGTH AND MOBILITY
TARGET MUSCLES	QUADS, GLUTES, HAMSTRINGS, ERECTORS, LATS, DELTS, OBLIQUES, TRICEPS, BICEPS

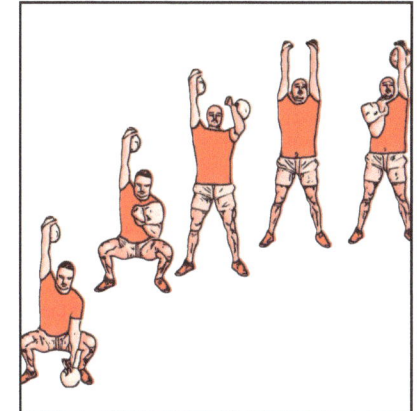

Start with two kettlebells and clean them into the rack position. Press one overhead while keeping the other racked. Perform an overhead squat, then lower the racked bell to the ground in a reverse-curling motion, then curl it back up to the rack. Stand and press the racked bell so that both bells are locked out overhead. Alternate arms for each rep, repeating the sequence. Maintain alignment throughout the movement and begin with light weights or bodyweight to learn proper technique and control.

▶ PROKETTLEBELL.COM/313

314. Surrenders

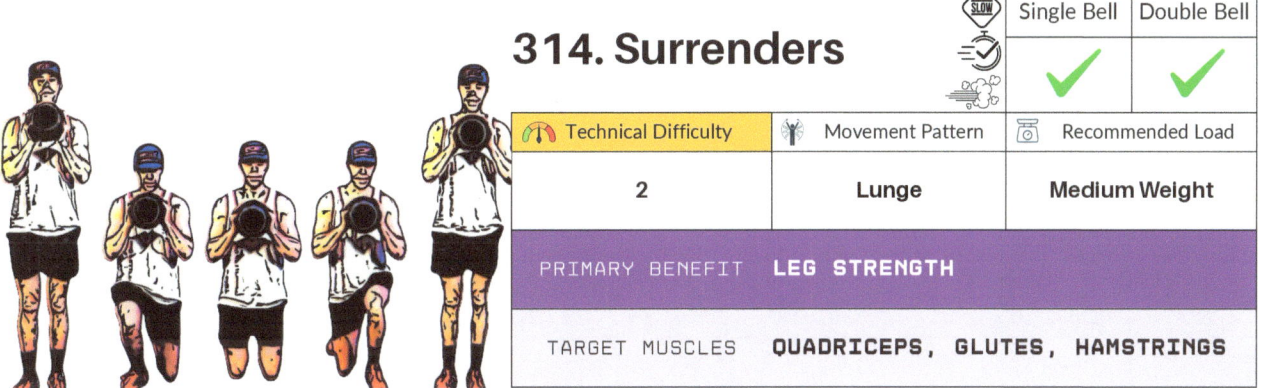

	Single Bell	Double Bell
SLOW	✓	✓

Technical Difficulty	Movement Pattern	Recommended Load
2	Lunge	Medium Weight

PRIMARY BENEFIT	LEG STRENGTH
TARGET MUSCLES	QUADRICEPS, GLUTES, HAMSTRINGS

Hold the kettlebell tightly at your chest. Kneel down on one knee, then the other, and return to standing by stepping up in reverse order. Alternate the lead leg or perform one side at a time. Use a mat if needed and keep your chest proud and core tight throughout the movement. ▶ PROKETTLEBELL.COM/314

315. Surrenders, Double Overhead

	Single Bell	Double Bell
SLOW	✗	✓

Technical Difficulty	Movement Pattern	Recommended Load
2	Compound	Light Weight

PRIMARY BENEFIT	FULL-BODY STRENGTH AND MOBILITY
TARGET MUSCLES	QUADRICEPS, GLUTES, HAMSTRINGS, ERECTORS, LATS, DELTOIDS, TRICEPS

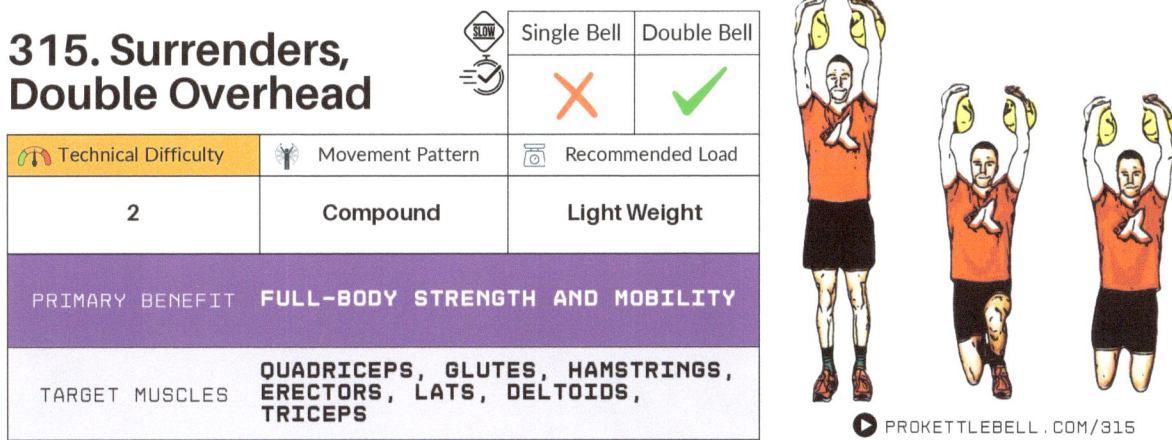

▶ PROKETTLEBELL.COM/315

Start with two light kettlebells, clean them into the rack position, and press them both overhead. Begin the surrender by kneeling with one leg, then the other, keeping the bells locked overhead. Stand up by leading with the leg that went down first. You can alternate legs or perform several reps on the same side before switching. Maintain core engagement and shoulder stability throughout the entire movement to protect joints and improve balance.

THRUSTERS & GETUPS

316. Handless Getup

	Single Bell	Double Bell
	✓	✗

Technical Difficulty	Movement Pattern	Recommended Load
3	Compound	Light Weight

PRIMARY BENEFIT	FULL-BODY STRENGTH AND MOBILITY
TARGET MUSCLES	QUADRICEPS, GLUTES, HAMSTRINGS, ERECTORS, OBLIQUES, LATS, DELTOIDS, TRICEPS

Here's a Turkish Get-Up variation that can be performed unweighted as a progression drill, or loaded for an added challenge once control and mechanics are solid.

Lie in a sit-up position with a kettlebell pressed overhead. Perform an armbar sit-up without using your hands. Transition your legs into a shin box position and then rise to a kneeling lunge. Stand up fully, maintaining the kettlebell overhead the entire time. Reverse the movement by stepping back into the lunge, lowering into the shin box, transitioning to a sit-up position, and returning to the ground. Train each phase separately for better control and stability.

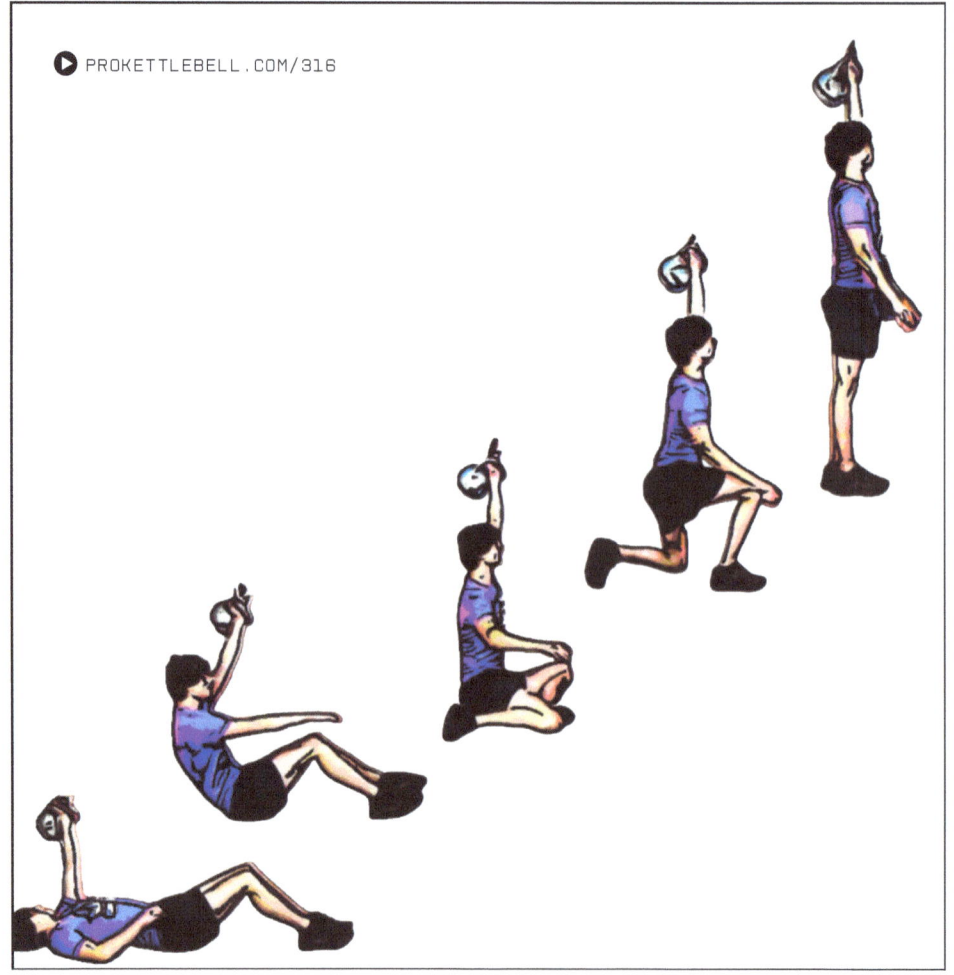

PROKETTLEBELL.COM/316

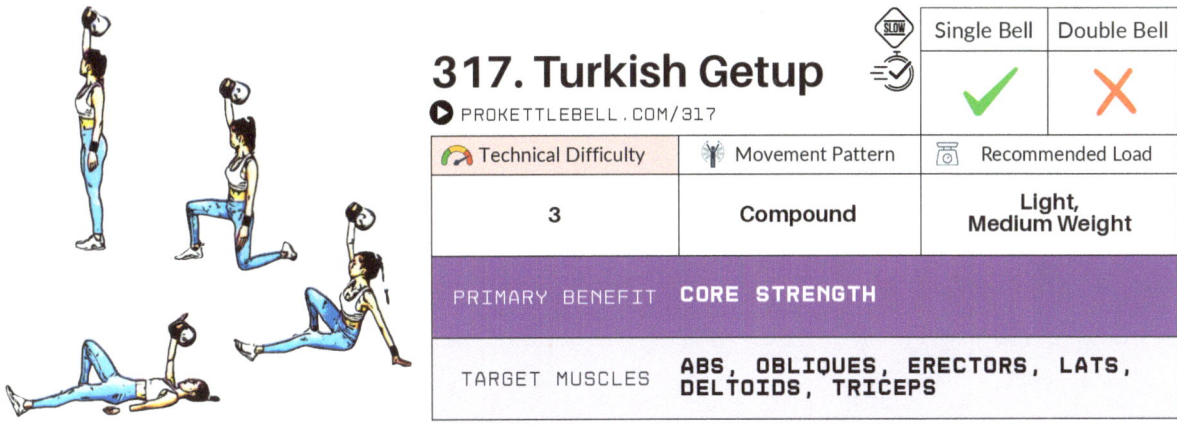

317. Turkish Getup
PROKETTLEBELL.COM/317

	Single Bell	Double Bell
	✓	✗

Technical Difficulty	Movement Pattern	Recommended Load
3	Compound	Light, Medium Weight

PRIMARY BENEFIT	CORE STRENGTH
TARGET MUSCLES	ABS, OBLIQUES, ERECTORS, LATS, DELTOIDS, TRICEPS

The Turkish Get-Up (TGU) is a full-body movement that blends strength, mobility, and control. The movement involves transitioning from lying on your back to standing up—and then returning—while holding a weight overhead. Beginners should start with a light object like a shot glass or water bottle cap to learn balance and alignment before progressing to weights. Drill the individual phases forward and backward prior to stringing them together.

Phase 1: Get into Position
- Lay on the floor on your side. Pull the kettlebell close, roll onto your back and press the kettlebell overhead until fully locked out above your shoulder.
- Bend the leg on the kettlebell side and keep your lats engaged to stabilize the weight and prepare for movement.

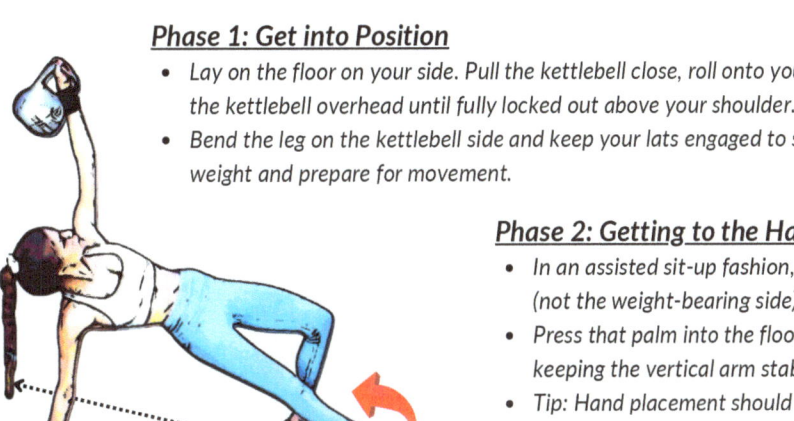

Phase 2: Getting to the Hand
- In an assisted sit-up fashion, roll onto your opposite elbow (not the weight-bearing side).
- Press that palm into the floor and straighten your arm, keeping the vertical arm stable.
- Tip: Hand placement should be at a 45-degree angle from your hip—not behind you. This ensures a good path for the next step.

Phase 3: Bridge and Sweep
- Bridge your hips high using your bent leg.
- Sweep the straight leg behind you into a half-kneeling position (this is the "Johnny sweep" move).
- Drop your hips down slightly for balance and square off into a proper kneeling lunge.

Phase 4: Stand Up
- Check your posture: weight over shoulder, shoulder over hip.
- Ensure your feet are wide enough apart to form a strong base.
- Drive up into a standing position—don't rush.

Phase 5: Stand Up
- Step back into your reverse lunge.
- Drop the knee carefully, then place your hand out to
- the side (not behind).
- Sweep your leg back through to the front.
- Lower your hips, then to your elbow, then your shoulders, and finally guide the weight down to your chest.
- Use your free hand to assist in rolling the weight off safely.

Whether you're a wrestler, a desk worker, or just building better movement habits, the TGU offers joint-friendly, progressive training that strengthens your foundation from the ground up. Start slow, stay precise, and build strength with intention.

THRUSTERS & GETUPS

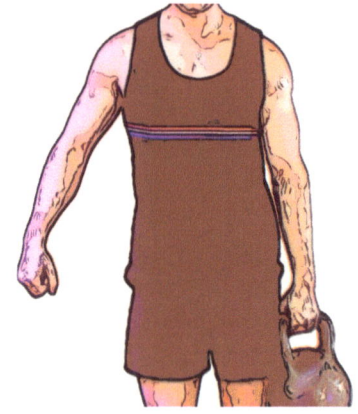

318. Farmer Carry

Technical Difficulty	Movement Pattern	Recommended Load
1	Compound	Heavy

	Single Bell	Double Bell
	✓	✓

PRIMARY BENEFIT — GRIP STRENGTH

TARGET MUSCLES — FOREARMS, TRAPS

To perform the farmer carry or farmer hold, begin by standing tall with a kettlebell in one or both hands, arms relaxed at your sides, and shoulders pulled back. Brace your core and maintain a neutral spine. For the carry, walk forward in a controlled manner, keeping your steps steady and upright posture intact. For the hold, simply stand still while maintaining your grip and posture. ▶ PROKETTLEBELL.COM/318

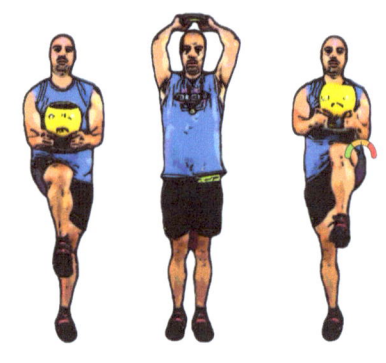

319. Pull-Over March

Technical Difficulty	Movement Pattern	Recommended Load
1	Pull	Medium, Heavy Weight

	Single Bell	Double Bell
	✓	✗

PRIMARY BENEFIT — UPPER BODY STRENGTH

TARGET MUSCLES — LATS, BICEPS, HIP FLEXORS

▶ PROKETTLEBELL.COM/319

This movement targets your lats, core, and hip flexors. Hold the kettlebell by the horns in a bottoms-up grip. Reach the kettlebell back behind your head while keeping your elbows tight and forearms parallel. From that extended position, pull the handle up to align with the top of your knee as you march in place, lifting your knees high to activate your hip flexors. Maintain a tall posture and slow, controlled movement throughout to keep constant tension on your muscles. You can perform this in place or travel forward with each march.

320. Racked Waiter Carry ▶ PROKETTLEBELL.COM/320

Technical Difficulty	Movement Pattern	Recommended Load
1	Compound	Medium Weight

	Single Bell	Double Bell
	✗	✓

PRIMARY BENEFIT — UPPER BODY STRENGTH AND MOBILITY

TARGET MUSCLES — ERECTORS, LATS, DELTOIDS, TRICEPS

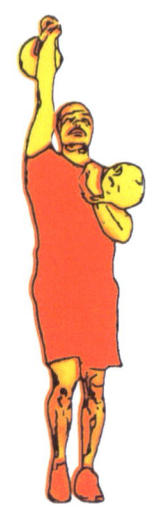

Begin with two kettlebells in the rack position, then press one overhead, making sure your bicep stays close to your cheek and the weight is stacked directly above your shoulder. Keep your shoulder packed, not shrugged. The second kettlebell remains in a secure rack position. Depending on space, you can stay still, march in place, or walk. Maintain even kettlebell weights and perfect alignment to avoid imbalances and maximize shoulder and core engagement.

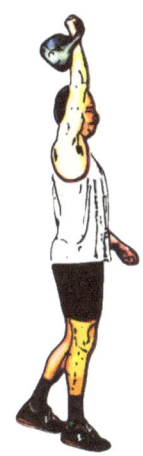

321. Walking One-Arm Waiter Carry

	Single Bell	Double Bell
	✓	✗

Technical Difficulty	Movement Pattern	Recommended Load
1	Compound	Medium Weight

PRIMARY BENEFIT	SHOULDER, ELBOW AND CORE STABILITY
TARGET MUSCLES	DELTOIDS, TRICEPS, LATS, OBLIQUES

Start with a kettlebell in the rack position, ensuring good hand insertion for overhead stability. Press the bell overhead with the bicep next to your cheek and the weight stacked over your shoulder. Walk forward in a steady, upright manner, keeping the arm locked and body upright without leaning. This exercise strengthens your shoulder, elbow, and core stability. Choose a walking style—regular, lunges, or other—as long as your form stays solid and the weight remains balanced. ▶ PROKETTLEBELL.COM/321

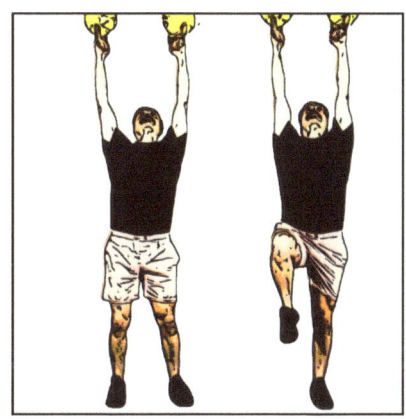

322. Bottoms-Up High Knees

	Single Bell	Double Bell
	✓	✗

Technical Difficulty	Movement Pattern	Recommended Load
2	Compound	Light Weight

PRIMARY BENEFIT	FULL-BODY STRENGTH
TARGET MUSCLES	HIP FLEXORS, ERECTORS, LATS, DELTOIDS, TRICEPS

Begin by cleaning a pair of kettlebells into a bottoms-up position, then press them directly overhead. Keep your eyes on the bells to help with balance. Start performing high knees, either in place or walking for an added challenge. Focus on keeping your core tight and the kettlebells stacked directly over your center. If needed, grip more toward the corners of the bells for better control. This full-body move challenges your grip, shoulders, and stabilizers throughout. ▶ PROKETTLEBELL.COM/322

323. Duck Walk

▶ PROKETTLEBELL.COM/323

	Single Bell	Double Bell
	✓	✗

Technical Difficulty	Movement Pattern	Recommended Load
2	Compound	Light, Medium Weight

PRIMARY BENEFIT	LOWER BODY STRENGTH AND MOBILITY
TARGET MUSCLES	QUADRICEPS, GLUTES, HAMSTRINGS, ERECTORS

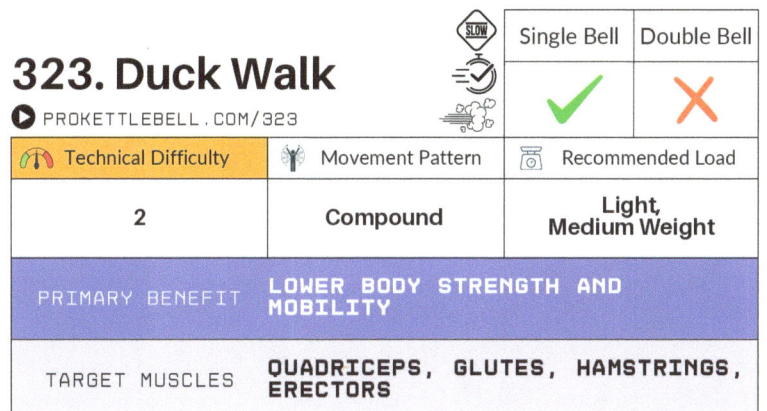

Place the kettlebell behind your shoulder blades, letting it rest securely. Lower into the deepest squat you can manage while keeping your heels down and knees tracking over your toes. Your feet will turn out slightly, and your back should remain flat throughout. From this squat, begin walking forward slowly, maintaining depth and posture. This movement targets leg and core strength, plus hip mobility. Extra credit if you add a little "quack" as you go.

Specialized
Movement Training

---------- Section Six ----------

Agility
Mobility

Specialty Exercises

1. Agility	
Slingshots	141
Soccer Drill	141
Kettlebell Touchdowns	141
Jump Turns	142
Overhead Lateral Shuffle Steps	142
Side-Step Figure-8s	142
Skaters	143
Step-Thru Figure-8s	143
Speed-Switch Slingshots	143
Walking Figure-8s	144

2. Mobility	
Good Morning	145
Groin Glider	145
Hip/Hamstring Opener	145
KB Knee Circles	146
Overhead Chair Twist	146
Seated Good Morning	146
Stagger Stance Good Morning	147
Dive-Bomber	147
Loaded Beast Sliders	147
Shin Boxes	148

324. Slingshots

	Single Bell	Double Bell
	✓	✗

Technical Difficulty	Movement Pattern	Recommended Load
1	Compound	Medium Weight

PRIMARY BENEFIT	COORDINATION AND TRUNK CONTROL
TARGET MUSCLES	FOREARMS, OBLIQUES, SPINAL ERECTORS, SHOULDERS

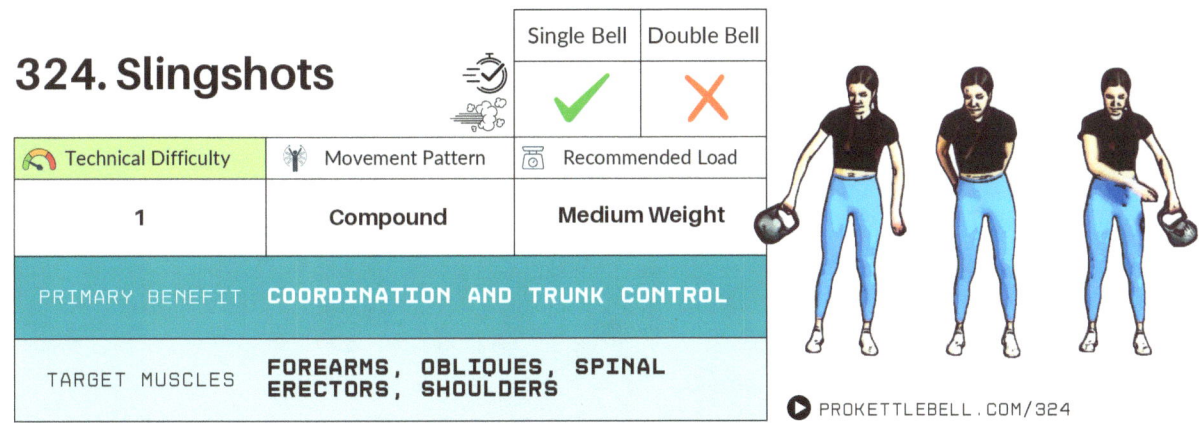

► PROKETTLEBELL.COM/324

Begin holding a kettlebell with a hook grip, fingers relaxed while the palm stays open. Swing the kettlebell in a circular path around your waist, smoothly switching hands in front and back of the body. Counterbalance naturally with your stance and hips while maintaining an upright posture and controlled trunk. Adjust speed, direction, and stance width as needed to reinforce coordination, grip strength, and rotational control.

325. Soccer Drill

	Single Bell	Double Bell
	✓	✗

Technical Difficulty	Movement Pattern	Recommended Load
1	Compound	Heavy Weight

PRIMARY BENEFIT	FOOT SPEED, AGILITY AND CONDITIONING
TARGET MUSCLES	CALVES, QUADRICEPS, GLUTES, HIP FLEXORS

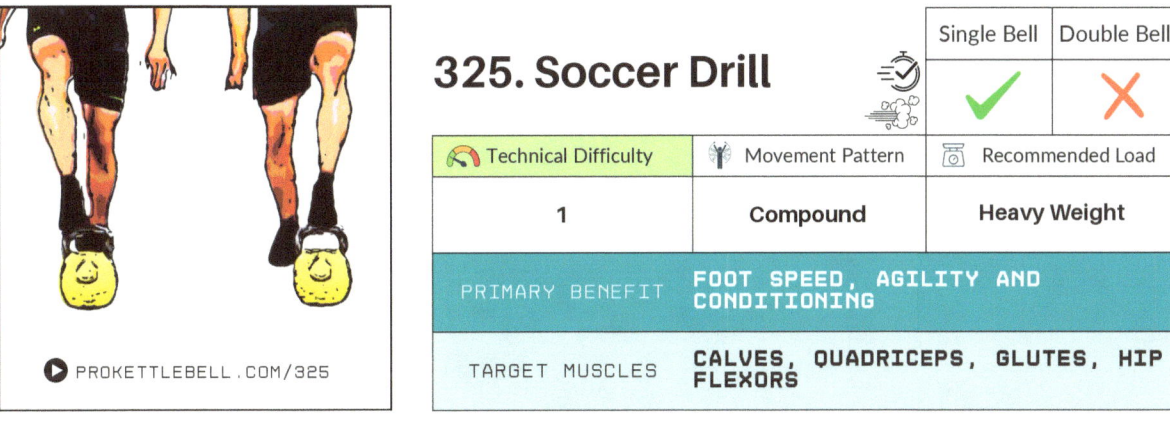

► PROKETTLEBELL.COM/325

The kettlebell soccer drill, or toe taps, challenges agility and cardiovascular endurance. Place a kettlebell upright with the handle facing up. Rapidly alternate tapping the top of the kettlebell with your toes, keeping one foot in the air at all times. Modify by slowing the pace or lowering the kettlebell height for accessibility. Ensure ample space and good body condition before performing this high-intensity, heart-pumping drill. Using a heavy weight prevents accidentally knocking the kettlebell over.

326. Touchdowns

► PROKETTLEBELL.COM/326

	Single Bell	Double Bell
	✗	✓

Technical Difficulty	Movement Pattern	Recommended Load
1	Compound	Any Weight

PRIMARY BENEFIT	LATERAL LEG STRENGTH, COORDINATION AND CONDITIONING
TARGET MUSCLES	GLUTES, HAMSTRINGS, QUADRICEPS, CALVES, SPINAL ERECTORS

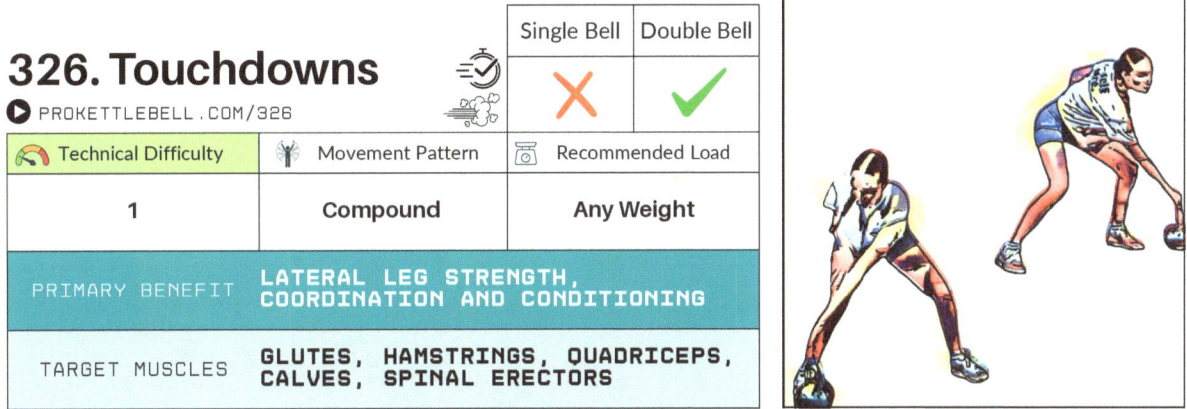

Set two kettlebells on the floor on either side of your body at a distance that matches your lateral step width. Begin in an athletic stance with hips pushed back, spine neutral, and chest tall. Step laterally and reach down to touch the kettlebell handle with your hand, either across the body or on the same side. Perform a quick shuffle step to switch foot positions and move to the opposite side, alternating hands with each rep. This is a favorite drill for developing lateral leg strength, coordination, and cardiovascular conditioning with a strong athletic emphasis.

AGILITY

327. Jump Turns

	Single Bell	Double Bell
	✓	✗

Technical Difficulty	Movement Pattern	Recommended Load
1	Compound	Light Weight

PRIMARY BENEFIT	ROTATIONAL LEG POWER AND LANDING CONTROL
TARGET MUSCLES	QUADRICEPS, GLUTES, HAMSTRINGS, CALVES, OBLIQUES

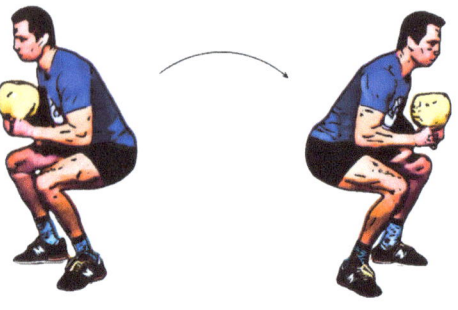

PROKETTLEBELL.COM/327

Hold a kettlebell tight to your chest with both hands while standing on a stable surface. Brace your core and perform a vertical jump, rotating your body in the air before landing softly and under control. Reset your balance before initiating the next repetition. Adjust the rotation angle—quarter turn, 90 degrees, or up to 180 degrees—based on skill level and kettlebell load. Keep the kettlebell close to your center of mass to maintain control and safe landing mechanics.

328. Overhead Lateral Shuffle Steps

	Single Bell	Double Bell
	✓	✓

Technical Difficulty	Movement Pattern	Recommended Load
2	Compound	Light Weight

PRIMARY BENEFIT	OVERHEAD STABILITY WITH LATERAL AGILITY
TARGET MUSCLES	QUADRICEPS, GLUTES, HAMSTRINGS, ADDUCTORS, ABDUCTORS, ERECTORS, LATS, DELTOIDS, TRICEPS

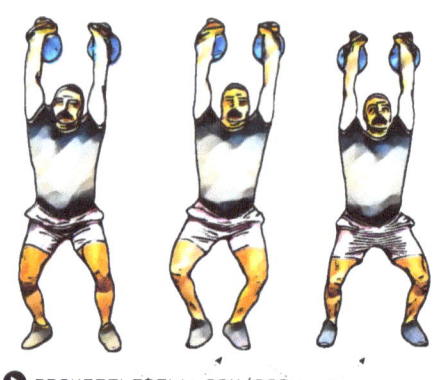

PROKETTLEBELL.COM/328

Hold two light to medium kettlebells locked out overhead with the arms fully extended and stacked over your shoulders and midfoot. Begin in a wide, athletic stance with an upright torso and braced core. Shuffle laterally by quickly switching foot positions, allowing the trailing foot to replace the lead foot with each step. Keep the kettlebells stable overhead and your ribs down as you move side to side. Maintain smooth, controlled footwork to reinforce lower-body agility, overhead stability, and full-body coordination.

329. Side-Step Figure-8s

	Single Bell	Double Bell
	✓	✗

Technical Difficulty	Movement Pattern	Recommended Load
2	Compound	Light, Medium Weight

PRIMARY BENEFIT	LATERAL LEG STRENGTH AND ROTATIONAL CORE CONTROL
TARGET MUSCLES	GLUTES, QUADRICEPS, HAMSTRINGS, ADDUCTORS, SPINAL ERECTORS, OBLIQUES

Step wide to the left and sit back into an athletic squat as you swing the kettlebell from front to back between your legs, passing it to your left hand (which grabs it from behind). After the pass, sling the kettlebell outside the body and quickly bring the left foot back to center. Step out to the right with the right leg to mirror the movement. The continuous hand-to-hand passes create a fluid figure-eight pattern. Maintain a long, upright spine and smooth, rhythmic movement to emphasize coordination, lateral strength, and core control.

PROKETTLEBELL.COM/329

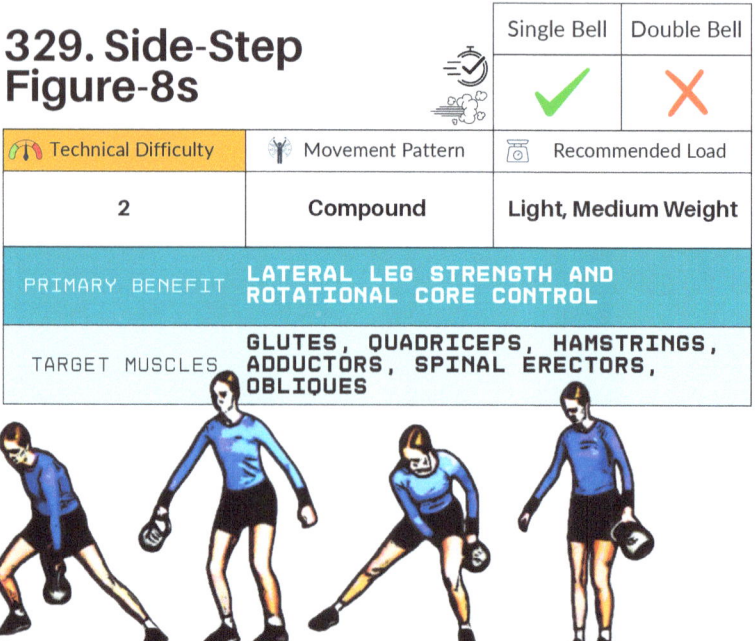

330. Skaters

PROKETTLEBELL.COM/330

	Single Bell	Double Bell
	✓	✗

Technical Difficulty	Movement Pattern	Recommended Load
2	Compound	Light, Medium Weight

PRIMARY BENEFIT	LATERAL POWER, AGILITY AND SINGLE-LEG CONTROL
TARGET MUSCLES	GLUTES, QUADRICEPS, HAMSTRINGS, CALVES, OBLIQUES, SPINAL ERECTORS

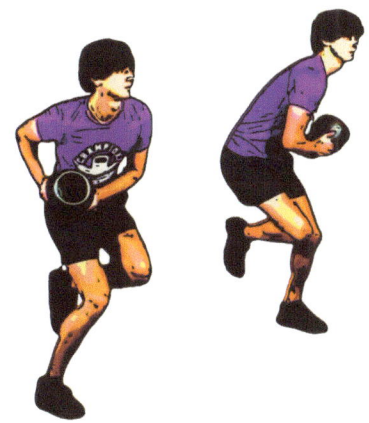

Hold a kettlebell with both hands close to your chest. Load one leg and explosively bound laterally to the opposite side, landing softly on the outside leg while the trailing leg crosses behind for balance. Keep the kettlebell close to your body and your torso stable as you move side to side. Emphasize controlled landings, lateral power, and single-leg stability. Adjust distance and tempo to match skill level.

331. Step-Thru Figure-8s

PROKETTLEBELL.COM/331

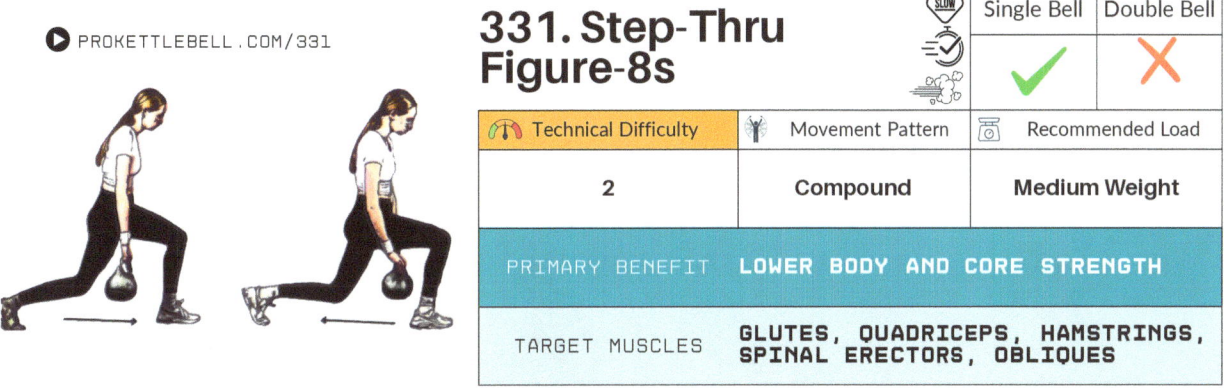

	Single Bell	Double Bell
	✓	✗

Technical Difficulty	Movement Pattern	Recommended Load
2	Compound	Medium Weight

PRIMARY BENEFIT	LOWER BODY AND CORE STRENGTH
TARGET MUSCLES	GLUTES, QUADRICEPS, HAMSTRINGS, SPINAL ERECTORS, OBLIQUES

Begin holding a kettlebell in one hand and step back into a reverse lunge on the same side. As you complete the lunge, pass the kettlebell through your legs to the opposite hand. Step forward past center into a forward lunge with the same working leg, switching hands again as the lunge is completed. The kettlebell switches hand-to-hand with each lunge while one leg remains the primary working leg and the opposite foot stays planted. Perform multiple repetitions before switching sides. Maintain an upright torso, smooth transitions, and a consistent rhythm to reinforce coordination and full-body control.

332. Speed-Switch Slingshots

	Single Bell	Double Bell
	✓	✗

Technical Difficulty	Movement Pattern	Recommended Load
3	Compound	Medium Weight

PRIMARY BENEFIT	SHOULDER INTEGRITY, UPPER BODY STRENGTH AND COORDINATION
TARGET MUSCLES	LATS, BICEPS, DELTOIDS, FOREARMS

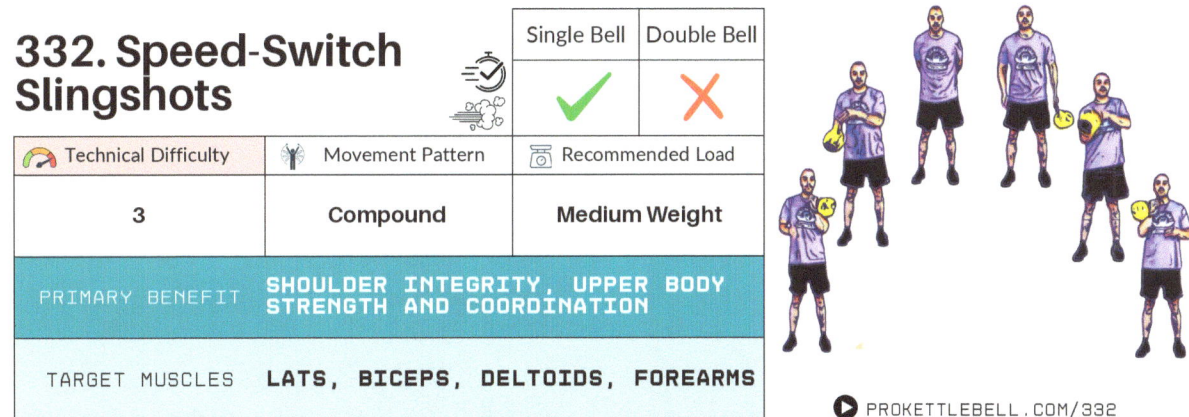

PROKETTLEBELL.COM/332

Start with the kettlebell in the rack position on the left side. Drop the handle into your right hand and swing the kettlebell behind your body. Switch hands behind you, sling the bell around to the front, and toss it into the rack position on the right side. Reverse the sequence and repeat. Use a relaxed grip to allow fast, fluid hand switches. Maintain balance, a neutral lumbar spine, and even weight distribution through both feet. This dynamic sequence develops arm strength, coordination, and dexterity.

AGILITY

333. Walking Figure-8s

Single Bell	Double Bell	
✓	✗	

Technical Difficulty	Movement Pattern	Recommended Load
3	Lunge + Hinge + Rotation	Light, Medium Weight
PRIMARY BENEFIT	LOCOMOTION-BASED CORE CONTROL AND COORDINATION	
TARGET MUSCLES	GLUTES, HAMSTRINGS, ADDUCTORS, SPINAL ERECTORS, OBLIQUES	

▶ PROKETTLEBELL.COM/333

Hold the kettlebell in one hand at your side. Step forward with the opposite leg, pass the kettlebell through your legs, switch hands, and continue walking while alternating the passing motion hand-to-hand with each step. Maintain an upright torso, flat lumbar, and take wider steps if needed to avoid bumping the kettlebell. This continuous movement targets lower-body strength and core control while challenging coordination.

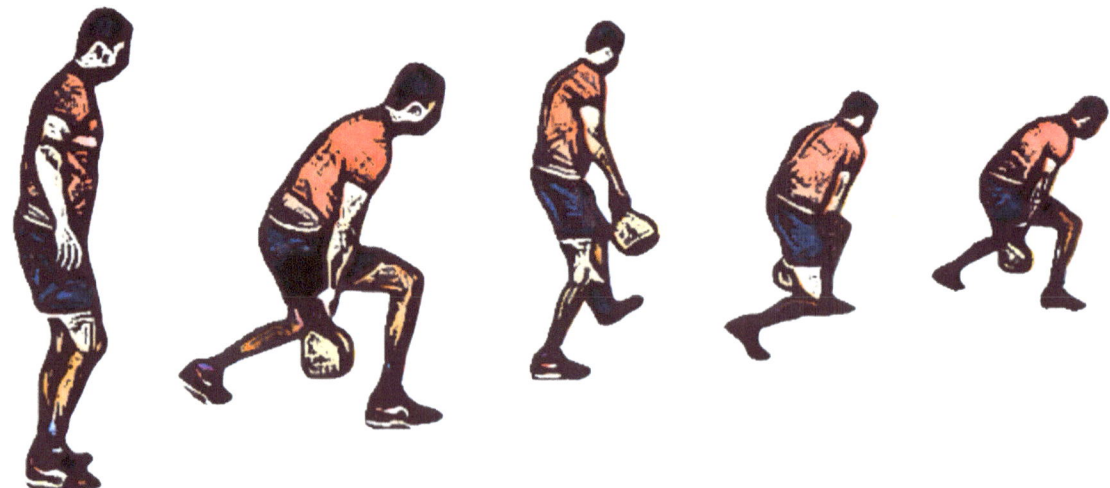

334. Good Morning

PROKETTLEBELL.COM/334

	Single Bell	Double Bell
SLOW	✓	✗

Technical Difficulty	Movement Pattern	Recommended Load
1	Hinge	Light Weight

PRIMARY BENEFIT	POSTERIOR-CHAIN STRENGTH
TARGET MUSCLES	GLUTES, HAMSTRINGS, SPINAL ERECTORS

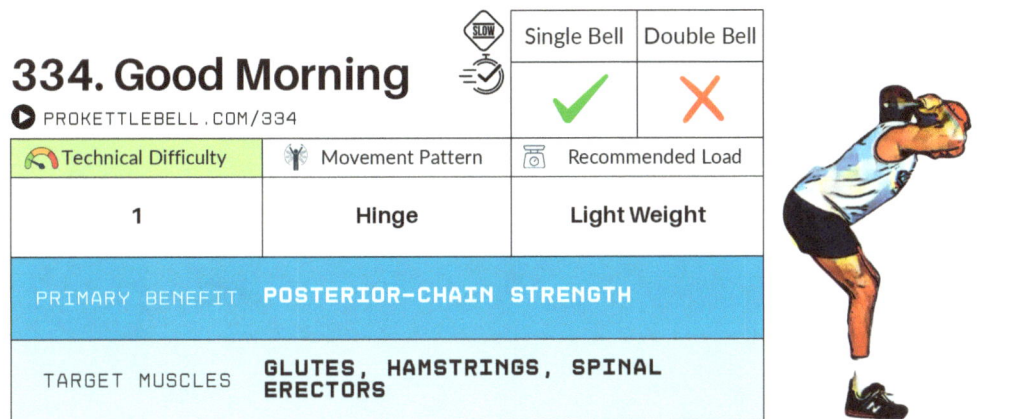

Position the kettlebell securely between your shoulder blades, gripping the handles firmly. Stand tall with feet hip-width apart and brace your core. Initiate the movement by hinging at the hips, keeping your chest lifted and spine neutral as your hips move backward. Lower under control to a comfortable range, then drive the hips forward and squeeze the glutes to return to standing. Maintain tension throughout and avoid rounding the back.

335. Groin Glider

PROKETTLEBELL.COM/335

	Single Bell	Double Bell
SLOW	✓	✗

Technical Difficulty	Movement Pattern	Recommended Load
1	Squat + Lateral	Medium Weight

PRIMARY BENEFIT	LATERAL HIP MOBILITY AND ADDUCTOR CONTROL
TARGET MUSCLES	ADDUCTORS, GLUTES, QUADRICEPS

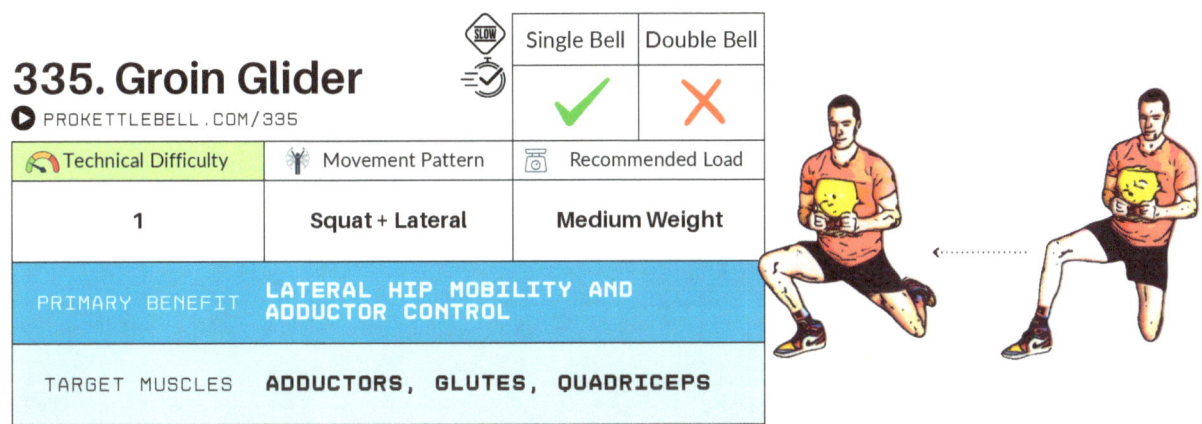

Begin in a kneeling position with a single kettlebell held securely close to your body. Place your front leg forward at roughly a 45-degree angle, adjusted for your mobility. Glide your hips laterally toward the extended leg, allowing a stretch through both groins. Move smoothly and use a light kettlebell to avoid overstretching. Repeat on both sides, keeping in mind that one side may feel tighter than the other. With consistent practice, balance between sides can improve, making this an excellent mobility warm-up.

336. Hip/Hamstring Opener

	Single Bell	Double Bell
SLOW	✓	✗

Technical Difficulty	Movement Pattern	Recommended Load
1	Lunge	Light, Medium Weight

PRIMARY BENEFIT	HIP AND HAMSTRING MOBILITY WITH POSITIONAL STRENGTH
TARGET MUSCLES	HAMSTRINGS, GLUTES, HIP FLEXORS, SPINAL ERECTORS

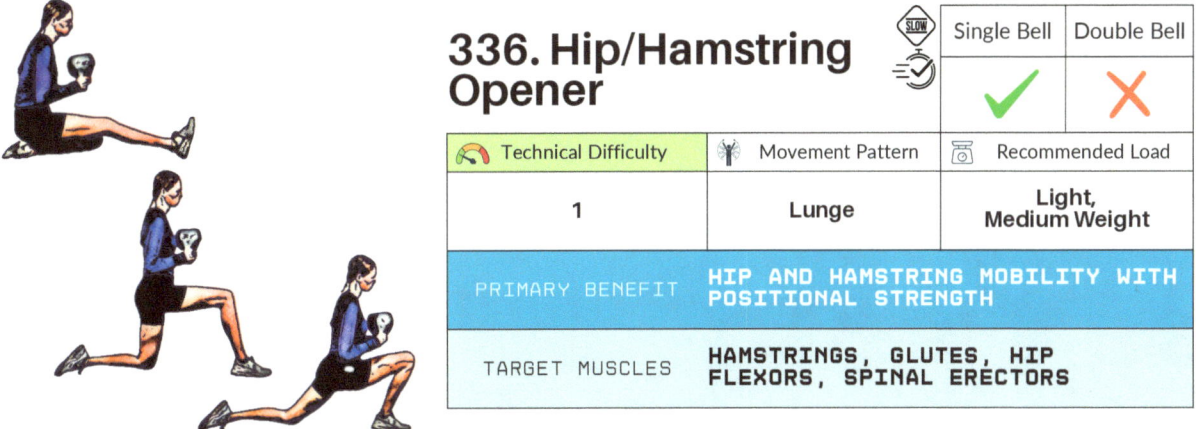

Start in a half-kneeling position with one leg forward at approximately 90 degrees and the rear knee on the ground. Hold a light kettlebell at your chest, ideally bottom-up by the horns. Maintain an upright torso as you shift forward to stretch the hip flexor of the rear leg. Then shift your hips back, straightening the front leg while sitting back toward the heel of the rear leg, keeping the hips level and spine neutral. Move smoothly between positions, using a load light enough to maintain control through the full range of motion. PROKETTLEBELL.COM/336

MOBILITY

337. KB Knee Circles

PROKETTLEBELL.COM/337

	Single Bell	Double Bell
SLOW	✓	✗

Technical Difficulty	Movement Pattern	Recommended Load
1	Squat	Light, Medium Weight

PRIMARY BENEFIT	LOWER-BODY JOINT MOBILITY, KNEE CONTROL
TARGET MUSCLES	QUADRICEPS, ADDUCTORS, GLUTES, HAMSTRINGS, CALVES

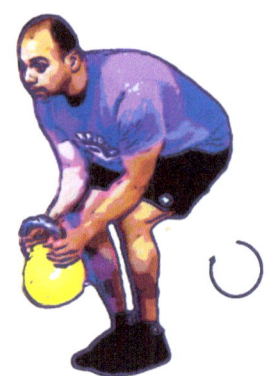

Stand with your feet close together, holding a kettlebell by the horns. Set into a shallow squat and rest your forearms lightly on your thighs while keeping your spine neutral. With ankles, knees, and hips aligned, draw smooth, controlled circles with your knees in one direction for the prescribed reps, then switch directions. Emphasize joint control and even pressure through the feet. This movement may also be performed unloaded.

338. Overhead Chair Twist

	Single Bell	Double Bell
SLOW	✓	✗

Technical Difficulty	Movement Pattern	Recommended Load
1	Compound	Light Weight

PRIMARY BENEFIT	FULL-BODY ROTATIONAL MOBILITY AND OVERHEAD STABILITY
TARGET MUSCLES	GLUTES, QUADRICEPS, HAMSTRINGS, SPINAL ERECTORS, OBLIQUES, LATS, DELTOIDS, TRICEPS

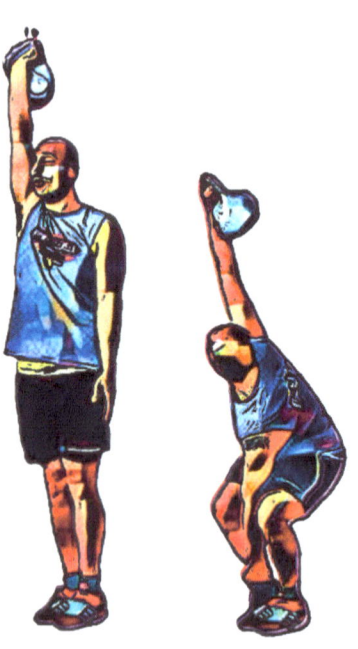

Hold a kettlebell stacked vertically overhead with one arm, aligned from shoulder to midfoot. Slowly rotate your torso, keeping your eyes up on the kettlebell as your free hand reaches toward the floor outside the opposite foot as you descend into a squat. Depth is secondary to stability and positioning. Move deliberately to engage mobility from the ankles through the shoulders. PROKETTLEBELL.COM/338

339. Seated Good Morning

	Single Bell	Double Bell
SLOW	✓	✗

Technical Difficulty	Movement Pattern	Recommended Load
1	Hinge	Light Weight

PRIMARY BENEFIT	POSTERIOR-CHAIN STRENGTH AND TRUNK CONTROL
TARGET MUSCLES	HAMSTRINGS, SPINAL ERECTORS, GLUTES, ABDOMINALS, OBLIQUES

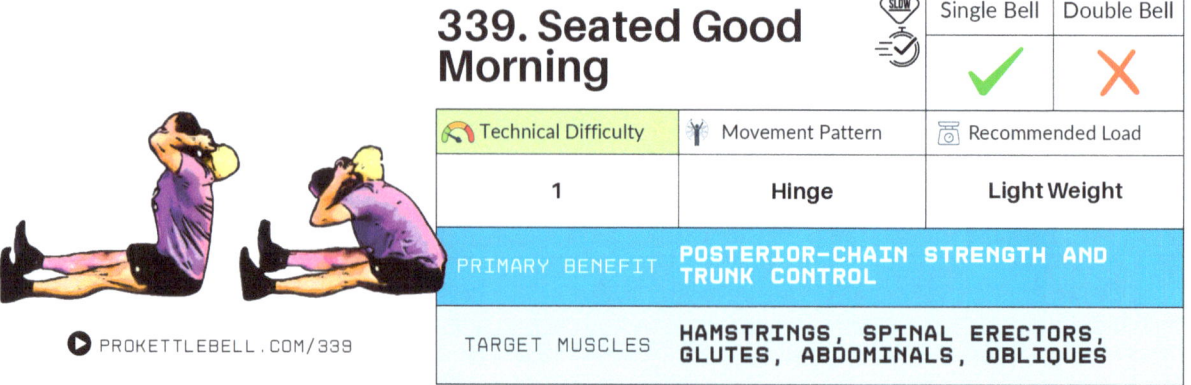

PROKETTLEBELL.COM/339

Sit on the ground with your legs extended straight in front of you or in a straddle position, holding a kettlebell behind your shoulders. Initiate the movement by hinging forward at the hips while maintaining a long, neutral spine. Lower under control to a comfortable depth, then engage your core and hip extensors to return to an upright position. Emphasize hamstring mobility and trunk control. Begin unloaded to establish proper form before adding weight.

340. Stagger Stance Good Morning

	Single Bell	Double Bell
SLOW	✓	✗

Technical Difficulty	Movement Pattern	Recommended Load
1	Hinge	Light Weight

PRIMARY BENEFIT BACK AND CORE STRENGTH

TARGET MUSCLES HAMSTRINGS, GLUTES, ERECTORS

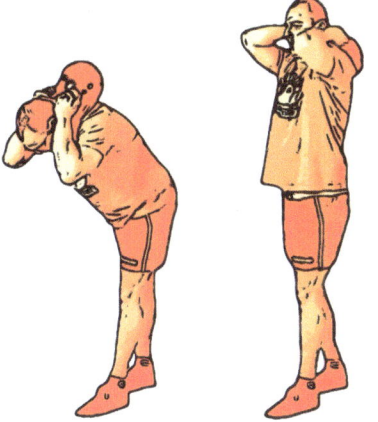

Take a narrow, staggered stance by starting with your feet together, then stepping one foot slightly back. Position the kettlebell behind your shoulders. With a flat back and minimal knee bend, hinge forward at the hips while keeping your shoulders square with your hips. Lower only as far as you can while maintaining a neutral spine and mostly straight legs, then return to standing by squeezing your glutes. If this variation feels uncomfortable, swap the load for a mobility stick or resistance band, or hold the kettlebell at your chest instead. ▶ PROKETTLEBELL.COM/340

341. Divebomber
▶ PROKETTLEBELL.COM/341

	Single Bell	Double Bell
SLOW	✗	✓

Technical Difficulty	Movement Pattern	Recommended Load
2	Compound	Heavy Weight

PRIMARY BENEFIT UPPER BODY STRENGTH AND MOBILITY

TARGET MUSCLES TRICEPS, DELTOIDS, LATS, PECTORALS, ABS, ERECTORS

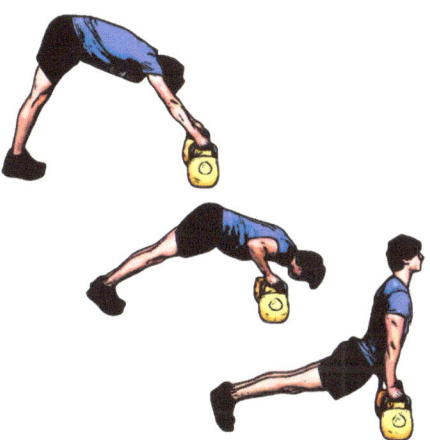

Begin in a downward dog position; hips high, with your feet on the floor and hands on kettlebells shoulder-width apart. Drive your heels to the ground, straightening and stretching the calves and hamstrings. Swoop your chest low, forward between the kettlebells, and slide into an upward-facing dog with hips close to the ground and chest lifted. Reverse the motion to return to the starting position. Perform this slowly and with control to build upper body strength and mobility through the spine and hips.

342. Loaded Beast Sliders

▶ PROKETTLEBELL.COM/342

	Single Bell	Double Bell
SLOW	✗	✓

Technical Difficulty	Movement Pattern	Recommended Load
2	Compound	Heavy Weight

PRIMARY BENEFIT CORE STRENGTH, HIP AND GROIN MOBILITY

TARGET MUSCLES ABS, ERECTORS, LATS, DELTOIDS, TRICEPS

Start in a plank position with hands on kettlebells placed directly beneath your shoulders. Shift your weight backward and slide your hips toward your heels, allowing your knees to splay outward and your feet to turn slightly out. This creates a crouched, loaded position that stretches the groin and lumbar area. Pause briefly before reversing the move by shifting your weight forward, sliding into a high plank and squeezing your body tight at the top. Alternate between these two positions with slow, controlled movement.

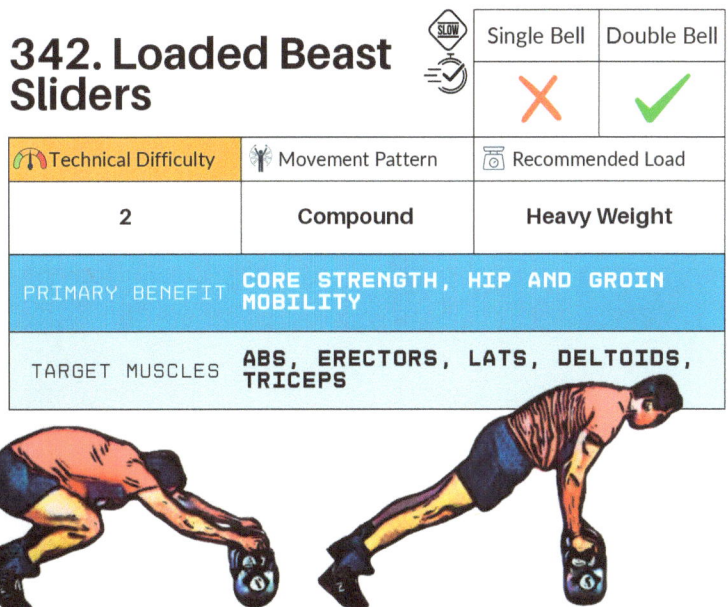

MOBILITY

343. Shin Boxes

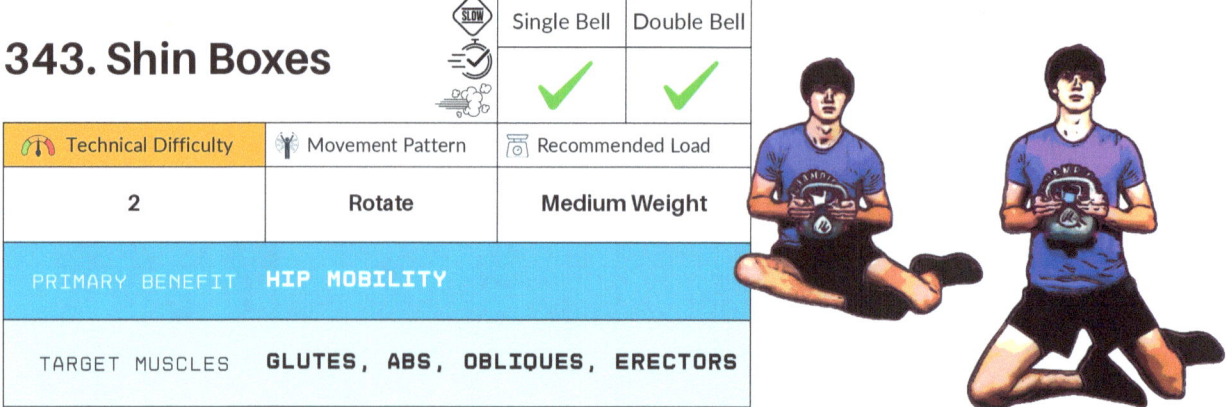

Technical Difficulty	Movement Pattern	Recommended Load
2	Rotate	Medium Weight

PRIMARY BENEFIT	**HIP MOBILITY**
TARGET MUSCLES	**GLUTES, ABS, OBLIQUES, ERECTORS**

Single Bell ✓   Double Bell ✓

Begin seated with one shin in front of your body and the other to the side, both legs maintaining contact with the floor and bent deeply to create 90-degree angles. Individual mobility will affect how this position appears, but do your best to maintain the shape. Hold a kettlebell securely at your chest, or in the rack or overhead position for variation and increased challenge. Squeeze your glutes to lift yourself from the ground and drive your hips forward into an upright kneeling posture. Hold the glute squeeze briefly at the top, then lower back to the ground slowly and under control. If needed, forego the kettlebell and use your hands for assistance during the lift. Complete multiple repetitions on one side before switching and mirroring the movement with the opposite leg forward.

▶ PROKETTLEBELL.COM/343

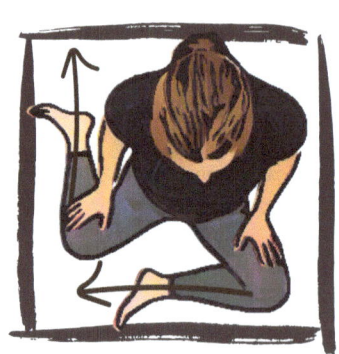

Shin Box

Specialty Movements
Complexes

―――――――― Section Seven ――――――――

Complexes

A *complex* is a continuous sequence of **two or more different kettlebell movements** performed **back-to-back with the same bell(s)** until the entire chain is complete.

Technical Difficulty Level–2		Technical Difficulty Level–3	
Alternating Clean + Ballistic Row	151	Curtsy Power Plank	163
Alternating Swing + Long Cycle	152	Double Clean + Double Half Snatch	164
KB Beast Makers	153	Double Clean + Jerk + Plank Row	165
Kettlebell Burpee	154	Double Jerk + Split Jerk	166
Clean + High Pull	155	Double Long Cycle + Half Snatch	167
Clean + Squat	156	Gunslinger + High Pull + Snatch	168
Dead Clean + Push Press + Windmill	157	Long Cycle + Squat Thrust	169
Dead Clean + Swing + Clean	158	The Mad Max	170
Dead Clean + Squat + Press	159	Over the Mountain	171
Outside Clean + Side Lunge + Press	160	Plyo Burpee	172
Stop Clean Thruster Press	161		
Swing + Clean + Thruster	162		

Every rep of the complex—or every round if you assign reps to each link—flows from one pattern to the next, demanding seamless transitions, full-body coordination, and sustained power output.

Hallmarks of a Complex

- **Single Load** – You'll never change kettlebells mid-set
- **Linked but Distinct Patterns** – Each link is a standalone exercise (clean, squat, press, etc.). Performed in order, they cover multiple movement patterns or planes.
- **Equal Work Per Side** – When the complex uses unilateral moves, you mirror the full chain on the opposite side (e.g., Alternating Clean + Ballistic Row).

Programming Notes

- **Rep Prescription:** Either "one rep = entire chain" (e.g., Clean + Squat + Press = 1) or assign specific reps to each link (3 cleans → 3 squats → 3 presses).
- **Goal Framing:** Use lighter loads for metabolic finishers or heavier loads/longer rests for strength-dominant sessions.

This combination builds posterior chain strength and pulling power by combining hang cleans with ballistic rows. It emphasizes explosive hip drive, grip strength, and upper back development while challenging coordination between alternating sides.

344. Alternating Hang Clean + Ballistic Row

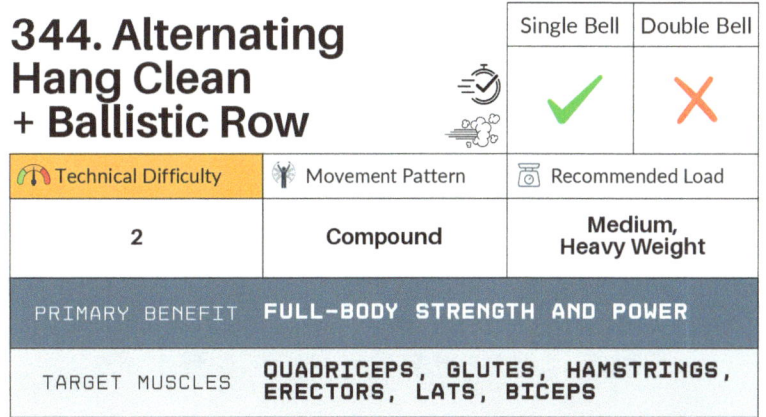

	Single Bell	Double Bell
	✓	✗

Technical Difficulty	Movement Pattern	Recommended Load
2	Compound	Medium, Heavy Weight

PRIMARY BENEFIT	FULL-BODY STRENGTH AND POWER
TARGET MUSCLES	QUADRICEPS, GLUTES, HAMSTRINGS, ERECTORS, LATS, BICEPS

Develop your posterior chain and introduce dynamic rhythm while targeting strength and endurance in back, glutes, and biceps.

▶ PROKETTLEBELL.COM/344

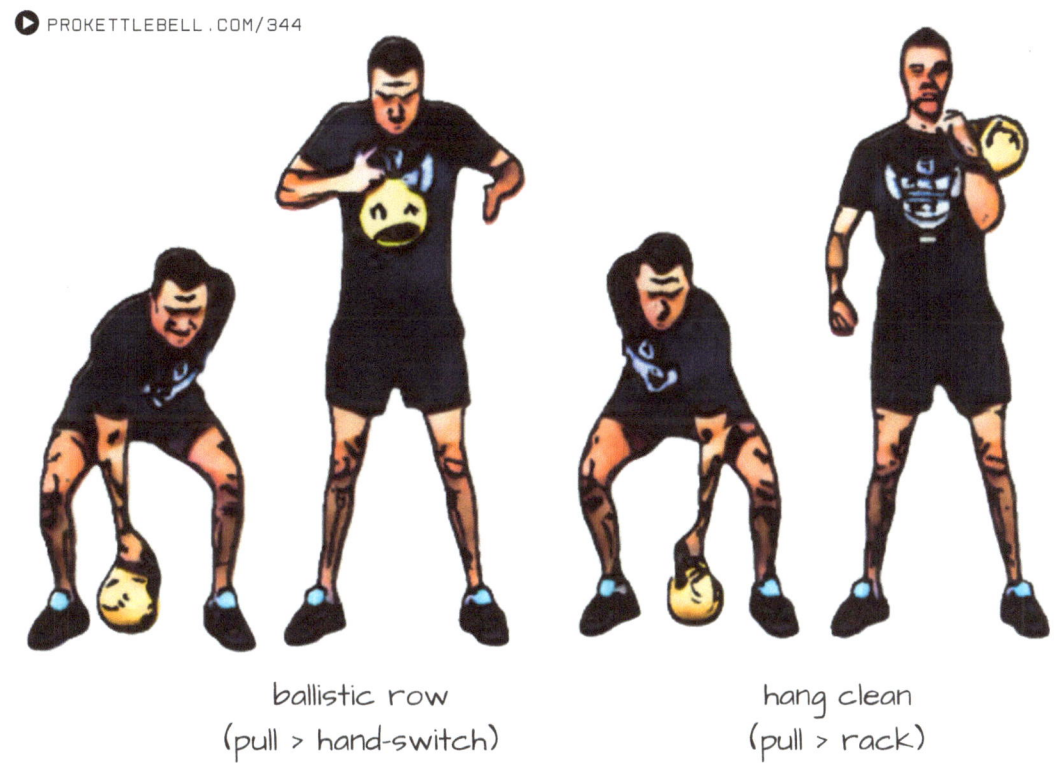

ballistic row
(pull > hand-switch)

hang clean
(pull > rack)

Directions:

1. **Hang Clean (Right):** Start with the kettlebell under your center of mass. With a straight arm and athletic stance, use leg drive to clean the kettlebell into the rack position on your right side.
2. **Ballistic Row (Right):** From the rack, immediately transition into a ballistic row, with a hand-switch at the top of the row.
3. **Hang Clean (Left):** From the hang postion (the bottom of the ballistic row), clean the kettlebell into the rack on your left side.
4. **Reverse and Repeat.**

345. Alternating Swing + Long Cycle

	Single Bell	Double Bell
	✓	✗

Technical Difficulty	Movement Pattern	Recommended Load
2	Compound	Heavy Weight

PRIMARY BENEFIT	FULL-BODY STRENGTH AND CONDITIONING
TARGET MUSCLES	QUADRICEPS, GLUTES, HAMSTRINGS, ERECTORS, OBLIQUES, LATS, BICEPS

PROKETTLEBELL.COM/345

This sequence blends endurance-based alternating swings with the full-body power of the long cycle (clean + jerk). The result is a conditioning-focused complex that hits nearly every muscle group with volume and intensity.

This hybrid improves timing, breathing control, and overhead mechanics. It's especially effective for high-volume training or building total-body endurance.

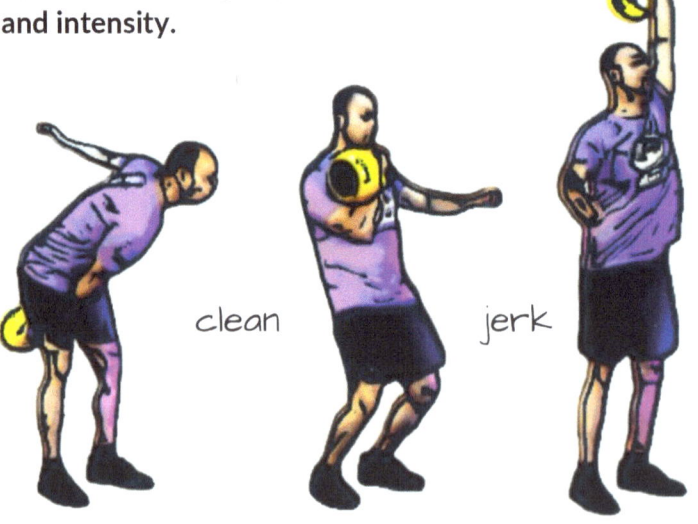
clean   jerk

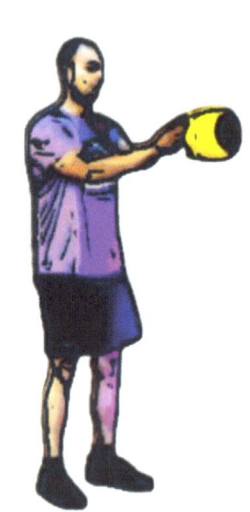
extra swing to switch hands

Directions:

1. *Alternating Swing:* Begin with a one-arm kettlebell swing using your left hand, switching to your right hand at the top.
2. *Clean (Right):* Complete the following swing by catching the bell into the rack position with your right arm.
3. *Jerk (Right):* Perform a jerk (see jerk directions for details).
4. *Switch Hands with a Swing:* Lower the kettlebell to the rack position, then drop it into a swing.
5. *Repeat Clean + Jerk (Left):* Continue the flow on the left side.

KB Beast Makers are a compound strength and conditioning drill that blend a ballistic deadlift, push-up, and renegade row. They build full-body strength, power, and grit under load. This complex hits strength, stability, and endurance. It's ideal for athletes and fitness enthusiasts looking for a single move to cover multiple movement patterns under fatigue.

346. KB Beast Makers

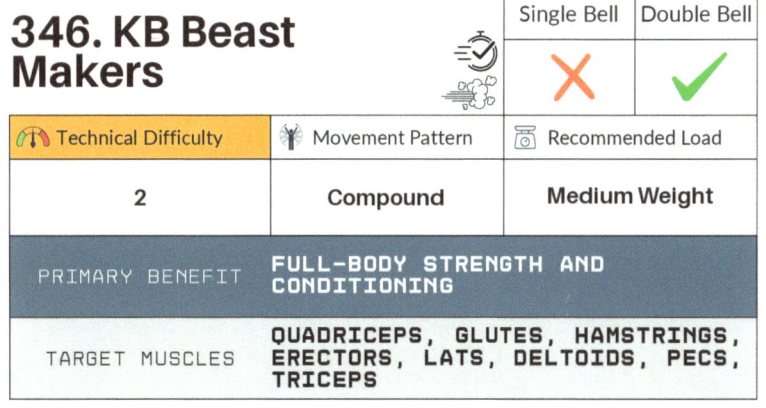

	Single Bell	Double Bell
	✗	✓

Technical Difficulty	Movement Pattern	Recommended Load
2	Compound	Medium Weight
PRIMARY BENEFIT	**FULL-BODY STRENGTH AND CONDITIONING**	
TARGET MUSCLES	**QUADRICEPS, GLUTES, HAMSTRINGS, ERECTORS, LATS, DELTOIDS, PECS, TRICEPS**	

▶ PROKETTLEBELL.COM/346

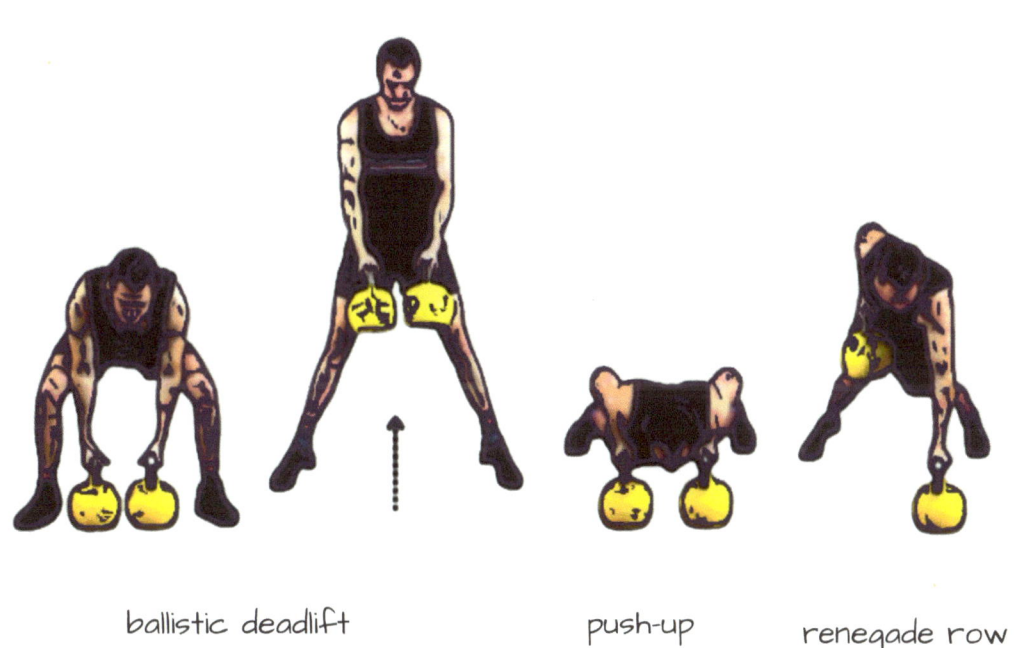

ballistic deadlift   push-up   renegade row

Directions:

1. **Ballistic Deadlift:** Stand with feet shoulder-width apart, straddling two kettlebells. Perform the deadlift explosively, so that you jump at the top of the lift, while keeping arms extended straight.
2. **Lower to Floor:** Land softly and place the kettlebells back between your feet.
3. **Push-Up:** Jump or step back into a plank and complete one solid push-up.
4. **Renegade Row (Right):** Row the right kettlebell to your ribcage with control.
5. **Push-Up:** Perform a second push-up, keeping tight form.
6. **Renegade Row (Left):** Row the left kettlebell, keeping hips square.
7. **Reset:** Hop or step forward, stand up, and repeat the sequence.

COMPLEXES

347. Kettlebell Burpee

	Single Bell	Double Bell
	✗	✓

Technical Difficulty	Movement Pattern	Recommended Load
2	Compound	Heavy Weight

PRIMARY BENEFIT	FULL-BODY STRENGTH AND EXPLOSIVENESS
TARGET MUSCLES	QUADRICEPS, GLUTES, HAMSTRINGS, ERECTORS, LATS, PECS, DELTOIDS, TRICEPS

Kettlebell Burpees are a fast-paced way to reinforce quality movement patterns under load while challenging your cardio-respiratory system and muscular endurance.

Complete a suitcase deadlift, squat thrust, and push-up for a kettlebell-enhanced burpee that strengthens your posterior chain, upper body, and core while keeping your heart rate high. It's a smart fusion of resistance and conditioning work.

▶ PROKETTLEBELL.COM/347

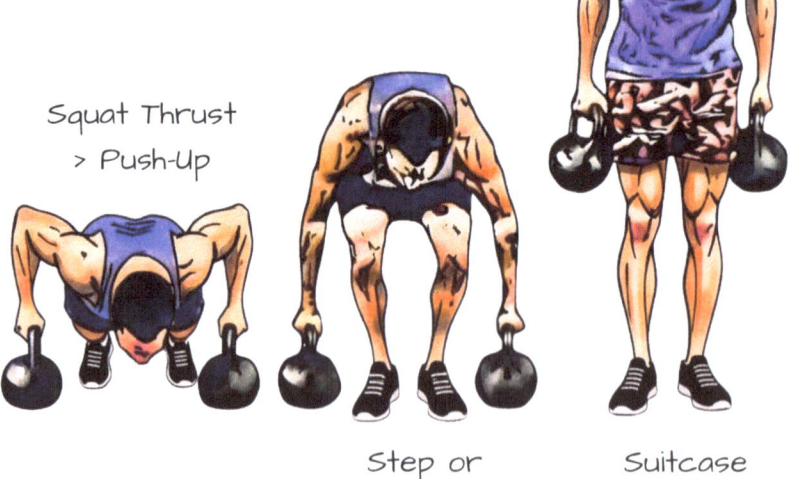

Squat Thrust > Push-Up

Step or Jump Forward

Suitcase Deadlift

Directions:

1. **Suitcase Deadlift:** Start with kettlebells beside your feet. Hinge at the hips and deadlift with good form.
2. **Lower to Ground:** Place the kettlebells down in the same spot with control.
3. **Kick Back:** Jump or step back into a push-up position.
4. **Push-Up:** Complete one push-up, maintaining a straight line from head to heels.
5. **Return to Feet:** Jump or step back to the starting position and reset for the next round.

348. Clean + High Pull

This combination is a great blend of vertical pulling strength and explosive clean mechanics. It helps refine coordination, pulling technique, and builds shoulder and upper back strength. It's ideal as a lead-up to snatches or as part of a complex conditioning circuit.

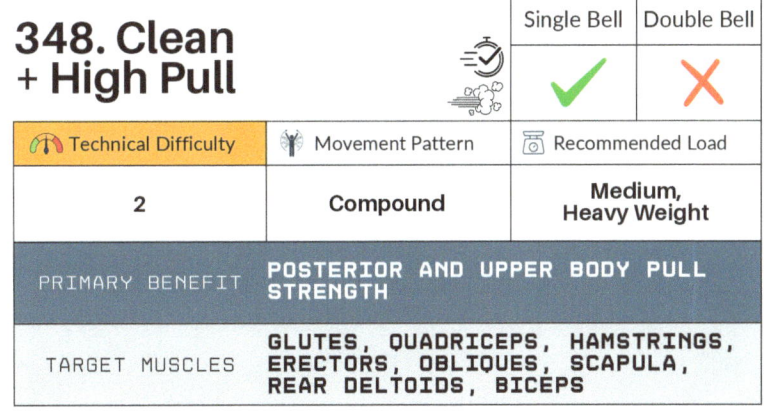

	Single Bell	Double Bell
	✓	✗

Technical Difficulty	Movement Pattern	Recommended Load
2	Compound	Medium, Heavy Weight

PRIMARY BENEFIT	POSTERIOR AND UPPER BODY PULL STRENGTH
TARGET MUSCLES	GLUTES, QUADRICEPS, HAMSTRINGS, ERECTORS, OBLIQUES, SCAPULA, REAR DELTOIDS, BICEPS

▶ PROKETTLEBELL.COM/348

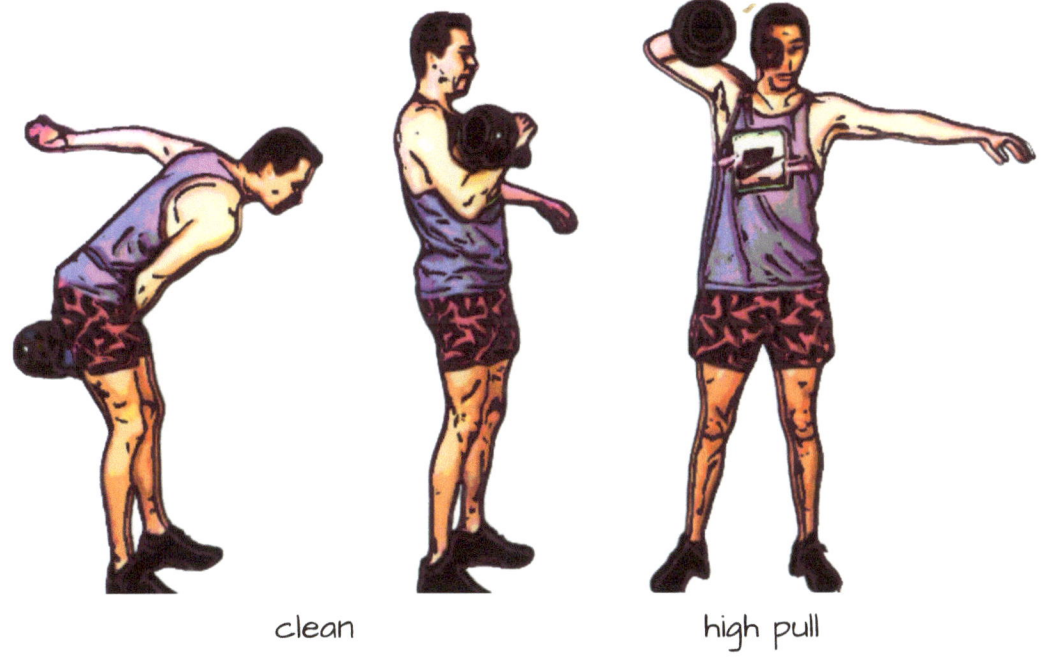

clean   high pull

Directions:

1. **Clean:** Start with a kettlebell on the floor and clean it into the rack using powerful hip extension and proper hand insertion.
2. **High Pull:** From the rack, drop the bell into a backswing. When the bell approaches the apex of its swing, pull by driving your elbow up and back at shoulder height, bringing the kettlebell closer to your body.
3. **Reset and Repeat:** After the high pull's descent, resume the flow with another clean.

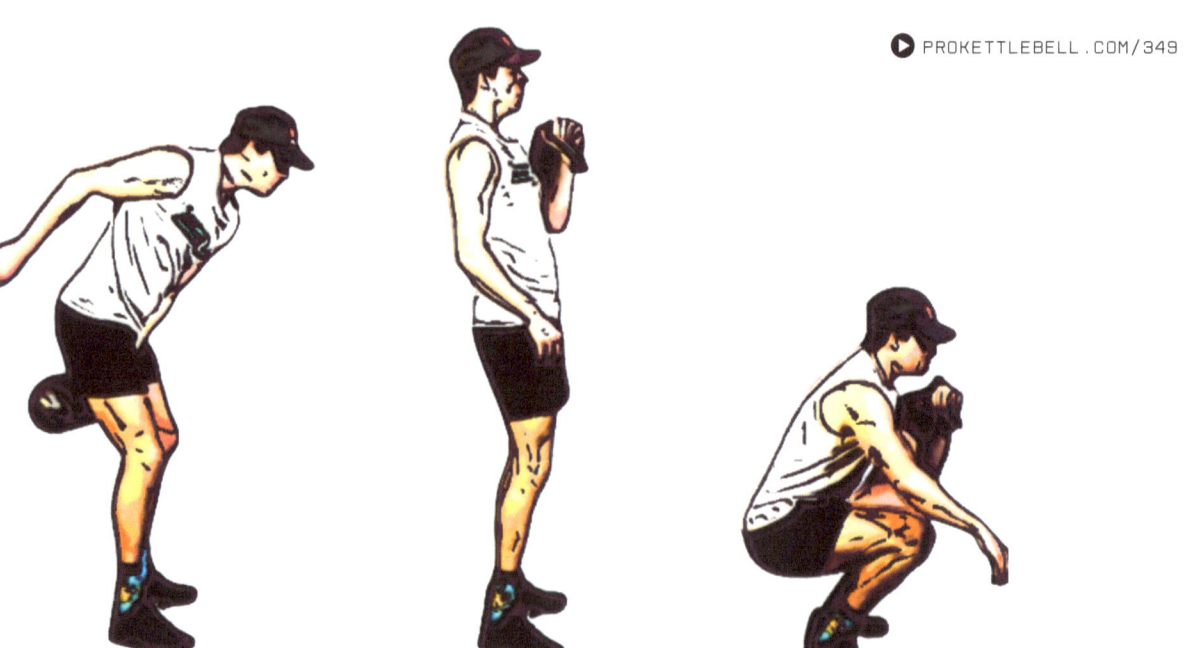

clean — rack squat

349. Clean + Squat

	Single Bell	Double Bell
	✓	✓

Technical Difficulty	Movement Pattern	Recommended Load
2	Squat	Medium, Heavy Weight

PRIMARY BENEFIT	CORE AND LEG STRENGTH
TARGET MUSCLES	GLUTES, HAMSTRINGS, QUADRICEPS, LATS, ERECTORS, BICEPS

Modify by performing multiple cleans and multiple squats during the sequence (for example, 5 cleans and 5 squats, then 4 cleans and 4 squats, all the way down to zero).

A classic combo for developing full-body coordination, Clean and Squat focuses on transferring energy from a dynamic pull into a stable front-loaded squat. It targets the legs, glutes, core, and reinforces rack position control.

Directions:

1. **Clean:** Begin with a single-arm clean into the rack, making sure the kettlebell lands softly.
2. **Squat:** From the rack, drop into a deep squat with heels grounded, chest tall, and spine neutral.
3. **Stand and Repeat:** Return to standing and repeat.
4. **Extra Credit:** Try it with double kettlebells to heighten the intensity.

▶ PROKETTLEBELL.COM/350

350. Dead Clean + Push Press + Windmill

	Single Bell	Double Bell
	✓	✗

🎛 Technical Difficulty	🐜 Movement Pattern	⚖ Recommended Load
2	Compound	Medium Weight

PRIMARY BENEFIT	FULL-BODY STRENGTH AND MOBILITY
TARGET MUSCLES	QUADRICEPS, GLUTES, ERECTORS, LATS, DELTOIDS, OBLIQUES, TRICEPS

This three-part combo builds strength, overhead mobility, and coordination. The dead clean builds power from the floor, the push press utilizes leg drive for overhead pressing, and the windmill strengthens the obliques and stabilizers.

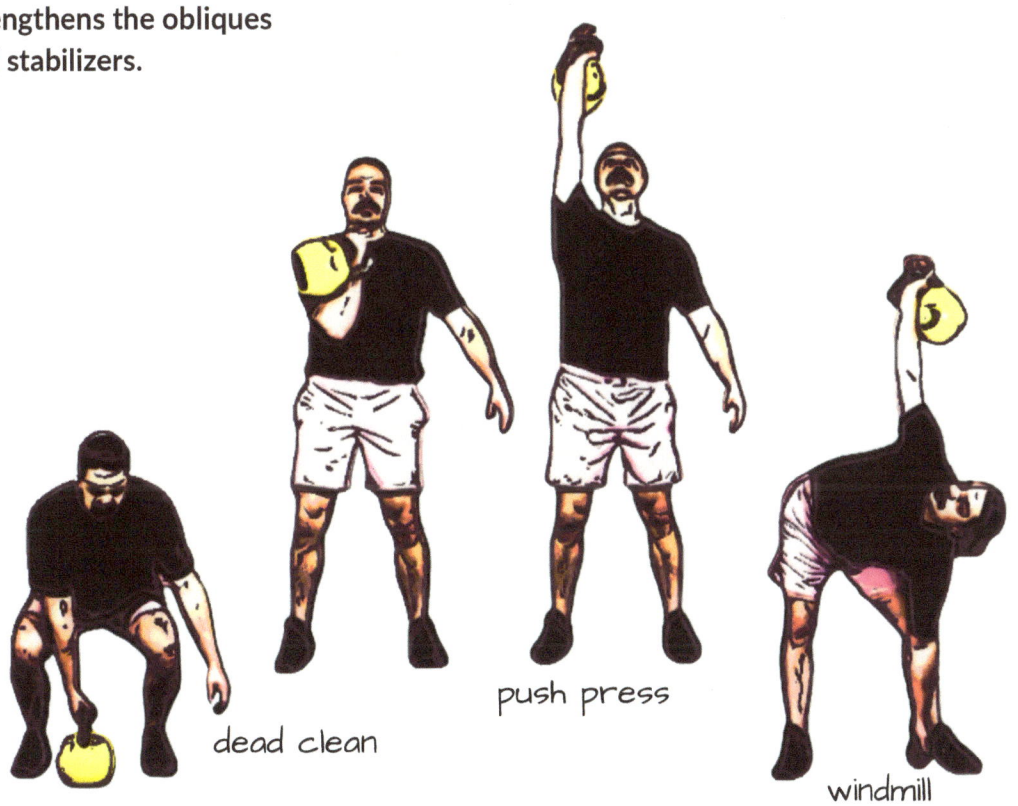

dead clean — push press — windmill

Directions:

1. **Dead Clean:** Start with the kettlebell between your feet and clean it with your left hand into the rack using mostly leg drive and hip extension.
2. **Push Press:** Use a small dip and drive through the legs to press the bell overhead, locking out fully.
3. **Windmill:** Slightly turn your right foot outward, then hinge sideways at the hips, reaching your free hand down your inner thigh while keeping the overhead arm locked and leg under the kettlebell straight.
4. **Return and Repeat:** Stand tall from the windmill, lower the bell to rack, then the floor to begin again.

COMPLEXES

This triple combo enhances kettlebell flow, power development, and technique. It blends foundational skills: the dead clean for explosive power, the swing for hip drive, and the clean for control and timing.

▶ PROKETTLEBELL.COM/351

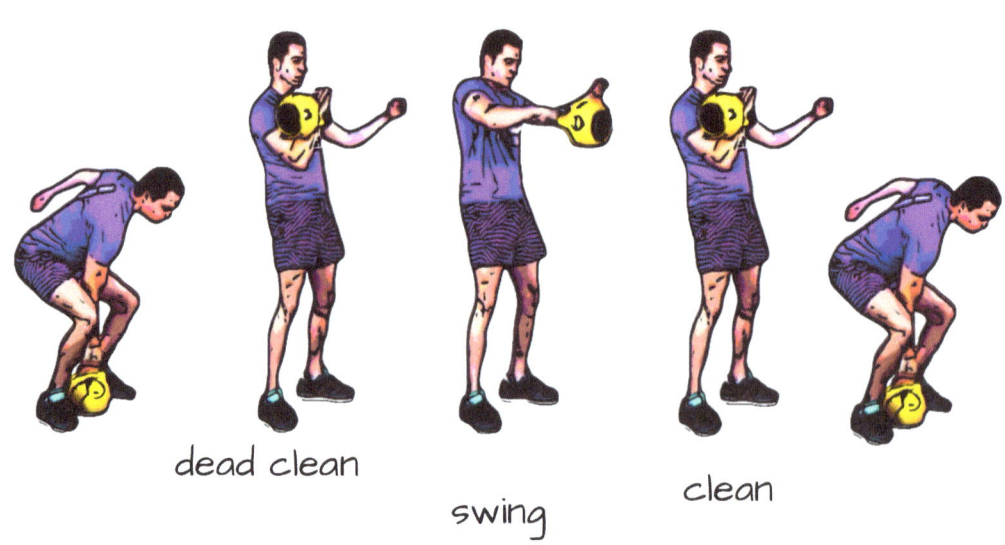

dead clean   swing   clean

351. Dead Clean + Swing + Clean

	Single Bell	Double Bell
	✓	✓

Technical Difficulty	Movement Pattern	Recommended Load
2	Compound	Heavy Weight

PRIMARY BENEFIT	FULL-BODY STRENGTH AND CONDITIONING
TARGET MUSCLES	QUADRICEPS, GLUTES, HAMSTRINGS, ERECTORS, LATS, BICEPS

This combination builds technical skill and reinforces clean mechanics under fatigue. It's ideal for kettlebell practitioners focused on flow, power, and precision.

Directions:

1. **Dead Clean:** Begin with the kettlebell on the floor between your feet. Clean it into the rack position.
2. **Swing:** Drop the bell to allow it to swing back between your legs and then project it forward into a one-hand swing.
3. **Clean:** After completing a full swing, perform another swing clean, making sure to shorten the arc and insert the hand quickly to facilitate a soft catch in the rack.
4. **Repeat:** Keeping a neutral spine, drop the bell back between your feet for the next rep.

352. Dead Clean + Squat + Press

	Single Bell	Double Bell
	✓	✓

Technical Difficulty	Movement Pattern	Recommended Load
2	Compound	Medium, Heavy Weight

PRIMARY BENEFIT	FULL-BODY STRENGTH
TARGET MUSCLES	QUADRICEPS, GLUTES, HAMSTRINGS, ERECTORS, LATS, BICEPS, DELTOIDS, TRICEPS

▶ PROKETTLEBELL.COM/352

This classic strength triad develops full-body control. The dead clean builds explosive power, the squat challenges lower-body strength under load, and the strict press finishes the rep with overhead stability and shoulder strength.

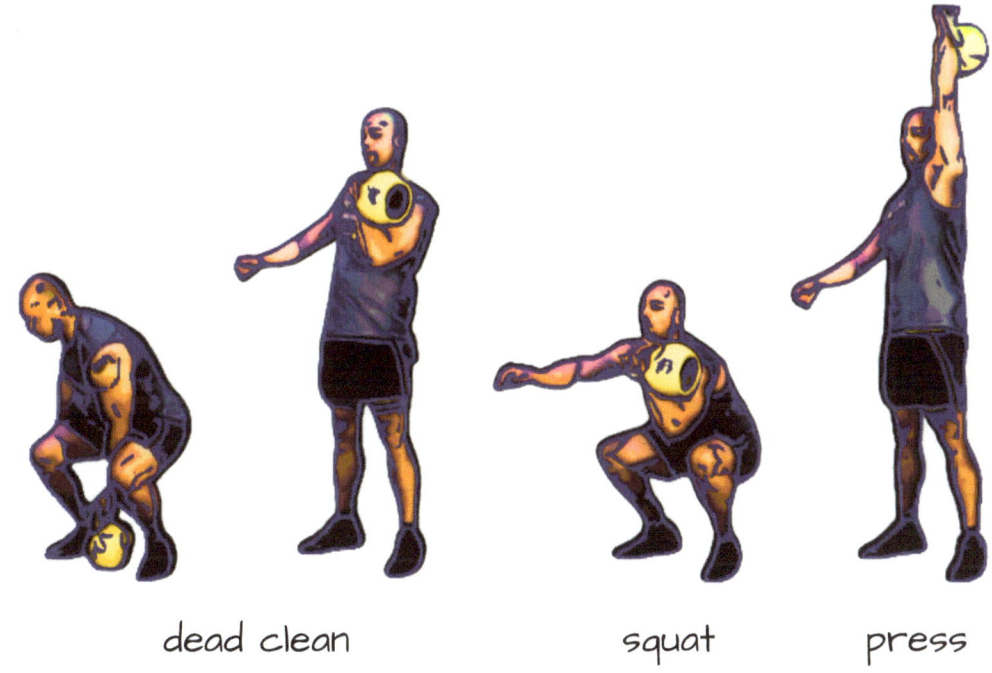

dead clean　　squat　　press

Directions:

1. **Dead Clean:** Start with the kettlebell between your feet. Explosively clean it to the rack with good posture.
2. **Squat:** Drop into a deep squat with the bell racked, keeping heels down and spine upright.
3. **Press:** Stand fully, then strict press the bell overhead without using leg drive.
4. **Reset and Repeat:** Lower the kettlebell under control and repeat the sequence.

This combination builds mobility, strength, and overhead stability in a lateral movement plane. It challenges your legs, glutes, core, and shoulders while also testing your balance and control. ▶ PROKETTLEBELL.COM/353

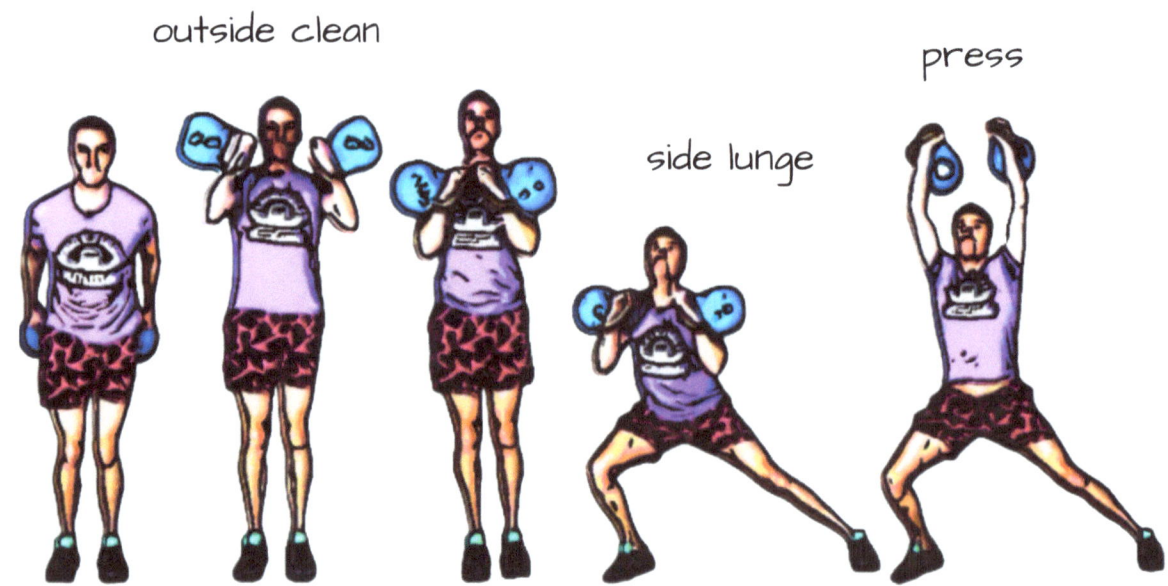

353. Outside Clean + Side Lunge + Press

	Single Bell	Double Bell
	✓	✗

Technical Difficulty	Movement Pattern	Recommended Load
2	Compound	Medium Weight

PRIMARY BENEFIT	FULL-BODY STRENGTH AND MOBILITY
TARGET MUSCLES	QUADRICEPS, GLUTES, HAMSTRINGS, ERECTORS, LATS, DELTOIDS, TRICEPS

A mobility-strength hybrid, this complex is perfect for enhancing lateral stability, overhead strength, and coordination under load.

Directions:

1. **Outside Clean:** Begin with two light kettlebells placed outside your feet. Clean them into the rack position using an outside path.
2. **Side Lunge:** Step out into a lateral lunge, keeping the kettlebells racked. Sink into the lunge as deep as mobility allows, maintaining stacked joints.
3. **Press:** From the bottom or mid-lunge position, press both kettlebells overhead while keeping balance and control.
4. **Return to Center:** Bring the kettlebells back to the rack, step to neutral stance, and re-clean if alternating sides.

160   PRO KETTLEBELL

354. Stop Clean Thruster Press

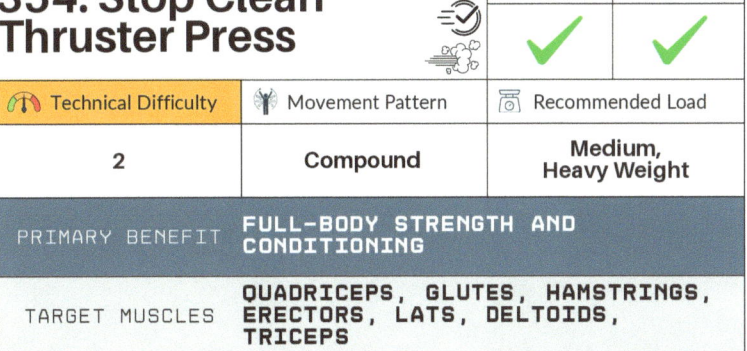

Technical Difficulty	Movement Pattern	Recommended Load
2	Compound	Medium, Heavy Weight
PRIMARY BENEFIT	FULL-BODY STRENGTH AND CONDITIONING	
TARGET MUSCLES	QUADRICEPS, GLUTES, HAMSTRINGS, ERECTORS, LATS, DELTOIDS, TRICEPS	

This complex stacks strength on strength. It begins with a clean, flows into a squat-to-press thruster, and finishes with a strict press—maximizing posterior chain recruitment and overhead pressing volume. The inclusion of both a thruster and strict press makes this ideal for focused strength and conditioning work.

▶ PROKETTLEBELL.COM/354

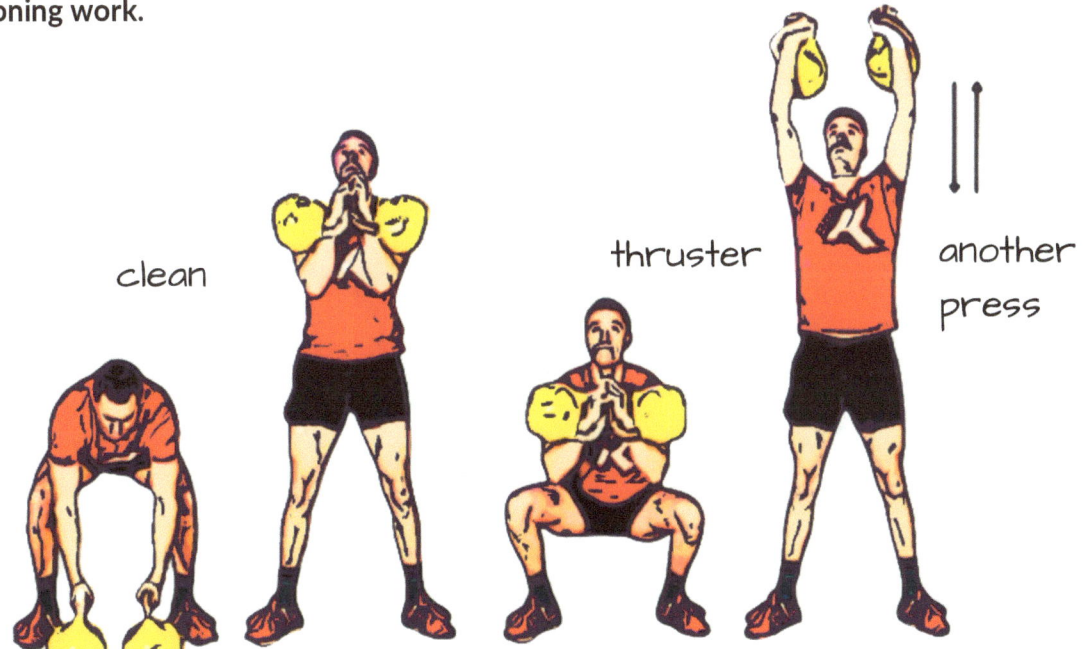

Directions:

1. **Double Clean:** Start with two kettlebells on the floor 12-18" in front of you. Clean them into the rack position.
2. **Thruster (Squat):** Drop into a deep squat, keeping your chest up and back flat.
3. **Thruster (Press):** Press the kettlebells overhead as you rise. Lockout, then lower the bells to the rack.
4. **Strict Press:** After returning to the rack, perform one strict overhead press without using your legs.
5. **Reset and Repeat:** Reverse the clean and swing the bells back to the floor.

PROKETTLEBELL.COM/355

Thruster Swings are a high-output, time-saving complex. They combine strength, power, and endurance, making them a staple for metabolic conditioning and athletic performance..

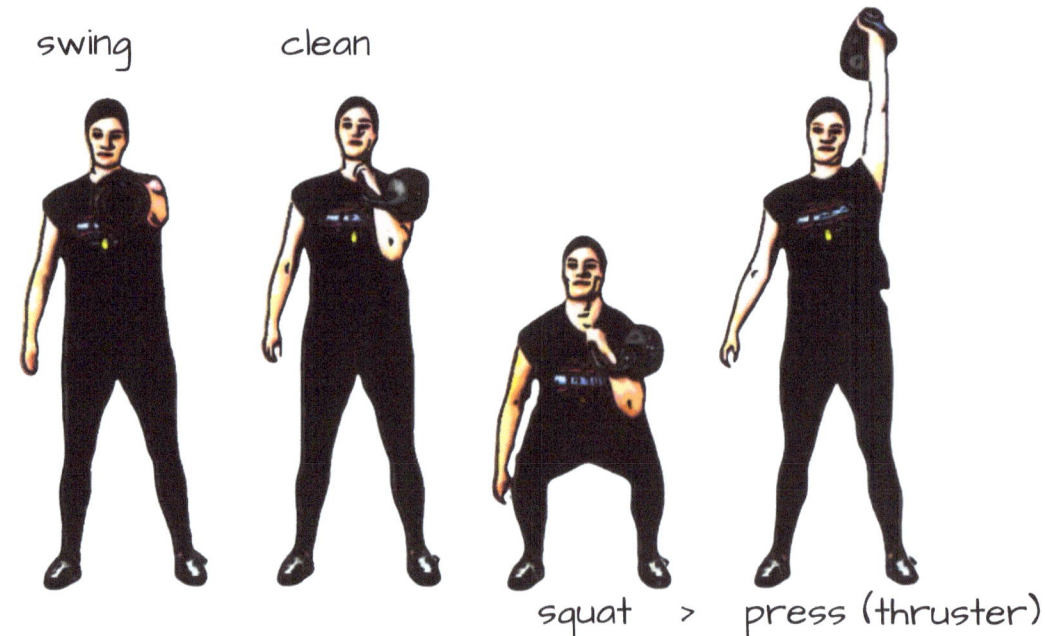

355. Swing + Clean + Thruster

	Single Bell	Double Bell
	✓	✓

Technical Difficulty	Movement Pattern	Recommended Load
2	Compound	Medium, Heavy Weight

PRIMARY BENEFIT	FULL-BODY STRENGTH AND CONDITIONING
TARGET MUSCLES	QUADRICEPS, GLUTES, HAMSTRINGS, ERECTORS, LATS, BICEPS, DELTOIDS, TRICEPS

This flow combines the power of a swing, control of a clean, and full-body explosiveness of a thruster. Whether using one or two kettlebells, it challenges conditioning and muscular endurance.

Directions:

1. **Swing:** Begin with a powerful hip hinge and swing the kettlebell up to chest height.
2. **Clean:** At the top of the next swing, clean the bell smoothly into the rack position.
3. **Thruster:** Drop into a front squat. As you rise, use the upward momentum to drive the bell(s) overhead into a press.
4. **Reset:** Lower the kettlebell back to the rack, then back to swing position to repeat. For doubles, perform the entire sequence with both bells.

The Curtsy Power Plank combines unilateral leg strength and core control into a single, flowing movement. It strengthens the glutes, quads, and deep core stabilizers while also helping to correct muscle imbalances between the legs.

356. Curtsy Power Plank

	Single Bell	Double Bell
	✗	✓
Technical Difficulty	Movement Pattern	Recommended Load
3	Compound	Heavy Weight
PRIMARY BENEFIT	LEG AND CORE STRENGTH	
TARGET MUSCLES	QUADRICEPS, GLUTES, HAMSTRINGS, ERECTORS, LATS, DELTOIDS, TRICEPS	

▶ PROKETTLEBELL.COM/356

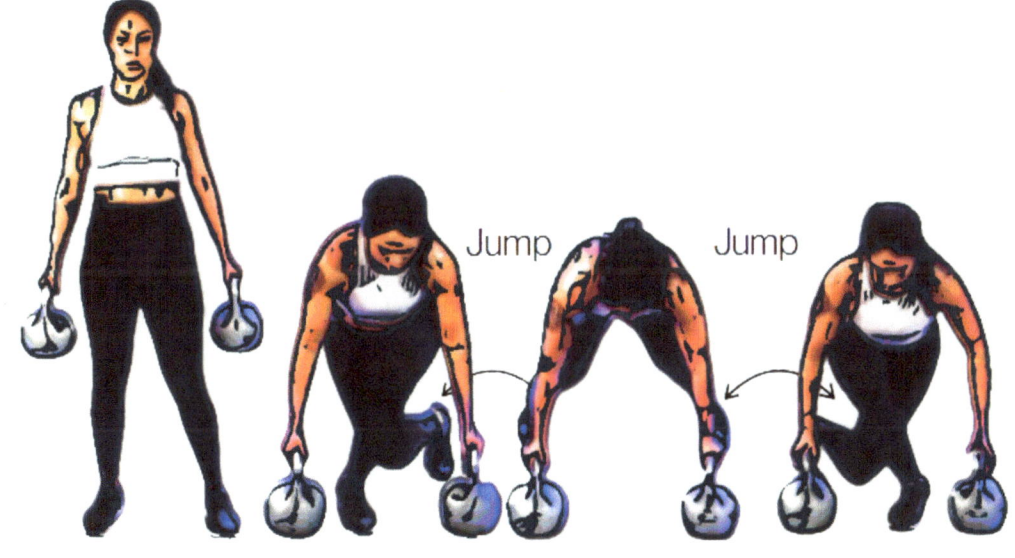

suitcase deadlift — curtsy plank — wide plank — curtsy plank other side

Directions:

1. **Suitcase Deadlift:** Stand between two medium-weight kettlebells and lift them using a suitcase grip, keeping your core braced and spine neutral.
2. **Curtsy Squat:** As you lower the bells to the floor, step one leg diagonally behind the other into a curtsy position, keeping most of your weight on the front leg.
3. **Plank Kick-Out:** At the bottom of the squat (and once your kettlebells are firmly on the ground) jump your feet back into a solid plank position, feet shoulder width or wider apart.
4. **Reverse the Kick-Out:** Step or hop your feet forward into the curtsy squat position again.
5. **Stand Tall:** Drive through your front heel to return to standing. Switch legs or repeat on the same side.

COMPLEXES

357. Double Clean + Double Half Snatch

	Single Bell	Double Bell
	✗	✓

Technical Difficulty	Movement Pattern	Recommended Load
3	Compound	Medium Weight

PRIMARY BENEFIT	FULL-BODY STRENGTH AND POWER
TARGET MUSCLES	QUADRICEPS, GLUTES, HAMSTRINGS, ERECTORS, LATS, DELTOIDS, TRICEPS

Power combo time.

Cleans set the rhythm, snatches bring the heat.

If your timing is sloppy, it exposes you. If your technique is dialed, it levels you up fast.

Tax the shoulders, lats, and core while training rhythm and explosiveness with this solid test of coordination and upper-body endurance.

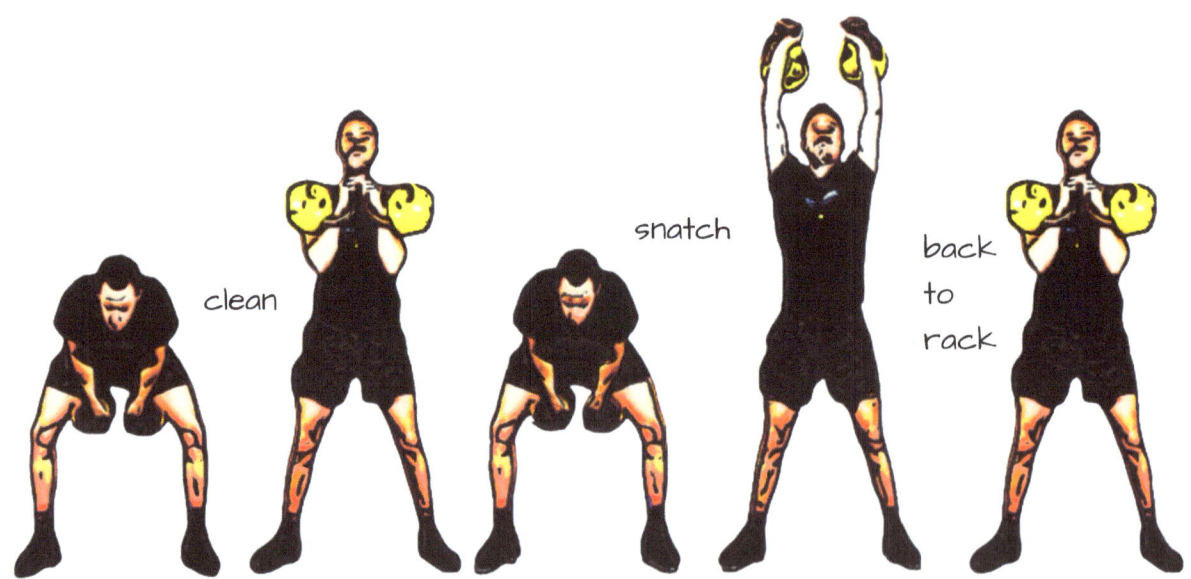

PROKETTLEBELL.COM/357

Directions:

1. **Double Clean:** Begin with kettlebells on the ground. Clean them into the front rack with clean mechanics.
2. **Double Half Snatch:** Swing both bells and punch them overhead simultaneously, locking them out smoothly.
3. **Return to Rack:** Lower both bells from overhead directly back into the rack position.
4. **Repeat:** Drop the bells for the next clean or cycle back directly from the rack.

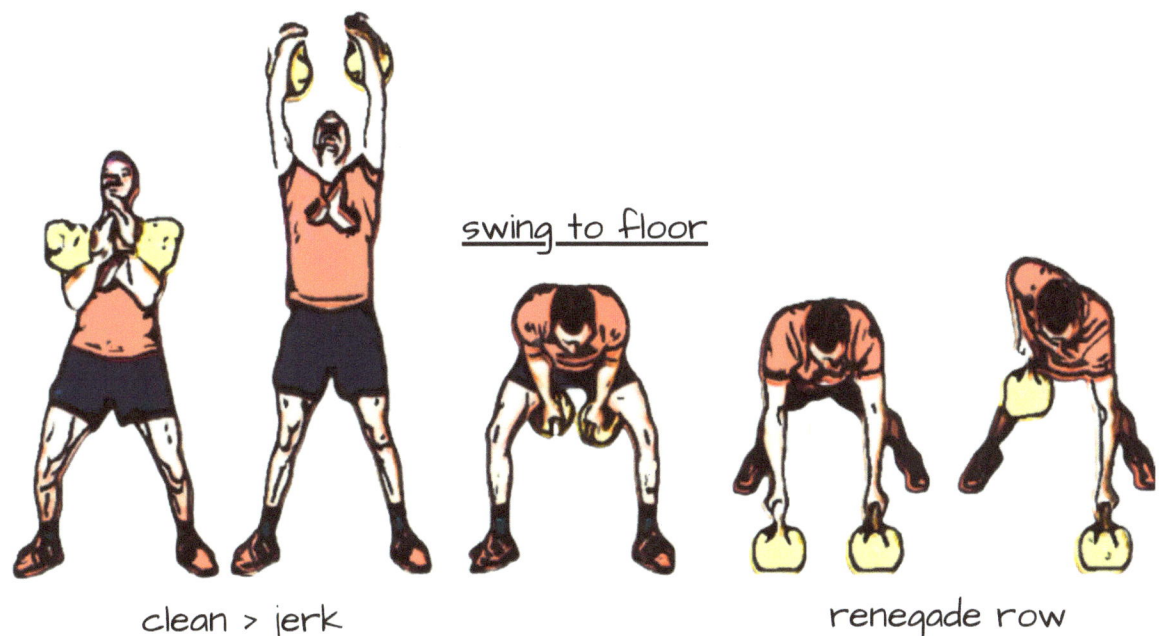

clean > jerk   swing to floor   renegade row

This powerful complex trains full-body strength, core control, and explosive movement. It links a clean, overhead press, and a grounded row into one fluid circuit.

358. Double Clean + Jerk + Renegade (Plank) Row

	Single Bell	Double Bell
	✗	✓

Technical Difficulty	Movement Pattern	Recommended Load
3	Compound	Medium, Heavy Weight

PRIMARY BENEFIT	FULL-BODY STRENGTH AND CONDITIONING
TARGET MUSCLES	QUADRICEPS, GLUTES, HAMSTRINGS, ERECTORS, LATS, BICEPS, PECS, DELTOIDS, TRICEPS

▶ PROKETTLEBELL.COM/358

Directions:

1. **Double Clean:** Begin with two kettlebells in front of you. Clean them into the front rack position.
2. **Double Jerk:** Dip and drive to explode the bells overhead, locking out with fixation.
3. **Return and Lower:** Bring the bells back to the rack and then to the ground.
4. **Plank Position:** Step or hop your feet back into a plank, hands on the bells.
5. **Renegade Row:** Row the left bell, then the right, keeping your core stable.
6. **Reset:** Step or hop to standing and repeat the sequence, alternating the row lead arm each round.

COMPLEXES

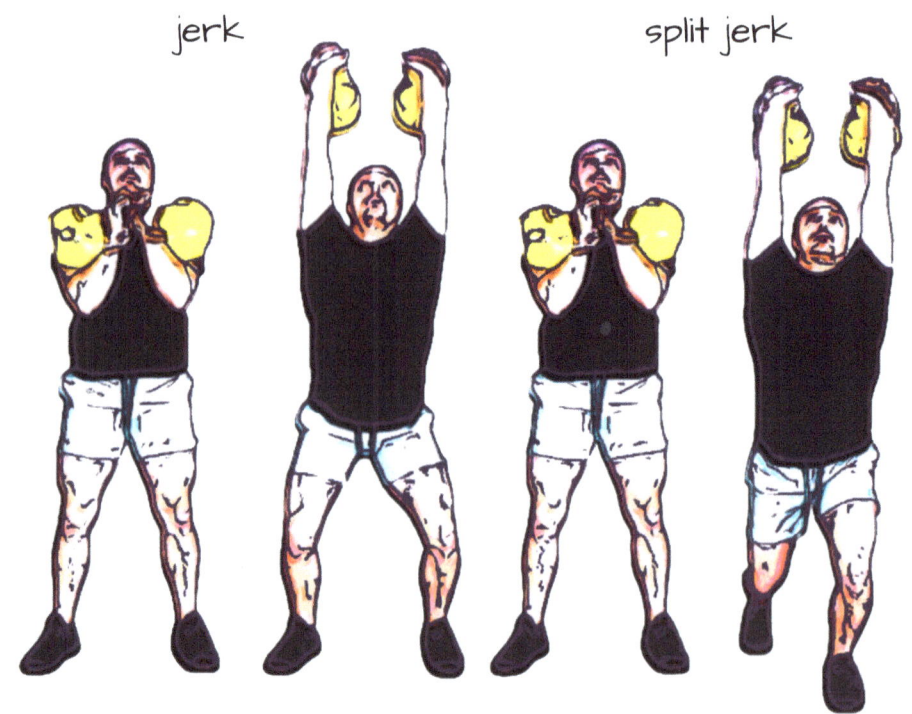

PROKETTLEBELL.COM/359

359. Double Jerk + Split Jerk

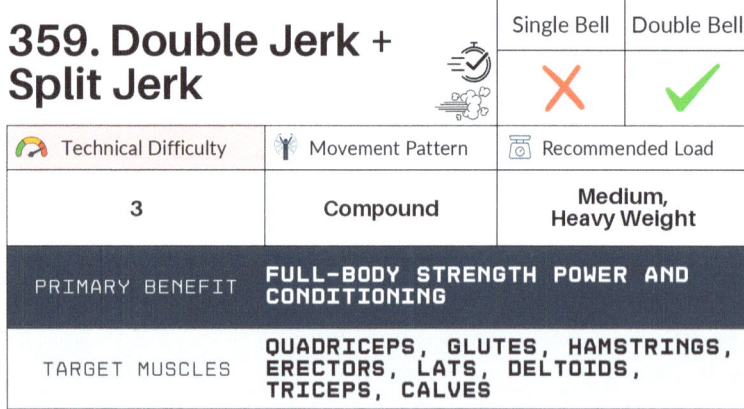

	Single Bell	Double Bell
	✗	✓

🌈 Technical Difficulty	🤸 Movement Pattern	⚖️ Recommended Load
3	Compound	Medium, Heavy Weight

PRIMARY BENEFIT	FULL-BODY STRENGTH POWER AND CONDITIONING
TARGET MUSCLES	QUADRICEPS, GLUTES, HAMSTRINGS, ERECTORS, LATS, DELTOIDS, TRICEPS, CALVES

This sequence is all about overhead control, lower body power, and technique. It trains both bilateral and unilateral stance stability under a loaded jerk, improving explosiveness and body positioning. It teaches leg drive, coordination, and dynamic control under load.

Directions:

1. *Double Clean to Rack:* Start by cleaning both kettlebells into a stable rack position.
2. *Double Jerk:* Perform a dip and drive to lock the bells overhead with feet parallel.
3. *Split Jerk:* After returning to the rack, perform a second dip and this time launch into a split stance, one leg moves forward, one back - catching the bells locked out overhead as you land softly.
4. *Return to Rack:* Bring the bells back down as are after you bring your feet back together.
5. *Repeat:* Each round, alternate your lead leg on each split jerk.

This compound sequence delivers full-body strength, conditioning, and technique refinement. While the double half snatch adds explosive overhead work, the long cycle provides advanced strength-conditioning. The complex develops timing, breathing patterns, and control under double overhead load.

360. Double Long Cycle + Half-Snatch

	Single Bell	Double Bell
	✗	✓

Technical Difficulty	Movement Pattern	Recommended Load
3	Compound	Medium Weight

PRIMARY BENEFIT	FULL-BODY STRENGTH AND POWER
TARGET MUSCLES	QUADRICEPS, GLUTES, HAMSTRINGS, ERECTORS, LATS, DELTOIDS, TRICEPS

▶ PROKETTLEBELL.COM/360

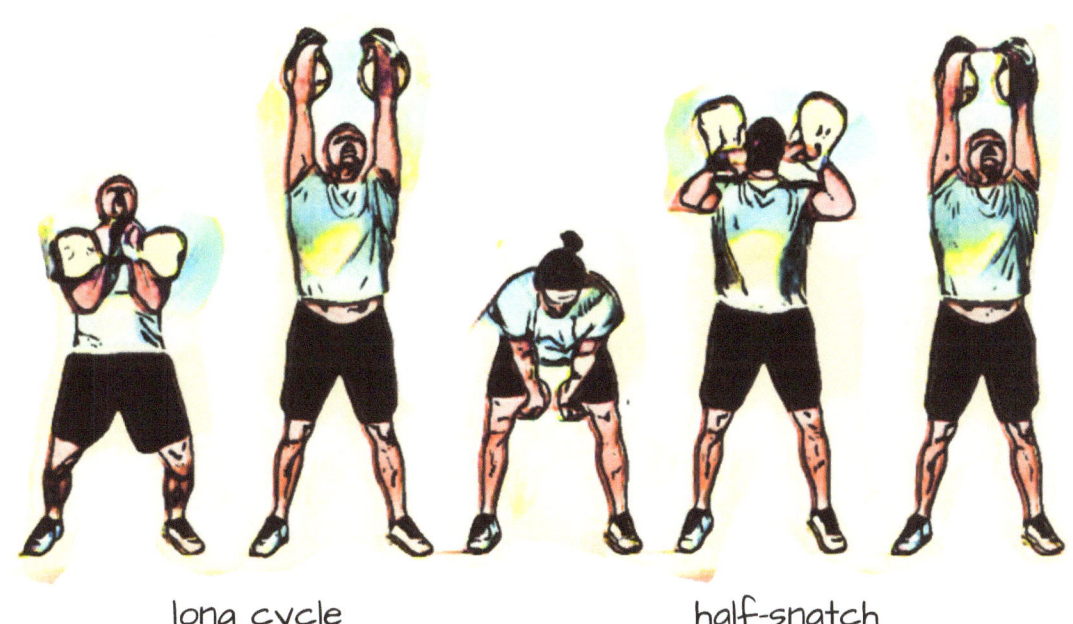

long cycle   half-snatch

Directions:

1. **Double Clean:** *Begin by cleaning two kettlebells into the rack.*
2. **Double Jerk:** *Dip and drive to press both bells overhead with strong fixation.*
3. **Return to Rack:** *Bring the bells back to the rack position with control.*
4. **Double Half Snatch:** *Swing both bells and snatch them overhead in a single motion. After fixation, lower to the rack—not the ground.*
5. **Reset and Repeat:** *Flow back into the clean to continue the sequence.*

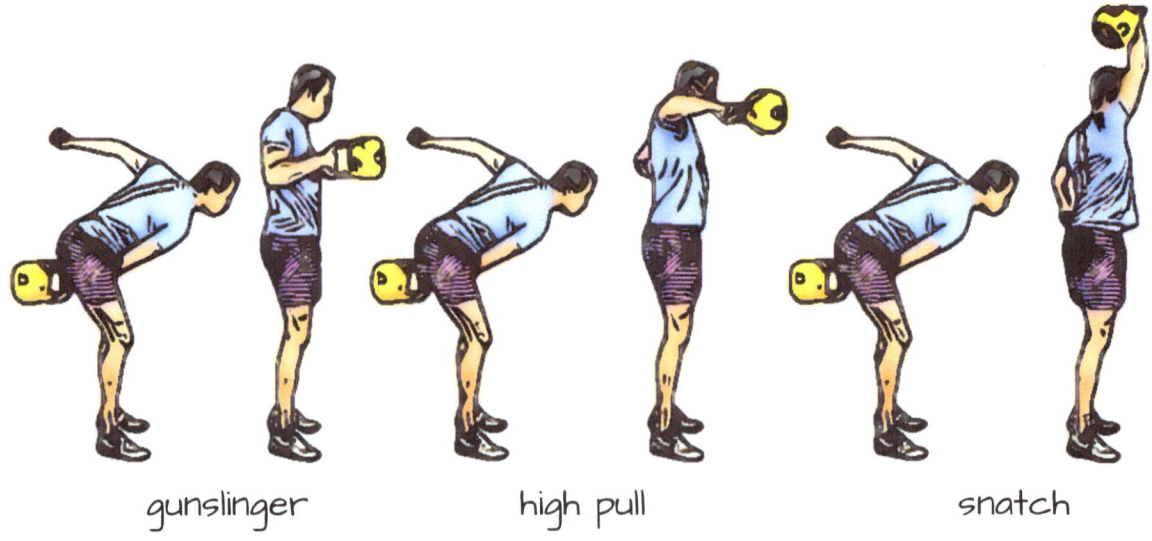

gunslinger   high pull   snatch

361. Gunslinger + High Pull + Snatch

	Single Bell	Double Bell
	✓	✗

Technical Difficulty	Movement Pattern	Recommended Load
3	Compound	Medium Weight

PRIMARY BENEFIT	FULL-BODY STRENGTH AND CONDITIONING
TARGET MUSCLES	QUADRICEPS, GLUTES, HAMSTRINGS, ERECTORS, LATS, DELTOIDS, TRICEPS

This trio builds serious upper-body power and precision. Each phase increases in complexity—from the controlled gunslinger, to the high pull, to the overhead snatch.

▶ PROKETTLEBELL.COM/361

This complex is a posterior chain and shoulder burner and an excellent progression series that strengthens pulling mechanics and overhead precision. It's great for improving snatch fluency and shoulder control.

Directions:

1. **Gunslinger:** Perform a swing with the elbow tucked, pulling the bell back quickly while keeping it close to the ribs.
2. **High Pull:** On the next swing, pull the kettlebell high with the elbow leading, bringing it level with your shoulder.
3. **Snatch:** Perform a full snatch by swinging and punching the bell directly overhead into a locked-out position.
4. **Reset and Repeat:** Return the kettlebell under control and repeat the sequence.

This complex combines the clean and jerk with a squat thrust. It targets power production and muscular endurance across the entire body as a full-body flow that trains lifting power, cardio, and movement efficiency. It's especially effective in high-rep or timed conditioning blocks.

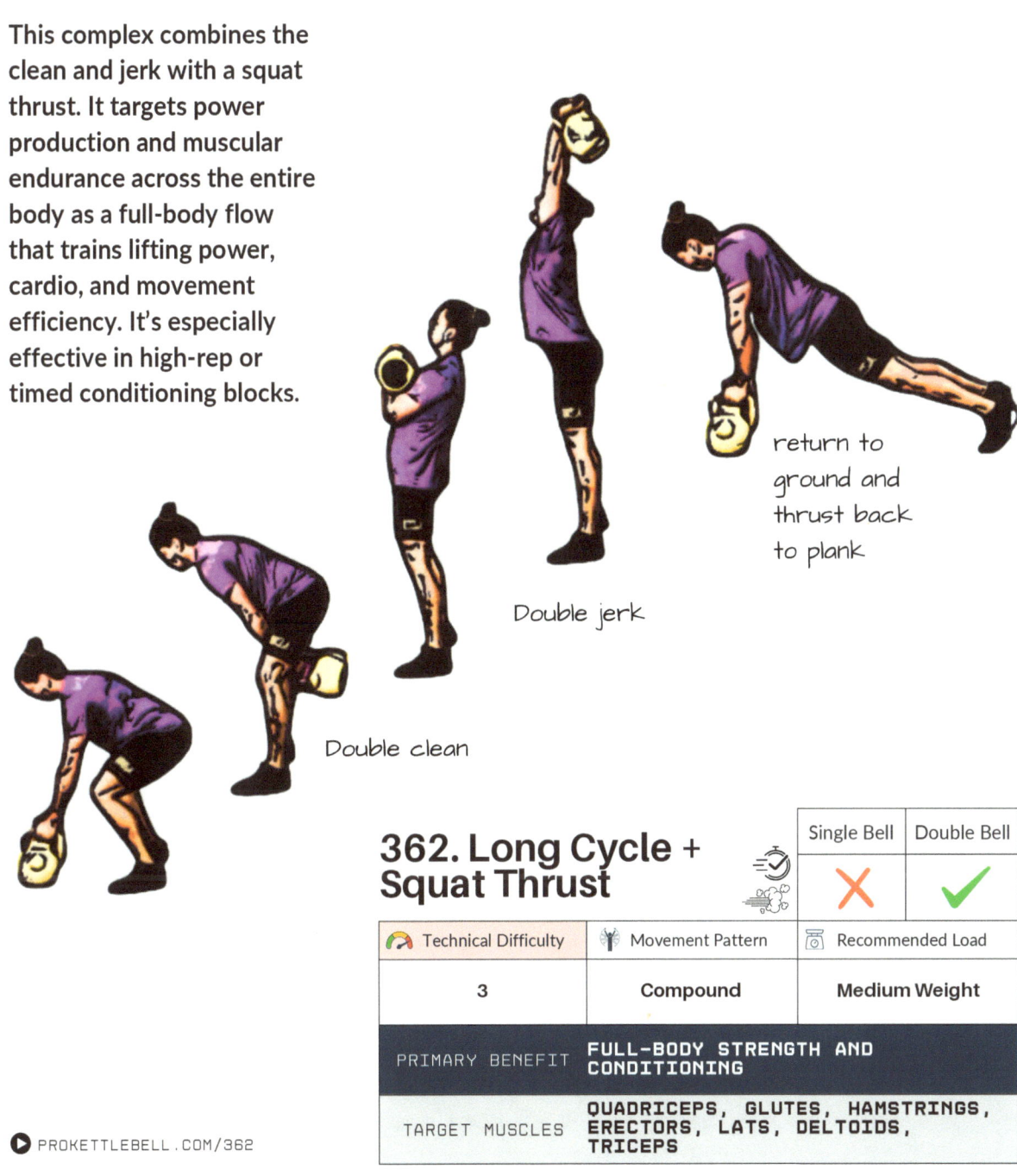

return to ground and thrust back to plank

Double jerk

Double clean

362. Long Cycle + Squat Thrust

	Single Bell	Double Bell
	✗	✓

Technical Difficulty	Movement Pattern	Recommended Load
3	Compound	Medium Weight

PRIMARY BENEFIT	FULL-BODY STRENGTH AND CONDITIONING
TARGET MUSCLES	QUADRICEPS, GLUTES, HAMSTRINGS, ERECTORS, LATS, DELTOIDS, TRICEPS

▶ PROKETTLEBELL.COM/362

Directions:

1. **Kettlebell Clean:** Begin with kettlebells in front of you. Use hip drive to clean them to the rack position.
2. **Jerk:** Dip slightly, then explosively drive the bells overhead. Lock out with control.
3. **Return to Floor:** Lower the kettlebells under control back to the ground.
4. **Squat Thrust:** Placing your hands on the kettlebells, jump your legs back into a plank.
5. **Return to Start:** Bring your feet forward, stand tall, and go right into the next clean. You can optionally add a push-up at the bottom for added challenge.

COMPLEXES

363. The Mad Max

	Single Bell	Double Bell
	✗	✓

🌈 Technical Difficulty	🧍 Movement Pattern	⚖️ Recommended Load
3	Compound	Medium Weight
PRIMARY BENEFIT	**FULL-BODY STRENGTH AND CONDITIONING**	
TARGET MUSCLES	**QUADRICEPS, GLUTES, HAMSTRINGS, ERECTORS, LATS, DELTOIDS, PECS, TRICEPS, BICEPS**	

▶ PROKETTLEBELL.COM/363

The Mad Max is a full-body complex designed to hit nearly every muscle group. It blends strength, conditioning, and core stability into one relentless sequence that builds resilience, coordination, and power - perfect for advanced trainees needing maximal effort in minimal time and space.

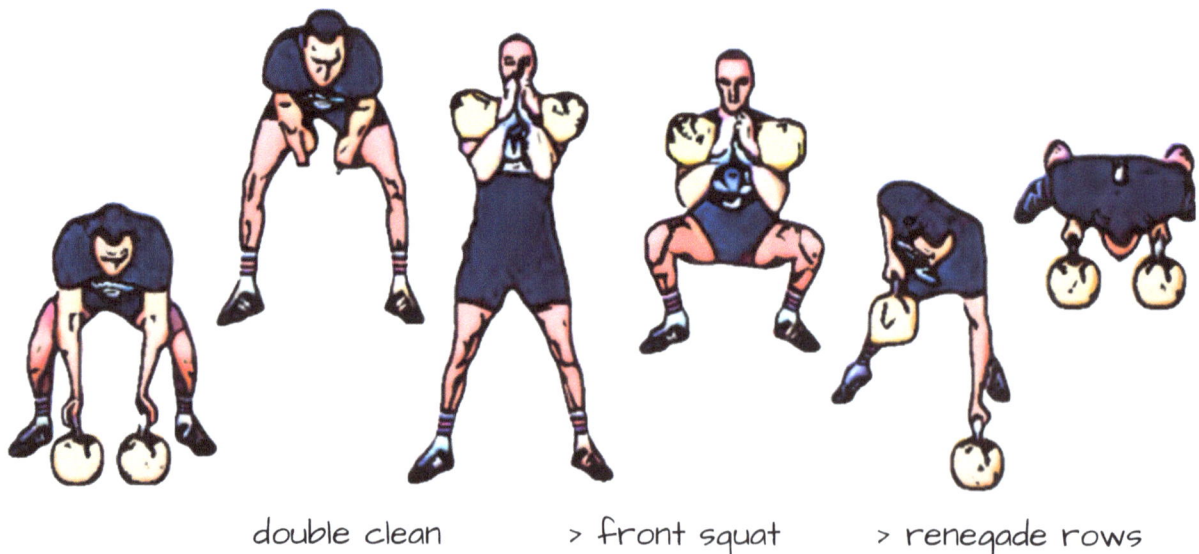

double clean   > front squat   > renegade rows

Directions:

1. *Clean to Rack:* Clean both kettlebells to the front rack position.
2. *Front Squat:* Lift your elbows and drop into a deep squat while keeping your torso upright.
3. *Stand Up & Lower:* Rise fully, then drop the kettlebells with control to the floor.
4. *Plank Setup:* Place your hands on the kettlebell handles and kick your legs back into a plank.
5. *Renegade Row (Right):* Row the right kettlebell toward your ribs without rotating.
6. *Renegade Row (Left):* Now perform a row on the left side (still keeping your hips still/no rotation).
7. *Push-Up:* Perform a narrow push-up, elbows tight to your torso.
8. *Reset:* Hop forward so the bells are between your feet. Reset and clean the bells to begin again.

364. Over the Mountain

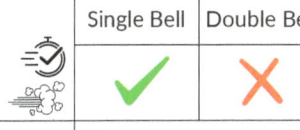

	Single Bell	Double Bell
	✓	✗

Technical Difficulty	Movement Pattern	Recommended Load
3	Compound	Medium Weight

PRIMARY BENEFIT	FULL-BODY STRENGTH, CONDITIONING AND COORDINATION
TARGET MUSCLES	QUADRICEPS, GLUTES, HAMSTRINGS, ERECTORS, LATS, DELTOIDS, OBLIQUES, TRICEPS, BICEPS

Over the Mountain is a dynamic complex with clean, thruster, and snatch transitions that challenge coordination, shoulder endurance, and flow under fatigue. It's a strong choice for athletes seeking variety and challenge.

▶ PROKETTLEBELL.COM/364

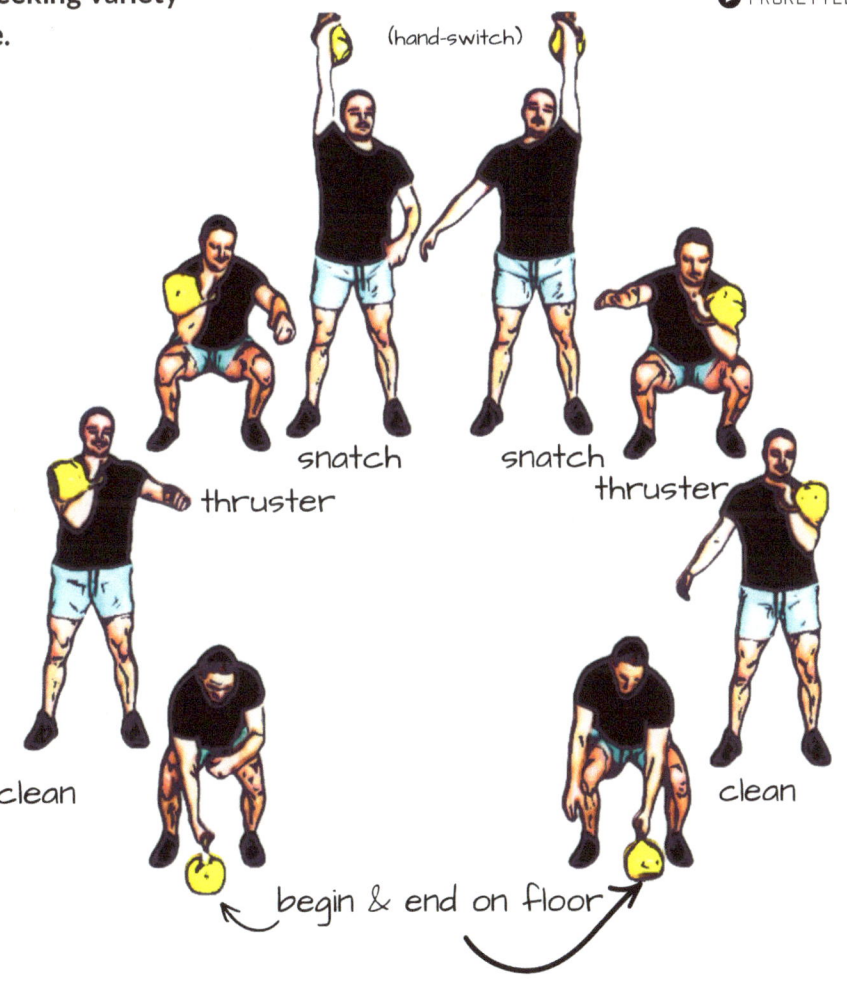

Directions:

1. **Clean (Right):** Start with a clean to rack on your right side.
2. **Thruster (Right):** Drop into a squat and use leg drive to stand and press the kettlebell overhead.
3. **Snatch (Right):** Bring the bell back to rack, then perform a full snatch on the same side.
4. **Switch Sides:** Pass it to the left hand with an alternating swing.
5. **Snatch (Left):** Perform a snatch with your left hand.
6. **Thruster (Left):** After fixation, bring the bell to rack and perform a thruster.
7. **Reverse Clean (Left):** After the thruster, swing the bell to the starting position and repeat.

COMPLEXES

365. Plyo Burpee

	Single Bell	Double Bell
	✓	✗

Technical Difficulty	Movement Pattern	Recommended Load
3	Compound	Heavy Weight

PRIMARY BENEFIT	FULL-BODY STRENGTH AND CONDITIONING
TARGET MUSCLES	QUADRICEPS, GLUTES, HAMSTRINGS, LATS, PECS, DELTOIDS, TRICEPS

Plyo Burpees combine explosive jumping with uneven push-ups to build upper-body strength, power, and reactive speed. They are excellent for conditioning and athletic agility.

Directions:

1. **Push-Up Setup:** Place a kettlebell handle-down and away on the ground and get into plank with one hand on the kettlebell, the other on the floor.
2. **Push-Up:** Lower your chest toward the floor and perform a push-up.
3. **Jump to Feet:** Explosively hop forward and rise to standing.
4. **Lateral Hop:** Immediately perform a lateral hop to the other side of the kettlebell.
5. **Push-Up:** Mirror the off-set push-up you performed on the other side.
6. **Reset:** Jump back to standing and continue the flow.

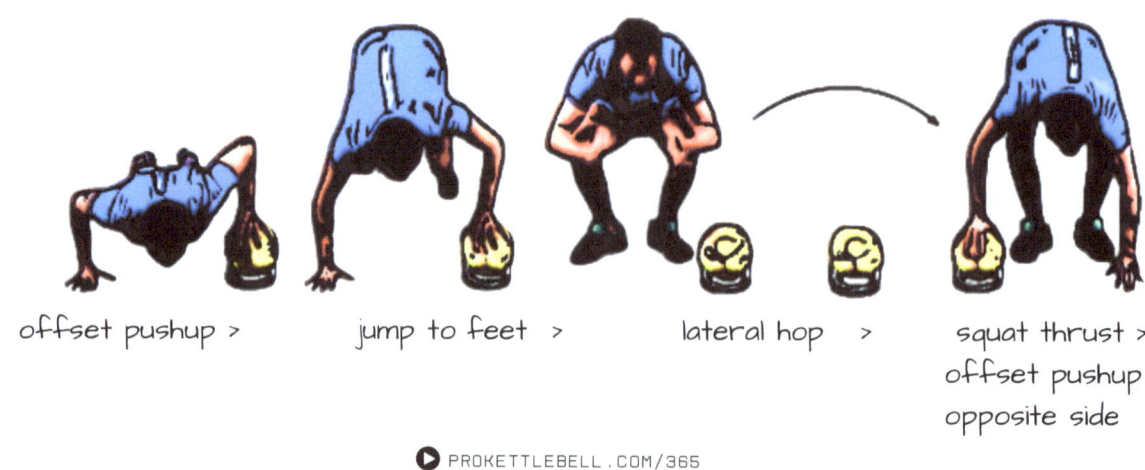

offset pushup > jump to feet > lateral hop > squat thrust > offset pushup opposite side

PROKETTLEBELL.COM/365

Plyo Burpees are a high-octane, muscle-shocking addition to any workout. They challenge coordination, increase work capacity, and build reactive strength through every rep.

Glossary

Kettlebell & Exercise Terminology

Ballistic: An explosive, fast movement (e.g., swing, snatch, clean).

Bottoms-Up: A grip where the kettlebell is held upside down by the handle, requiring extra grip and wrist stability.

Brace: Engage your core and lock your ribs down to stabilize the spine.

Clean: A movement that brings the bell from the floor or swing path into the racked position.

Complex / Flow: A series of movements performed without putting the kettlebell down.

Compound Exercise: A move that works multiple joints or muscle groups simultaneously.

Dead (from the floor): A lift that begins with the bell at rest on the ground.

Girevoy / Girevik: Russian for kettlebell lifting / kettlebell lifter.

Grind: A slow, controlled strength movement (e.g., strict press, heavy deadlift).

Hang: A still position where the kettlebell is held between the legs with a straight arm, not touching the ground.

Hike: The initial backward pull of the kettlebell (like hiking a football) in a swing or snatch.

Hinge: A hip-dominant movement like a swing or deadlift. The spine stays neutral as the hips push back.

Horns: The sides of the handle that connect the bell to the body.

Long Cycle: One of the competitive kettlebell sport lifts, it combines a clean and a jerk.

Offset Load: A unilateral or uneven load position that forces the core to stabilize.

Pack the Shoulder: Draw the shoulder blade down and in, preventing shrugging and instability.

Push / Pull / Rotate / Carry / Hold: Categories of movement patterns used to balance total-body training.

Rack Position: Kettlebell is held at chest height with the elbow tucked near the ribs and wrist straight: a foundation for cleans, pressing, squatting, or pausing.

Single Bell / Double Bell: Refers to using one or two kettlebells during a movement.

Slingshot: A movement where the kettlebell is passed around the body in a circular motion.

Speed-Switch: A transition where the rep starts in one hand and finishes in the other by releasing the bell and throwing it directly into the insertion point of the opposite hand, just prior to racking. It skips the swing phase.

Stop: A deliberate pause between repetitions to reset position or tension before continuing.

Swing-to-Snatch / Clean-to-Press: Indicates one exercise transitions directly into the next.

Tempo: The speed at which a rep is performed. Used for progression or variation.

Window: The open space between the horns and handle of the kettlebell.

Alphabetical Exercise Index

21-Curls	30
21-Deadlifts	121
3-Position Drill (2-Hand)	116
Ab Circles	73
Ab Squat	47
Alternating Clean + Ballistic Row	149
Alternating Lateral Swing	94
Alternating Press	16
Alternating Snatch	113
Alternating Stop Row	28
Alternating Swing	94
Alternating Swing + Long Cycle	149
Anchored Leg Raise	74
Anchored Plow	83
Anchored Racked Sit-Ups	73
Anchored Side Cycles	81
Anchored Wiper Crunch	73
Armbar Bicycles	74
Armbar Reverse Crunch	74
Armbar Sit-Up	81
Armbar Sit-Up + Press	82
Assisted Hang Snatch	110
Axe Chops	30
Backward Gunslingers	99
Ballistic Deadlift	121
Ballistic Row	28
Barn Door Fly	30
Battering Ram Swings	95
Bear Crawl Pull	129
Bent Over Gurney Row	28
Boat Pose Kicks	75
Bottoms Up-Cleans	103
Bottoms-Up Floor Press	16
Bottoms-Up High Knees	136
Bottoms-Up Press	16
Bottoms-Up Side Lunge	59
Bottoms-Up Snatch	110
Bottoms-Up Squat	47
Bottoms-Up Thruster	130
Bottoms-Up Thruster Twist	131
Bridge Crush Press	17
Bridge Pull Over	31
Bulgarian Back Squat	47
Bumps	116
Butt Kicker Sit-up	75
Cheat Curls	31
Clean + High Pull	151
Clean and Squat	151
Cleans, One-Arm	103
Cleans, Two-Arm	103
Clock Lunges	56
Concentration Curls	31
Conventional Two-Hand Deadlift	121
Cossack Squat	48
CPR Crunch	75
Crab Kick Dips	87
Cross Curl Press	32
Cross Curls (High Fives)	32
Cross Squat	48
Cross-Overs	86
Crouching Pull Across	86
Curtsy Cleans	104
Curtsy Power Plank	155
Curtsy Snatch	113
Curtsy Squat	48
Curtsy Toss	54
Diamond Cutter Push-Ups	25
Dive-Bomber	145
Dead Clean + High Knee	104
Dead Clean + Push Press + Windmill	152
Dead Clean + Squat + Press	153
Dead Clean + Swing + Clean	152
Dead Clean, One-Arm	104
Deadlift + Jump Squat	43
Deck Squat	49
Deck Squat Thruster	132
Decline Kettlebell Push-Ups	26
Deep Lunge Press	59
Diagonal Deadlifts	122
Diagonal Lunge Pull	66
Double 3-Position Drill	117
Double Alternating Sideways V Ups	83
Double Bridge Press	17
Double Clean + Double Half Snatch	155
Double Clean + Jerk + Plank Row	156
Double Deadlift + Renegade Row	126
Double Half-Snatch	113
Double Hand-Insertion Drill	110
Double Jerk + Split Jerk	156
Double Kettlebell Plank Jacks	127
Double Long Cycle + Half Snatch	157
Double Lunge Jump Rows	66
Double Overhead Squat	49
Double Overhead Surrenders	133
Double Rack Curtsy Squat	49
Double Rack Squat	43
Double Rack Squat Slider	50
Double Reverse Fly	38
Double Seated Press	17

Alphabetical Exercise Index

Exercise	Page	Exercise	Page
Double Snatch	114	Horn Clean + Press	102
Double Step Thru Press	18	Horn Clean + Squat Pulse	102
Double Swings, Outside & Inside	97	Horn Clean + Tip Toe Squat	105
Double Tip Toe Rack Squat	43	Horn Clean > Walkout Push-Up	101
Double Windmill	89	Horn Clean Squat Jack	105
Dropslingers	95	Horn Hold Reverse Lunge	56
Duck Walk	136	Hug Lunges	56
Dynamic Ribbons	38	Iron Cross Circle Press	24
Escape Punch	76	Jefferson Deadlift	122
Farmer Carry / Farmer Hold	135	Jerk, One-Arm	117
Figure 4 Chair Squat	50	Jerk, Two-Arm	117
Figure 4 Glute Bridge	68	Jerk, Two-Hand	116
Figure 4 Squat	50	Jump Turns	140
Figure 8 Clean	109	KB Beast Makers	150
Figure 8 Reverse Lunge	66	KB Kick Thru Push-Ups	26
Figure 8s	93	KB Knee Circles	144
Figure-8 Half-Snatch	114	KB Mountain Climb Twist	85
Figure-8 Snatch	114	KB Mountain Climbers	85
Fireman Clean	101	KB Shoulder Touches	85
Fireman Squats	44	KB Side Plank	87
Flat Kettlebell Fly	32	KB Touch + Spiderman Plank	127
Flat Lat Pullover	39	KB Touchdowns	139
Float Swing	95	Kettlebell Burpee	150
Floor Press	18	Kettlebell Dips	34
Floor Pullover	33	Kettlebell Kayaks	77
Floor-to-Kettlebell Plank	127	Kettlebell Leg Extensions	68
Frogger Sit-Up	76	Kettlebell Lunge Jumps	59
Front Press	18	Kettlebell Lunge Unders	60
Front Raise	33	Kettlebell Skull Crushers	34
Front Raise Rotations	33	Kickstand Deadlift	123
Front Raise Squat	44	Kneeling Clean	106
Goblet Squat	44	Kneeling Crab Press	22
Goblet Toss	51	Kneeling Curl + Press	35
Goblet Toss Thruster	132	Kneeling Outside Cleans	106
Golden Arches	76	Kneeling Press	19
Good Morning	143	Kneeling Windmill	88
Gorilla Cleans	105	Kneeling Windmill > Side Plank	88
Groin Glider	143	L-Sit	84
Gunslinger	93	L-Situp	78
Gunslinger + High Pull + Snatch	157	Lat-Pull Swings	96
Gurney Deadlifts	122	Lateral Frog Squats	51
Half-Snatch	111	Lateral Kettlebell Plank Walks	129
Halo Situp	77	Lateral Lunge Row	60
Halos	34	Lateral Lunge Slingers	60
Handless Getup	133	Lateral Lunges (Goblet Hold)	57
High Pull	96	Lawn Mower Pull	39
Hip/Hamstring Opener	143	Lo/Hi Swing-to-Snatch	111
Hollow Hold Crunch	77	Loaded Beast Sliders	145
Horn Clean	101	Loaded Jump Squat	51

Alphabetical Exercise Index

Loaded Stationary Lunge	57
Loaded Stop Squat	45
Long Cycle + Squat Thrust	158
Long Cycle	118
Low Windmill	89
Lunge Pulse	57
Lunge Twist	61
Lunge Twist, Hammer Grip	61
Lunging Halo	61
Marching Glute Bridge	68
Military Press (Strict Press)	19
Motorcycles	129
Narrow Kettlebell Pushups	25
Narrow/Wide Goblet Squats	52
Narrow/Wide Thrusters	131
Offset (Uneven) Push-Ups	25
One-Arm Row	29
One-Arm Squat Swing	100
Outside Clean + French Press	106
Outside Clean + Sd Lunge + Press	153
Outside Swing + Clean	107
Over the Mountain	159
Overhead Chair Twist	144
Overhead Curtsy Squat	52
Overhead Lateral Shuffle Steps	140
Overhead Lunge	58
Overhead Squat, Two-Hand	45
Overhead Walking Lunge	62
Palm Press	19
Peekaboo Squats	52
Pendulum Deadlift	126
Pistol Squat	55
Plank Palm Taps	128
Plank Push n' Pull	128
Plyo Burpee	159
Plyo Push-Up	27
Press + Overhead Squat	53
Pull Over Squats	45
Pull-Over Tucks	78
Pull-Over March	135
Pull-Under	86
Push Press	22
Rack Position	15
Rack Squat, One-Arm	46
Rack Step-Thru Lunge	62
Racked Circle Press	23
Racked Deadlift	123
Racked Lunge Hops	67
Racked Trunk Twists	78
Racked Waiter Carry	135
Renegade Row	29
Reverse Curls	35
Reverse Jump Squat	53
Reverse Lunge Cleans	107
Reverse Lunge Snatch	111
Ribbon	35
Rolling Push-Ups	27
Romanian Deadlifts	123
Romanian Suitcase Deadlift	124
Rotating Deadlift	124
Rotational Swings (Golf Swing)	96
Russian Twist	79
Scoop Swings	97
Seated Good Morning	144
Seated Ribbons	36
Seated Twister Press	20
Seated Wood Chopper	36
See Saw Press	22
Semi Squat	53
Shin Boxes	146
Shinbox Press	23
Shotgun Reverse Lunge	67
Shrugs	36
Shuffle Lunge	62
Side Lunge Ribbons	63
Side Lunge Toss	63
Side Lunge Twist	58
Side Plank Pull-Unders	128
Side-Hop Swing	100
Side-Step Figure-8s	140
Sideways V-Up	82
Single Back Squat	46
Single Hand Outside Swing	93
Single Kettlebell Inside Swing	97
Single Leg Ribbons	39
Single-Arm Staggered Swing	98
Single-Leg Gurney Deadlift	124
Sit-Up Getup	79
Sit-Up Twist	79
Skaters	141
Sledgehammer Cleans	102
Slider Push-Ups	27
Slingshot Curtsy Press	23
Slingshot Reverse Lunge	63
Slingshot Side Lunge	67
Slingshot Squat Variations	54
Slingshot Thruster	131
Slingshots	139

Alphabetical Exercise Index

Snatch	112
Soccer Drill	139
Speed-Switch Front Squat	55
Speed-Switch Long Cycle	118
Speed-Switch Slingshots	141
Speed-Switch Snatch	113
Speed-Switch Swing n' Clean	109
Split Jerk	118
Split Lunge Dead Clean	107
Split Lunge Jumps	64
Split Stance Dead Clean	108
Squat Curl	46
Squat Pulse Lunge Jumps	64
Squat Sliders	54
Stagger Stance Good Morning	145
Standing Chest Press	20
Star Pullover	80
Stationary Lunge Press, 2-Hand	58
Steam Rollers	26
Step Thru Sumo Turns	64
Step Ups	69
Step-Out Stop Swings	98
Step-Thru Figure-8s	141
Stop Clean	108
Stop Clean Thruster Press	154
Stop Snatch	112
Stop Snatch + Overhead Squat	112
Stop Swing	98
Stop Swing Switch-Snatch	115
Straddle Press, Two-Hand	20
Strict Press (Side Hold)	21
Suitcase Deadlift	125
Sumo Deadlift	125
Superman Press	21
Surrenders	133
Survival/Hang Snatch	115
Swing + Clean + Thruster	154
Swing + High Knee	99
Swinging Bottoms-Up Lunges	99
Tactical Lunge	65
The Mad Max	158
Thruster	130
Thruster Twist, Double	131
Thruster Twist, Single	130
Tik-Tok Deadlifts	125
Toe Lifts	69
Tricep Extension	37
Turkish Getup	134
Turkish Kick n' Sit	83
Turkish Planks	87
Turkish Sit-Up	82
Twisted Pull-Over	80
Twisted Punch	80
Two Hand Swing	94
Two-Hand Anyhow	132
Two-Hand Sprays	37
Upright Row	29
Vertical Halos	37
Walking Figure-8s	142
Walking Hang Cleans	108
Walking Lunge Row	65
Walking Lunges (Horn Hold)	65
Walking One-Arm Waiter Carry	136
Walking Swings, Two-Hand	100
Warrior Press	24
Weighted Wall Sit	69
Wheel Turns	38
Windmill	88
Windmill Cleans	89
Wiper Press	21
Wood Chopper Sit-Up	81

CIRCUIT CITY FULL-BODY WORKOUT

FULL-BODY		
Approx. Length	Single Bell	Double Bell
≤40-Minutes	✓	Some Optional

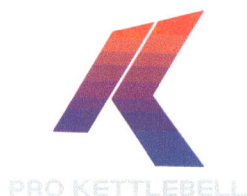

PRO KETTLEBELL

Section One (1)

Exercise
Tactical Lunge — Alternating legs, 5 lunges each side
Halos — 5 per direction, then switch
Romanian Deadlift — 10 slow-medium paced lifts *Optional: double kettlebells*

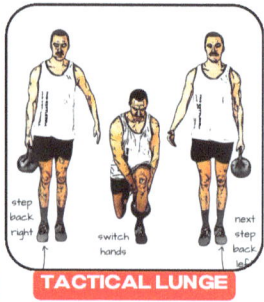
TACTICAL LUNGE
Alternating reverse lunges, pass the bell under the knee each rep.

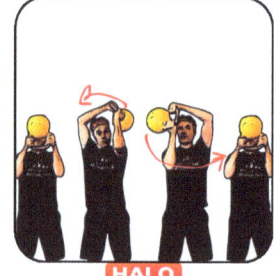
HALO
Circle your head, keeping it high.

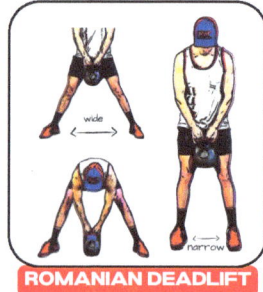
ROMANIAN DEADLIFT
Adjust your stance to keep your legs as straight as possible.

Section Two (2)

Exercise
Uneven Push-Ups — 5 push-ups per side
Wood Chopper Sit-Ups — 5 per side using minimal momentum
Strict Press — 5 slow-paced presses per side *Optional: double kettlebells*

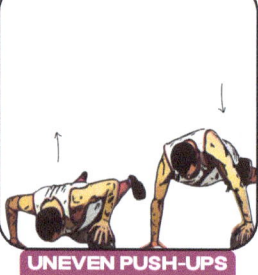
UNEVEN PUSH-UPS
One hand on, one hand off, from knees or toes.

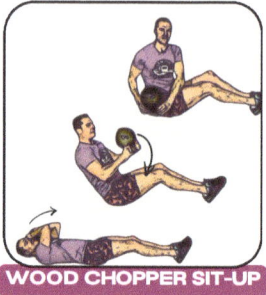
WOOD CHOPPER SIT-UP
Cross-body sit-up from shoulder to opposite hip.

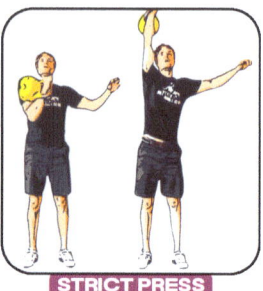
STRICT PRESS
Avoid elbow flare & keep lower body still, with tension.

Section Three (3)

Exercise
Tricep Extensions — 10 controlled, concurrent reps
Lateral Lunge Row — 5 concurrent prior to switching sides
Ballistic Deadlifts — 10 quick lifts, straight posture at top. Rise onto your toes if you can't jump *Optional: double kettlebells*

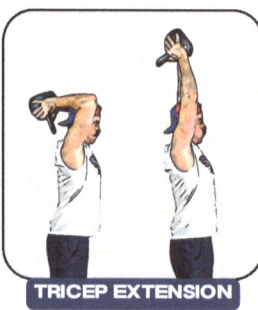
TRICEP EXTENSION
Lower and raise slowly, lock out the elbows at the top.

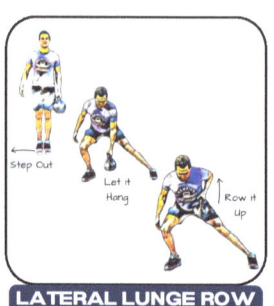
LATERAL LUNGE ROW
Lunge to the side, hinge forward and row w/flat back.

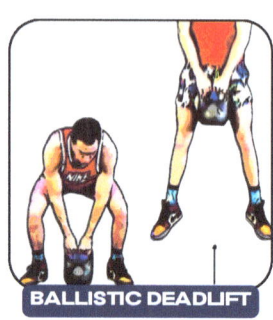
BALLISTIC DEADLIFT
A jumping deadlift. Back and arms straight, landing softly.

WARM-UP	Time
Hip Swings	1'
Toe Touches	1'
Air Squats	30"
Shoulder Circles	30"
Jumping Jacks	1'
Push-Ups	30"

- PERFORM 10 REPS OF EACH EXERCISE IN THE SECTION, IN ORDER.
- COMPLETE 3 ROUNDS BEFORE MOVING TO THE NEXT SECTION.
- TRY TO RESERVE BREAKS TO BETWEEN SECTIONS OR ROUNDS, NOT DURING THEM.

COOL-DOWN	Time
Forward Bend	30"
Standing Quad Stretches	1'
Figure-4 Glute Stretches	1'
Scorpion	1'
Lo/Hi Cobras	1'
Child's Pose	30"

PRO KETTLEBELL
LAST MAN STANDING WORKOUT

PERFORM 10 REPS OF EACH EXERCISE IN THE SECTION, IN ORDER.
REPEAT AND COMPLETE AS MANY ROUNDS AS POSSIBLE FOR THE PRESCRIBED TIME
PERIOD BEFORE MOVING TO THE NEXT SECTION.

SECTION 1: 3-MINUTE AMRAP

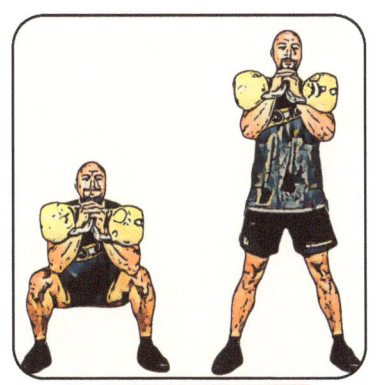
RACK SQUATS
Doubles

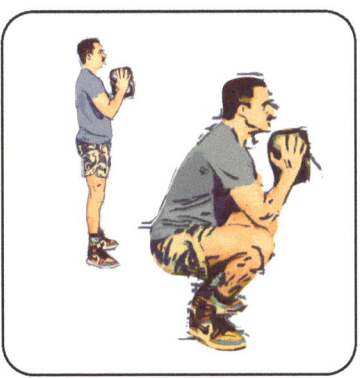
GOBLET SQUATS
(Single Bell Modifier for Section 1)

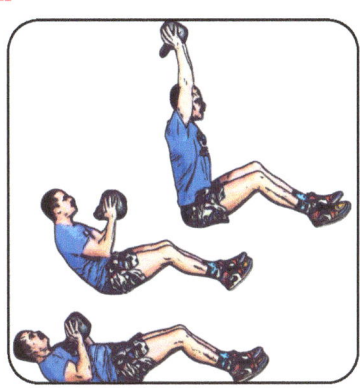
SITUP GETUPS
Single Bell

SECTION 2: 4-MINUTE AMRAP

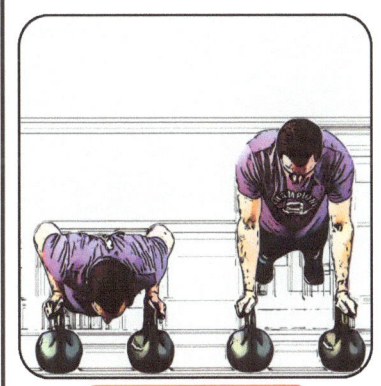
KB PUSH-UPS
Doubles OR → Regular Push-Ups

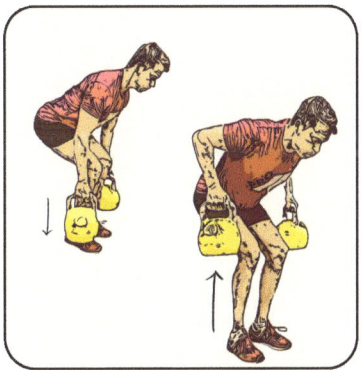
BENT-OVER ROWS
Single or Doubles

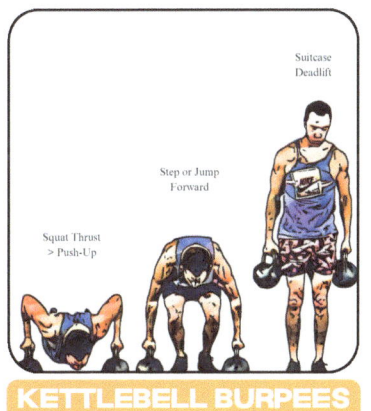
KETTLEBELL BURPEES
Doubles OR → Body-Weight Burpees

SECTION 3: 5-MINUTE AMRAP

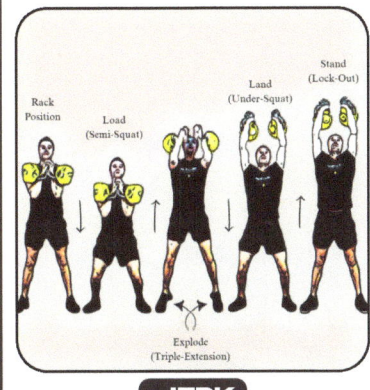
JERK
Single or Doubles

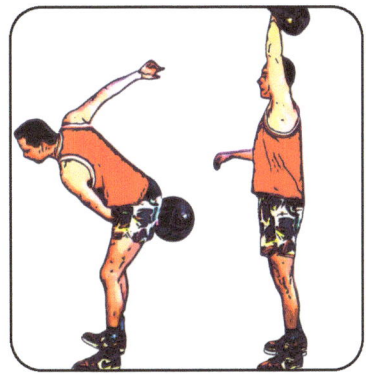
SNATCH
Single

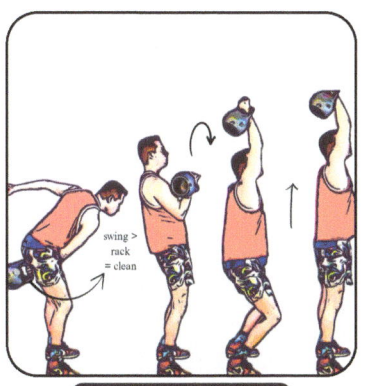
LONG CYCLE
Single or Doubles

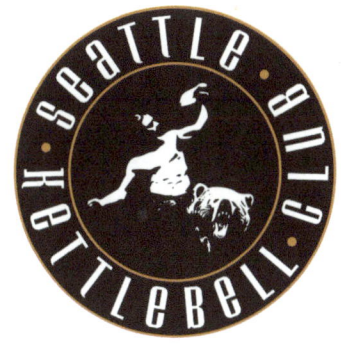

ACKNOWLEDGEMENTS

This book rests on the shoulders—and forearms, quads, and chalk-covered hands—of a remarkable community.

Seattle Kettlebell Club members and staff: your years of sweat-stained effort and comradery forged the foundation of this collection. Your reps echo in these pages.

To our first mentors in kettlebell lifting, **Mikhail Marshak** and **Tom Corrigan**—thank you for lighting the fuse and your continued support.

A special nod to the crew behind the "**Kettlebell 365**" video collection—**Reuben, Sheena, Alexa, Ayden, Natalie, Christiana, Henry, Vinay,** and **Buffy**. Your ability to grit through multiple takes with a smile enabled us to turn an idea into a living library. **Deb, Jen,** and **Aleksander,** thanks for stepping up and getting the digital library to the finish line.

To everyone named—and the many unsung colleagues, training partners, mentors, Pro Kettlebell customers, and family who cheer us on—your relentless support is incredible. This book is yours as much as ours.

Lift long and prosper!

Continue Your Kettlebell Practice

Train with world-class kettlebells. Grab the same high-performance kettlebells we use every day at *prokettlebell.com*.

Follow-along with structured workouts. Visit our website for the latest video workouts, books and resources.

Pursue professional certification. Join one of the most comprehensive online certification programs available. Visit *training.prokettlebell.com* for upcoming dates.

Follow us online

Linktr.ee/prokettlebell

Happy with this book?

Amazon Review Link

If so, we would be so thankful if you left us a review!

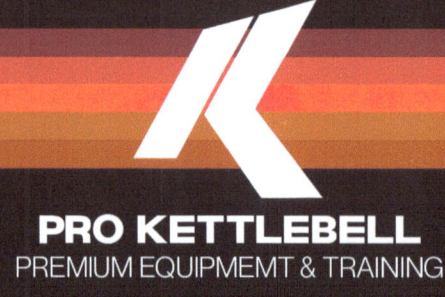

PRO KETTLEBELL
PREMIUM EQUIPMEMT & TRAINING

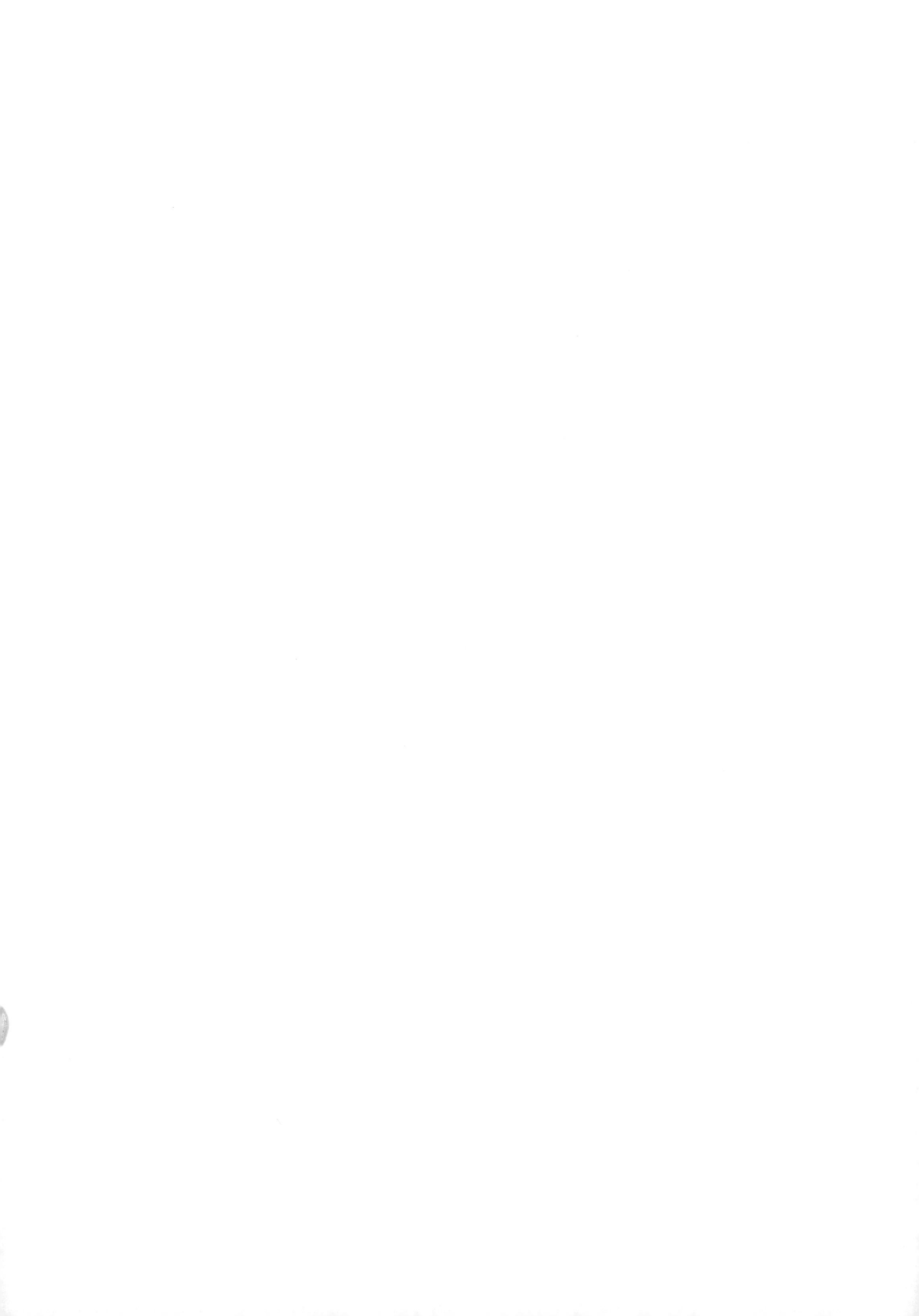

www.ingramcontent.com/pod-product-compliance
Lightning Source LLC
Chambersburg PA
CBHW061155030426
42337CB00002B/16